Williams
GYNECOLOGY
SECOND EDITION
STUDY GUIDE

Williams
GYNECOLOGY
SECOND EDITION
STUDY GUIDE

Claudia L. Werner, MD
Medical Director of Dysplasia Services
Co-Director Vulvology Clinic
Parkland Health and Hospital System, Dallas, Texas
Associate Professor, Department of Obstetrics and Gynecology
University of Texas Southwestern Medical Center at Dallas

Elysia Moschos, MD
Associate Professor, Department of Obstetrics and Gynecology
University of Texas Southwestern Medical Center at Dallas

William F. Griffith, MD
Medical Director, Intermediate Care Center Director, Vulvology Clinic
Co-Director, Dysplasia Services
Parkland Health and Hospital System, Dallas, Texas
Associate Professor, Department of Obstetrics and Gynecology
University of Texas Southwestern Medical Center at Dallas

Victor E. Beshay, MD
Assistant Professor, Department of Obstetrics and Gynecology
University of Texas Southwestern Medical Center at Dallas

David D. Rahn, MD
Assistant Professor, Department of Obstetrics and Gynecology
University of Texas Southwestern Medical Center at Dallas

Debra L. Richardson, MD, FACOG
Assistant Professor, Department of Obstetrics and Gynecology
University of Texas Southwestern Medical Center at Dallas

Barbara L. Hoffman, MD
Associate Professor, Department of Obstetrics and Gynecology
University of Texas Southwestern Medical Center at Dallas

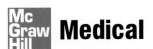 **Medical**

New York   Chicago   San Francisco   Lisbon   London   Madrid   Mexico City
Milan   New Delhi   San Juan   Seoul   Singapore   Sydney   Toronto

Williams Gynecology Second Edition Study Guide

Copyright © 2012 by The McGraw-Hill Companies, Inc. All rights reserved. Printed in China. Except as permitted under the United States copyright Act of 1976, no part of this publication may be reproduced or distributed in any form or by any means, or stored in a data base or retrieval system, without the prior written permission of the publisher.

1 2 3 4 5 6 7 8 9 0 CTP/CTP 17 16 15 14 13 12

ISBN 978-0-07-175091-2
MHID 0-07-175091-6

This book was set in Adobe Garamond by Aptara, Inc.
The editors were Alyssa Fried and Peter J. Boyle.
The production supervisor was Catherine H. Saggese.
Project management was provided by Indu Jawwad, Aptara, Inc.
The designer was Alan Barnett.
The illustration manager was Armen Ovsepyan.
China Translation & Printing, Ltd., was printer and binder.

Cataloging-in-publication data for this book is on file at the Library of Congress.

International Edition
ISBN 978-0-07-180055-6; MHID 0-07-180055-7
Copyright © 2012. Exclusive rights by The McGraw-Hill Companies, Inc., for manufacture and export. This book cannot be re-exported from the country to which it is consigned by McGraw-Hill. The International Edition is not available in North America.

McGraw-Hill books are available at special quantity discounts to use as premiums and sales promotions, or for use in corporate training programs. To contact a representative please e-mail us at bulksales@mcgraw-hill.com.

To our mentors and patients, who inspire us to strive for excellence in gynecology, and
To our families, whose love and support make this possible

CONTENTS

SECTION 3

FEMALE PELVIC MEDICINE AND RECONSTRUCTIVE SURGERY

SECTION 4

GYNECOLOGIC ONCOLOGY

SECTION 5

ASPECTS OF GYNECOLOGIC SURGERY

SECTION 6

ATLAS OF GYNECOLOGIC SURGERY

PREFACE

The *Williams Gynecology Second Edition Study Guide* is designed to assess comprehension and retention of information presented in the second edition of *Williams Gynecology*. The questions for each section have been selected to emphasize the key points from each chapter. In total, 1244 questions have been created from the 44 chapters. Questions are in a multiple-choice format, and one single best answer should be chosen for each. With this edition, we have also included more than 200 full-color images as question material. In addition, clinical case questions have been added to test implementation of content learned. At the end of each chapter, answers are found, and a page guide directs readers to the text section that contains the answer. We believe that our more clinical approach translates into a more accurate test of important clinical knowledge.

Claudia L. Werner, MD
Elysia Moschos, MD
William F. Griffith, MD
Victor E. Beshay, MD
David D. Rahn, MD
Debra L. Richardson, MD
Barbara L. Hoffman, MD

BENIGN GENERAL GYNECOLOGY

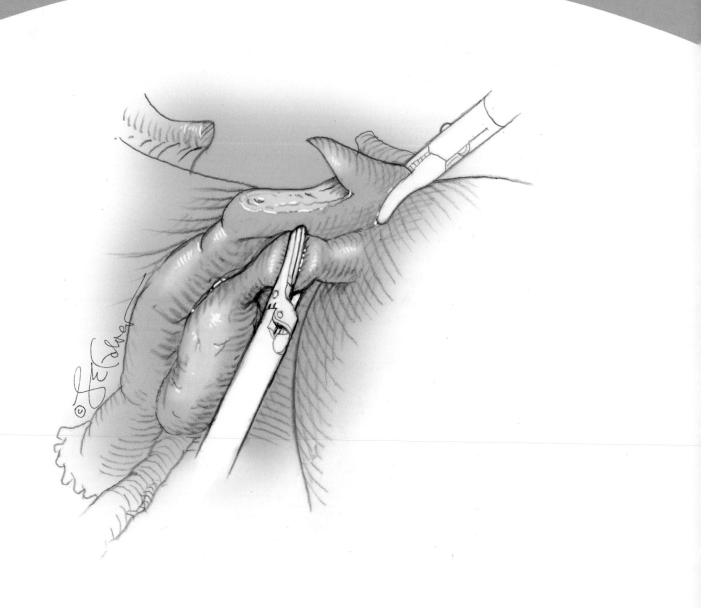

CHAPTER 1

Well Woman Care

1–1. A 15-year-old adolescent female who is sexually naïve comes to your office for the recommended initial reproductive health visit. She has no complaints related to her reproductive health. Which of the following is **NOT** indicated during this encounter?

a. Pelvic examination

b. Establishment of rapport

c. Stage of adolescence evaluation

d. Reproductive health care needs assessment

1–2. The American Cancer Society (ACS) has published guidelines for the conduct of the clinical breast examination. Which of the following components of the examination is no longer recommended?

a. Axillary lymph node palpation

b. Inspection for skin abnormalities

c. Breast palpation with the patient supine

d. Inspection with patient's arms raised overhead

1–3. In the past, expressing the nipples for the detection of discharge, as shown here, was a standard part of breast examination. This examination component is currently recommended selectively for which of the following indications?

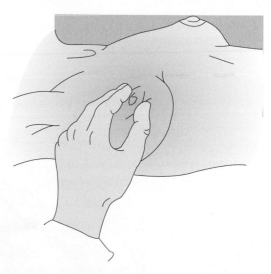

Reproduced, with permission, from Kawada C: Gynecologic history, examination, & diagnostic procedures. In DeCherney AH, Nathan L (eds): CURRENT Diagnosis & Treatment Obstetrics & Gynecology, 10th ed. New York, McGraw-Hill, 2007, Figure 33-1.

a. Breast pain (mastalgia)

b. Current breastfeeding with fever

c. Spontaneous nipple discharge in a nonlactating woman

d. Bilateral milky discharge that is present only when expressed by the patient

1–4. Which of the following components of the routine pelvic examination is more often performed for specific indications rather than routinely?

a. Vulvar inspection

b. Rectovaginal examination

c. Bimanual palpation of the uterus and adnexa

d. Speculum examination of the cervix and vagina

1-5. Assuming that childhood immunizations have been administered correctly, which vaccination warrants repeat dosing at 10-year intervals in adults?

a. Hepatitis B

b. Pneumococcal

c. Herpes zoster

d. Tetanus-diphtheria

1-6. All adults (up to age 64) should be screened regardless of risk factors for which sexually transmitted disease according to the American College of Obstetricians and Gynecologists (ACOG) and the Centers for Disease Control and Prevention (CDC)?

a. Hepatitis B virus

b. *Treponema pallidum*

c. *Chlamydia trachomatis*

d. Human immunodeficiency virus (HIV)

1-7. Your patient is a 32-year-old whose previous pregnancy resulted in the birth of a child with anencephaly. A sonographic example of anencephaly is shown here. She is currently using oral contraceptive pills to prevent pregnancy. She intends to have another child in the future, but is uncertain when. What is your recommendation for oral folic acid supplementation?

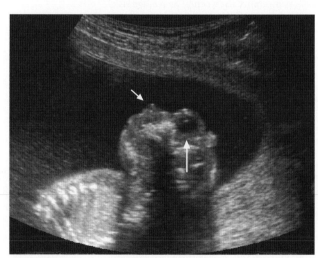

Arrows point to the nose and orbit. Reproduced, with permission, from Cunningham FG, Leveno KJ, Bloom SL, et al (eds): Fetal imaging. In Williams Obstetrics, 23rd ed. New York, McGraw-Hill, 2010, Figure 16-1.

a. Folic acid, 4 mg orally daily beginning now

b. Folic acid, 4 mg orally daily as soon as a pregnancy test is positive

c. Folic acid, 400 μg orally daily beginning 1 month prior to discontinuation of contraception

d. A diet with an increased percentage of foods high in folic acid is sufficient in the United States

1-8. According to current ACOG guidelines (2009), how often should a 26-year-old woman with HIV be screened for cervical cancer, assuming she has no symptoms or physical findings of cervical cancer (as seen below)?

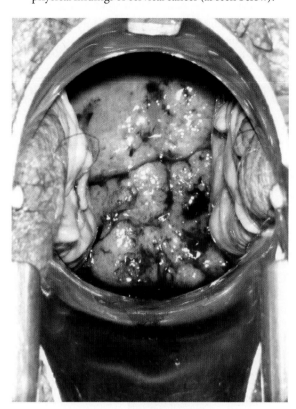

a. Annually

b. Every 2 years

c. Every 3 years

d. Every 5 years

1-9. Routine screening for endometrial cancer in asymptomatic women at average risk is not recommended. However, a woman with a strong family history of which disorder should be offered an endometrial biopsy annually beginning at age 35?

a. Adult-onset diabetes

b. Premenopausal breast cancer

c. Gastric or pancreatic cancer

d. Hereditary nonpolyposis colon cancer (Lynch syndrome)

1-10. Which of the following is currently recommended for ovarian cancer screening in women at average risk?

a. Pelvic examination

b. Pelvic sonography every 2 to 3 years

c. Annual cancer antigen (CA125) level measurement

d. Annual cancer antigen (CA125) level measurement and pelvic sonography

1-11. Which of the following are recommended for breast cancer screening by current ACOG guidelines?

a. Self breast examination

b. Periodic clinical breast exam starting at age 19

c. Screening mammography every 1 to 2 years for women ages 40 to 49 years

d. All of the above

1-12. Which of the following statements is **INCORRECT** regarding colon cancer and colon cancer screening in asymptomatic woman at average risk?

a. Screening colonoscopy, if negative, should be repeated every 5 to 7 years.

b. Colon cancer is ranked third among the leading causes of cancer death in women.

c. Several organizations recommend that women of average risk begin screening at age 50 years.

d. Annual fecal immunochemical testing (FIT) is more specific (fewer false positive results) than the fecal occult blood test (FOBT), which uses a guaiac paper-based oxidation reaction.

1-13. Skin cancer screening includes assessment of lesions for which of the following characteristics?

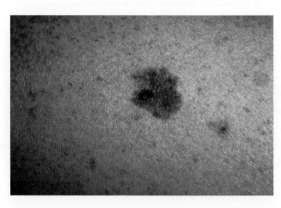

Reproduced, with permission, from Berger TG: Dermatologic disorders. In McPhee SJ, Papadakis MA (eds): CURRENT Medical Diagnosis & Treatment 2011. New York, McGraw-Hill, 2011, Figure 6-3.

a. Asymmetry

b. Border irregularity

c. Size greater than 6 mm diameter

d. All of the above

1-14. At what age do current guidelines for osteoporosis prevention recommend initiation of screening with this modality for women at average risk?

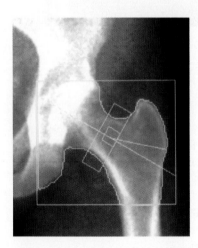

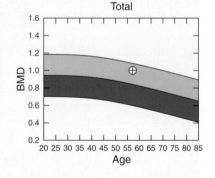

DXA Results Summary:

Region	Area (cm²)	BMC (g)	BMD (g/cm²)	T-Score	Z-Score
Neck	4.59	3.79	0.827	−0.2	1.0
Troch	8.57	6.65	0.775	0.7	1.5
Inter	14.62	17.48	1.196	0.6	1.2
Total	27.79	27.92	1.005	0.5	1.3
Ward's	1.12	0.71	0.639	−0.8	1.0

Total BMD CV 1.0%, ACF = 1.028, BCF = 0.998, TH = 6.508
WHO Classification: Normal
Fracture Risk: Not Increased

Reproduced, with permission, from Bradshaw KD: Menopausal transition. In Schorge JO, Schaffer JI, Halvorson LM, et al (eds): Williams Gynecology, 1st ed. New York, McGraw-Hill, 2008, Figure 21-10A.

a. 45

b. 55

c. 65

d. 75

1-15. Most U.S. women are overweight or obese. Which of the following statements is **FALSE** regarding the body mass index (BMI) as a clinical tool?

  a. A normal BMI in adults ranges from 18.5 to 24.

  b. For adolescents, BMI is expressed as a percentile.

  c. The calculation of BMI includes age, weight, and height.

  d. The BMI reflects risk of obesity-related medical conditions.

1-16. Bariatric surgery has become a more commonly used adjunct to other weight-loss strategies. Which of the following is an **INCORRECT** statement regarding recommendations for bariatric surgery?

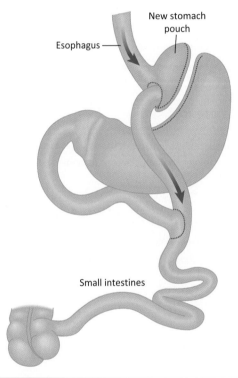

Reproduced, with permission, from Hoffman BL, Horsager R, Roberts SW, et al: Obesity. In Williams Obstetrics, 23rd Edition Study Guide, New York, McGraw-Hill, 2011, Figure 43-22.

  a. Pregnancy should be delayed for 12 to 18 months following bariatric surgery.

  b. Gastric banding is now the only recommended bariatric surgery method and has replaced the procedure shown here.

  c. Patients with comorbid conditions can be considered for bariatric surgery at BMIs of 35 or more.

  d. If no comorbid conditions are present, bariatric surgery may be selected for patients with BMIs of 40 or more.

1-17. The effect of obesity on the effectiveness of various contraceptive methods is not fully understood. Which contraceptive method has been determined most conclusively to be less effective in women weighing more than 90 kg?

  a. Subdermal contraceptive rod

  b. Depot medroxyprogesterone acetate

  c. Combination hormone contraceptive patch

  d. Combination hormone oral contraceptive pills

1-18. An appropriately sized blood pressure cuff is necessary for the accurate measurement of blood pressure and screening for hypertension. At minimum, what percentage of the arm above the elbow should the air bladder of the cuff encircle?

  a. 40%

  b. 60%

  c. 80%

  d. 100%

1-19. Prehypertension increases the risk of developing hypertension at a later time. Respectively, what are the lower limits of systolic and diastolic blood pressure measurements (mm Hg) that define prehypertension?

  a. 120, 80

  b. 135, 85

  c. 140, 90

  d. 145, 95

1-20. Identifiable causes of hypertension include the regular use of all **EXCEPT** which of the following agents?

  a. Licorice

  b. Valproic acid

  c. Combination oral contraceptives

  d. Nonsteroidal anti-inflammatory agents

1-21. Upon diagnosing hypertension, which of the following tests are recommended to further investigate possible causes and comorbidities?

  a. Urinalysis and serum creatinine

  b. Thyroid function and blood glucose

  c. Electrocardiogram and lipid profile

  d. All of the above

1-22. What fasting venous blood glucose value is the threshold for diagnosis of diabetes mellitus in adults?

  a. >120 mg/dL

  b. >125 mg/dL

  c. >140 mg/dL

  d. >145 mg/dL

SECTION 1

1-23. The clinical usefulness of diagnosing the metabolic syndrome is not fully understood at present. What waist circumference in females is the threshold value for one of metabolic syndrome's current diagnostic criteria?

   a. 35 inches (88 cm)

   b. 40 inches (101 cm)

   c. 45 inches (114 cm)

   d. 50 inches (127 cm)

1-24. Which lipoprotein category appears most strongly correlated with atherogenesis?

   a. Triglycerides

   b. Total cholesterol level

   c. Low-density lipoprotein cholesterol

   d. High-density lipoprotein cholesterol

1-25. The U.S. Preventive Services Task Force recommends a minimum of how many minutes of moderate-intensity activity per week, performed in episodes of at least 10 minutes?

   a. 60

   b. 90

   c. 120

   d. 150

1-26. The U.S. Preventive Services Task Force does not recommend routine screening for thyroid dysfunction in women. However, the American Thyroid Association recommends that women be screened with a serum thyroid-stimulating hormone level measurement every 5 years beginning at what age?

   a. 35 years

   b. 40 years

   c. 50 years

   d. 65 years

1-27. In a recent meta-analysis (Wu and colleagues, 2006), which of the following agents was associated with superior rates of smoking cessation after 1 year?

   a. Bupropion

   b. Varenicline

   c. Nicotine replacement agents

   d. None of the above was superior

References

American College of Obstetricians and Gynecologists: Cervical cytology screening. Practice Bulletin No. 109, December 2009

Wu P, Wilson K, Dimoulas P, et al: Effectiveness of smoking cessation therapies: a systematic review and meta-analysis. BMC Public Health 6(1):300, 2006

Chapter 1 ANSWER KEY

Question number	Letter answer	Page cited	Header cited
1–1	a	p. 2	Medical History and Physical Examination
1–2	d	p. 3	Breast Inspection
1–3	c	p. 3	Breast Palpation
1–4	b	p. 6	Rectovaginal Examination
1–5	d	p. 8	Vaccination, Table 1-1
1–6	d	p. 11	Table 1-2
1–7	a	p. 7	Contraception
1–8	a	p. 7	Cervical Cancer
1–9	d	p. 7	Endometrial Cancer
1–10	a	p. 7	Ovarian Cancer
1–11	d	p. 14	Table 1-4
1–12	a	p. 10	Colon Cancer
1–13	d	p. 11	Skin Cancer
1–14	c	p. 11	Osteoporosis

Question number	Letter answer	Page cited	Header cited
1–15	c	p. 13	Obesity
1–16	b	p. 16	Bariatric Surgery
1–17	c	p. 16	Bariatric Surgery
1–18	c	p. 19	Chronic Hypertension
1–19	a	p. 19	Chronic Hypertension
1–20	b	p. 19	Table 1-13
1–21	d	p. 20	Laboratory Tests and Other Diagnostic Procedures
1–22	b	p. 21	Table 1-16
1–23	a	p. 22	Table 1-18
1–24	c	p. 23	Dyslipidemia
1–25	d	p. 24	Exercise
1–26	a	p. 25	Thyroid Disease
1–27	b	p. 29	Smoking Pharmacotherapy

Techniques Used for Imaging in Gynecology

2–1. Which sonographic feature, as demonstrated here, is characteristic of cysts?

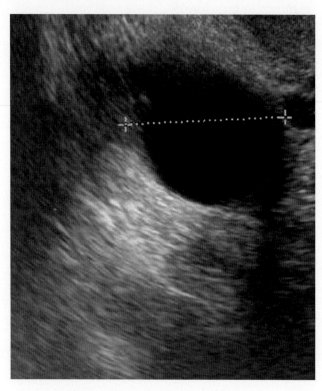

a. Acoustic window

b. Acoustic shadowing

c. Acoustic enhancement

d. Tip of the iceberg sign

2–2. Characteristics of the Doppler technology illustrated below include all **EXCEPT** which of the following?

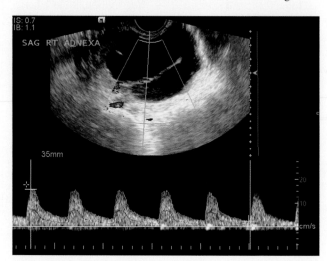

a. Scaling of color

b. More sensitive to low flow velocities

c. Directionality of blood flow with dual colors

d. Quantitative measurement of impedance to red blood cell velocity

2–3. Which of the following statements is true when performing saline infusion sonography?

a. SIS is best performed within the first 10 days of the menstrual cycle.

b. Touching the uterine fundus when advancing the catheter should be avoided as it can cause pain and false-positive results.

c. The uterine isthmus and endocervical canal should be evaluated as the catheter is withdrawn under sonographic visualization.

d. All of the above

2-4. Ovarian volume is one of the criteria for the sonographic diagnosis of polycystic ovaries. What is the formula to calculate ovarian volume, where A, B, and C are the ovarian diameters in centimeters?

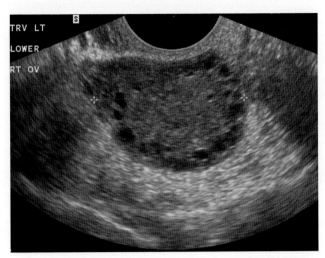

Reproduced, with permission, from Hoffman BL: Pelvic mass. In Schorge JO, Schaffer JI, Halvorson LM, et al (eds): Williams Gynecology, 1st ed. New York, McGraw-Hill, 2008, Figure 17-11.

    a. $(A \times B \times C)/\pi$
    b. $(A \times B \times C)/3$
    c. $(\pi/6) \times (A \times B \times C)$
    d. $[(A \times B \times C)/3 + 2.54]/0.7$

2-5. The sonographic appearance of the endometrium during the menstrual cycle correlates with the phasic changes in its histologic anatomy. Which phase of the cycle is depicted with the classic trilaminar appearance as shown below?

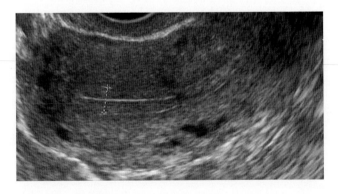

    a. Menstrual
    b. Secretory
    c. Proliferative
    d. Periovulatory

2-6. Sonographic features of adenomyosis, as depicted below, include all **EXCEPT** which of the following?

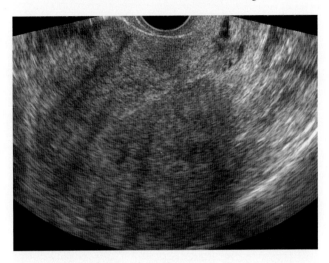

    a. Hypoechoic linear striations
    b. Anechoic areas within the myometrium
    c. Well-defined endometrial–myometrial junction
    d. Asymmetrically thickened and heterogeneous myometrium

2-7. Saline infusion sonography (SIS) may be used to evaluate which of the following clinical situations?

    a. Evaluating endometrial thickness in women taking tamoxifen and who have bleeding
    b. Determining whether an intrauterine device (IUD) is embedded
    c. Defining endometrial lesions such as polyps and submucosal fibroids
    d. All of the above

2-8. Which sonographic characteristic has been proven most important in distinguishing between a hemorrhagic cyst and an endometrioma?

    a. Retracting clot
    b. Fluid-debris levels
    c. Increased through-transmission
    d. Change in the internal structure over time

2-9. The classic sonographic features of the neoplasm shown here include which of the following?

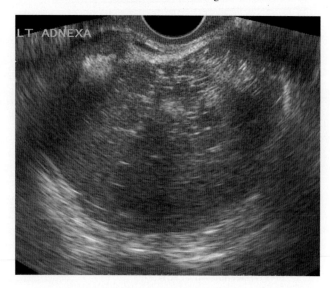

LT ADNEXA

a. Hyperechoic linear echoes

b. Cystic areas with round echogenic mural nodules

c. Hyperechogenic mass with "tip of the iceberg" sign

d. All of the above

2-10. Morphologic scoring systems used to predict the probability of malignancy of an ovarian mass include which of the following parameters?

a. Tumor size

b. Presence of a solid component

c. Color content of the tumor using color Doppler

d. All of the above

2-11. Which of the following statements regarding the use of sonography in the evaluation of pelvic inflammatory disease (PID) is true?

a. In early disease, most cases show anatomic changes.

b. Sonographic changes of the fallopian tubes are the least specific landmarks of PID.

c. The ovary can become involved as the disease progresses, creating a tuboovarian complex or abscess.

d. Large studies evaluating the sensitivity and specificity of sonography in this clinical setting are abundant.

2-12. What is the single most important sonographic finding for exclusion of an ectopic pregnancy?

a. Complex adnexal mass

b. Free fluid in the cul-de-sac

c. Identification of an intrauterine pregnancy

d. Ectopic pregnancy cannot be diagnosed sonographically

2-13. Uses of sonography in the evaluation and treatment of infertility include which of the following?

a. Endometrial cavity evaluation

b. Monitoring of folliculogenesis in normal and stimulated cycles

c. Demonstration and characterization of congenital uterine anomalies

d. All of the above

2-14. In gynecology, three-dimensional (3-D) sonography aids in the assessment of which of the following conditions?

a. IUD identification and positioning

b. Diagnosis of congenital müllerian anomalies

c. Calculation of ovarian volume and antral follicle counts

d. All of the above

2-15. All of the following statements are true regarding compression sonography of the lower extremities **EXCEPT** which one?

a. Normal venous sonography findings do not necessarily exclude pulmonary embolism.

b. Impaired visibility, noncompressibility, and the typical echo pattern of a thrombosed vein confirm the diagnosis.

c. Compression sonography, combined with color Doppler, is the initial test currently used to detect deep-vein thrombosis.

d. Compression sonography is as accurate in the diagnosis of distal (calf vein) thromboses as in proximal (popliteal or femoral vein) thromboses.

2-16. Your patient, who underwent hysterectomy 3 months ago, complains of urine leakage from her vagina. You suspect she has developed a vesicovaginal fistula. Which of the following radiologic tests is the most appropriate to order in her evaluation?

a. Intravenous pyelography (IVP)

b. Voiding cystourethrography (VCUG)

c. Computed tomography (CT) of the pelvis

d. Positive pressure urethrography (PPUG)

2–17. Which of the following is **NOT** a contraindication to this radiologic technique?

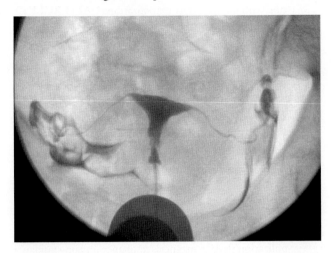

Reproduced, with permission, from Halvorson LM: Evaluation of the infertile couple. In Schorge JO, Schaffer JI, Halvorson LM, et al (eds): Williams Gynecology, 1st ed. New York, McGraw-Hill, 2008, Figure 19-5A.

  a. Pregnancy

  b. History of PID

  c. Iodine allergy

  d. Acute pelvic infection

2–18. Which of the following statements regarding bone densitometry methods is true?

  a. Dual-energy x-ray absorptiometry (DEXA) is the best technique for axial osteopenia evaluation.

  b. Quantitative computed tomography (QCT) is best at evaluating the bone mineral density in the high-turnover cortical bone.

  c. Quantitative sonography (QUS) is a recently validated alternative technique to dual-energy x-ray absorptiometry (DEXA).

  d. Dual-energy x-ray absorptiometry (DEXA) is a three-dimensional technique that can distinguish between cortical and trabecular bone.

2–19. Computed tomography (CT) is well suited to diagnose which of the following gynecologic surgical complications?

  a. Small bowel obstruction

  b. Ureteral disruption or obstruction

  c. Abdominal-pelvic abscesses or hematomas

  d. All of the above

2–20. Which of the following statements is true regarding imaging techniques for the evaluation and surveillance of gynecologic malignancies?

  a. Sonography is the most frequently used modality for this purpose.

  b. CT is more sensitive in the detection of intraperitoneal metastases rather than bulky metastases.

  c. There are few data to support use of positron emission tomography (PET) imaging in gynecologic malignancies.

  d. Magnetic resonance (MR) imaging is now often preferable to CT because MR does not use radiation and provides multiplanar views of the pelvis.

2–21. Which of the following statements is true regarding magnetic resonance (MR) imaging?

  a. Relaxation time properties are the factors principally responsible for contrast among tissues.

  b. Water-containing organs, such as the bladder, will appear bright on T1-weighted images and dark on T2-weighted images.

  c. Images are constructed based on the radiofrequency signal emitted by oxygen nuclei after they have been "excited" by radiofrequency pulses.

  d. MR contrast, such as gadolinium, is given in concentrations and doses significantly higher than that used in CT imaging and is unsafe in patients with mildly compromised renal function.

2–22. Contraindications to this imaging modality include all **EXCEPT** which of the following?

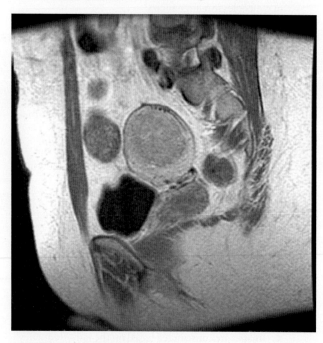

Image contributed by Dr. Samuel C. Chao.

a. Intrauterine device

b. Cochlear implant copper

c. Intracranial aneurysm clips

d. Internal cardiac pacemaker or defibrillator

2–23. Uses of magnetic resonance (MR) imaging in gynecology include all **EXCEPT** which of the following?

a. Diagnosis of adenomyosis

b. Initial evaluation of suspected gynecologic disease

c. Detailed characterization of congenital müllerian anomalies

d. Evaluation of endometrial lesions when sonography is nondiagnostic in a patient who is a poor surgical candidate

2–24. All of the following statements are true regarding the use of magnetic resonance (MR) imaging in conjunction with uterine artery embolization (UAE) **EXCEPT** which of the following?

a. Postprocedural evaluation of UAE is more accurately made by sonography.

b. MR imaging is the diagnostic method of choice for preoperative evaluation for UAE.

c. Leiomyomas with negligible enhancement and high signal intensity on T1-weighted sequences do not respond well to UAE.

d. Hypervascularity, which is seen as bright signal on T2-weighted images after contrast, correlates with a good predicted response to UAE.

2–25. In comparison to myomectomy or uterine artery embolization (UAE), magnetic resonance imaging guidance of focused ultrasound (MRgFUS) therapy for the treatment of leiomyomas has been shown to have which of the following attributes?

a. Is more cost-effective

b. Has fewer major adverse events

c. Stabilizes leiomyoma size over time

d. Gradually improves patient symptoms

Chapter 2 ANSWER KEY

Question number	Letter answer	Page cited	Header cited	Question number	Letter answer	Page cited	Header cited
2–1	c	p. 33	Physics	2–15	d	p. 48	Compression Sonography of Lower Extremities
2–2	b	p. 35	Doppler Technology	2–16	b	p. 49	Voiding Cystourethrography and Positive Pressure Urethrography
2–3	d	p. 35	Saline Infusion Sonography (SIS)				
2–4	c	p. 36	Reproductive Tract Organs	2–17	b	p. 50	Hysterosalpingography
2–5	c	p. 37	Endometrium	2–18	a	p. 50	Bone Densitometry
2–6	c	p. 39	Adenomyosis	2–19	d	p. 52	Imaging Following Gynecologic Surgery
2–7	d	p. 40	Saline Infusion Sonography (SIS)	2–20	d	p. 52	Gynecologic Malignancy, Positron Emission Tomography Imaging
2–8	d	p. 41	Lesion Characterization				
2–9	d	p. 41	Lesion Characterization	2–21	a	p. 52	Magnetic Resonance Imaging, Technique
2–10	d	p. 41	Malignant Characteristics				
2–11	c	p. 42	Acute Infection, Tuboovarian Infection	2–22	a	p. 53	Safety
2–12	c	p. 43	Ectopic Pregnancy	2–23	b	p. 54	Use in Gynecology
2–13	d	p. 44	Infertility	2–24	a	p. 54	Leiomyoma
2–14	d	p. 46	Three-Dimensional Sonography	2–25	b	p. 54	Leiomyoma

CHAPTER 3

Gynecologic Infection

3-1. Vaginal flora of a normal, asymptomatic reproductive-aged woman includes multiple anaerobic, aerobic, and facultative bacterial species. Anaerobes predominate over aerobic species by approximately what factor?

    a. 5

    b. 10

    c. 50

    d. 100

3-2. Normal colonization of the vaginal mucosa by bacteria serves what main physiologic function?

    a. Unknown

    b. Produces lubrication

    c. Stimulates epithelial differentiation

    d. Facilitates production of beneficial antibodies

3-3. In normal, healthy women, bacterial species can be recovered from what locations?

    a. Endocervix

    b. Endometrial cavity

    c. Peritoneal fluid of cul-de-sac

    d. All of the above

3-4. What is the typical range of normal vaginal pH?

    a. 3.0 to 3.5

    b. 4.0 to 4.5

    c. 5.0 to 5.5

    d. 6.0 to 6.5

3-5. The rise in vaginal pH observed after menopause is correlated with which of the following?

    a. Low serum estradiol levels

    b. Decrease in vaginal cellular glycogen content

    c. High serum follicle-stimulating hormone levels

    d. All of the above

3-6. Which of the following is **NOT** one of the three clinical diagnostic criteria for bacterial vaginosis described by Amsel and associates (1983)?

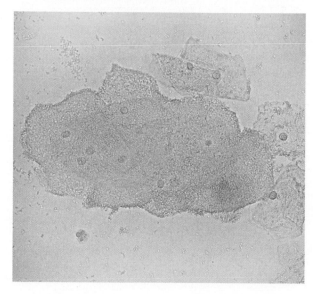

Photograph contributed by Dr. Lauri Campagna and Mercedes Pineda, WHNP.

    a. Abnormally high vaginal pH

    b. Presence of an abnormal discharge and erythema of the vagina

    c. Clue cells seen on vaginal saline preparation by light microscopy (shown here)

    d. Characteristic fishy odor release with addition of potassium hydroxide to vaginal secretions

3-7. Bacterial vaginosis is associated with which of the following?

    a. Postabortal endometritis

    b. Pelvic inflammatory disease

    c. Posthysterectomy pelvic infection

    d. All of the above

3-8. Which of the following is **NOT** one of the three treatment options proposed by the Centers for Disease Control and Prevention (CDC) (2010) for the treatment of bacterial vaginosis in nonpregnant women?

    a. Oral clindamycin

    b. Oral metronidazole

    c. Intravaginal clindamycin

    d. Intravaginal metronidazole

3–9. Recurrence of altered vaginal flora and symptoms is common (up to 30 percent) after initial treatment of bacterial vaginosis with antibiotics and can be frustrating for the patient. Which of the following has been consistently shown to decrease recurrence rates?

   a. Treatment of male partners

   b. Use of acidifying vaginal gels

   c. Douching with lactobacillus-rich products such as live culture yogurt

   d. None of the above

3–10. Which of the following is **NOT** a β-lactamase inhibitor?

   a. Sulbactam

   b. Probenecid

   c. Tazobactam

   d. Clavulanic acid

3–11. In addition to exfoliative dermatitis (shown here), which of the following are potential manifestations of a reaction to penicillins?

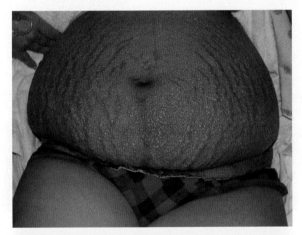

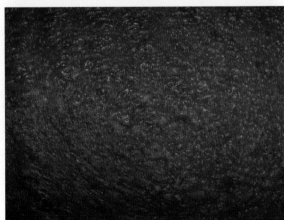

Photographs contributed by Dr. Meadow Good.

   a. Drug fever

   b. Interstitial nephritis

   c. Liver function abnormalities

   d. All of the above

3–12. Which of the following is treated most effectively with a member of the penicillin family of antibiotics?

   a. Syphilis

   b. Breast cellulitis

   c. *Actinomyces* infections related to intrauterine device (IUD) use

   d. All of the above

3–13. Which of the following antibiotic groups is best suited for prophylaxis against postoperative pelvic infections?

   a. Carbapenems

   b. Penicillins

   c. Cephalosporins

   d. Aminoglycosides

3–14. Serious toxicities of aminoglycosides include all **EXCEPT** which of the following?

   a. Ototoxicity

   b. Nephrotoxicity

   c. Hepatotoxicity

   d. Neuromuscular blockade

3–15. Your patient has a serious posthysterectomy pelvic infection. She relates a history of anaphylaxis (type I allergic reaction) after use of oral penicillin and a lesser allergic reaction (hives and pruritis) after being given a cephalosporin intravenously. Which of the following antibiotics poses the greatest risk of allergic reaction for this patient?

   a. Imipenem

   b. Doxycycline

   c. Ciprofloxacin

   d. Trimethroprim-sulfamethoxazole

3–16. Clindamycin is least useful for the treatment of which of the following?

   a. Pelvic abscess

   b. Pyelonephritis

   c. Bacterial vaginosis

   d. Soft tissue infections

3–17. Which of the following is **NOT** a potential adverse effect of vancomycin administration?

   a. Ototoxicity

   b. "Red man" syndrome

   c. Back and chest muscle spasms

   d. *Clostridium difficile* colitis

3–18. Metronidazole is commonly used to treat trichomonal infections and bacterial vaginosis. When prescribed, patients should be warned against concurrent ingestion of which of the following due to an increased incidence of associated side effects?

   a. Alcohol

   b. Benzodiazapines

   c. Grapefruit juice

   d. Monoamine oxidase inhibitors

3–19. Fluoroquinolones are contraindicated in children, adolescents, and breast-feeding women due to possible adverse effects on the development of which of the following tissues?

   a. Bone

   b. Liver

   c. Cartilage

   d. Dental enamel

3–20. Your patient is a healthy 30-year-old with a 2-cm vulvar abscess but with significant surrounding edema (shown here). She is otherwise healthy. You decide to start her on oral antibiotics while awaiting bacterial culture results following incision and drainage. Which of the following tetracyclines offers the least activity against methicillin-resistant *Staphylococcus* infections?

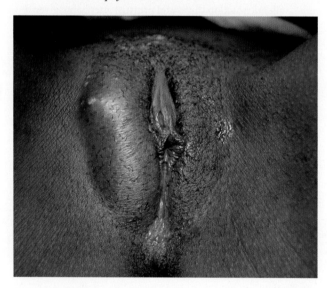

Photograph contributed by Dr. Kathryn Grande.

   a. Doxycycline

   b. Minocycline

   c. Tetracycline

   d. All of these are equally effective

3–21. You prescribe oral doxycycline to your patient for the treatment of mucopurulent cervicitis. You should caution her against which of the following while she takes this medication due to the increased potential for an adverse reaction?

   a. Sun exposure

   b. Alcohol consumption

   c. Contemporaneous use of muscle relaxants

   d. Standing upright quickly from sitting or lying positions

3–22. Your patient is a 28-year-old with her first episode of painful vulvar lesions, which first appeared as "blisters." Which of the following statements regarding this type of infection is true?

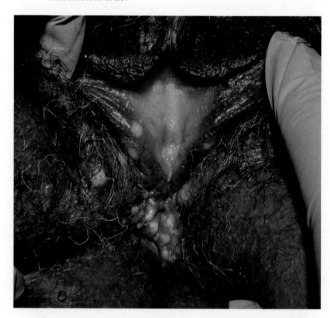

Photograph contributed by Dr. Thoa Ha.

   a. Antibody testing is more sensitive than viral culture.

   b. Men manifest a higher proportion of active cases than women.

   c. More than 90 percent of genital infections caused by this pathogen will be diagnosed during the initial infection.

   d. The average immune response to this infection lowers the risk of subsequent human immunodeficiency virus (HIV) infection.

3-23. Your patient is a 45-year-old woman with confirmed primary syphilis. She has a history of respiratory distress and hives with past penicillin use. She refuses to undergo skin testing to confirm her penicillin allergy and to complete subsequent desensitization. What is the best alternative oral antibiotic regimen?

a. Doxycycline

b. Azithromycin

c. Erythromycin

d. Ciprofloxacin

3-24. Your patient is a 32-year-old recently diagnosed elsewhere with HIV/acquired immunodeficiency syndrome (AIDS). She is currently not taking any medications. She presents with genital lesions that have been present for 1 week. She reports having had a single sore 4 months ago that was not painful and subsided without treatment after approximately 2 weeks. Which of the following tests specific to these lesions do you expect to be positive?

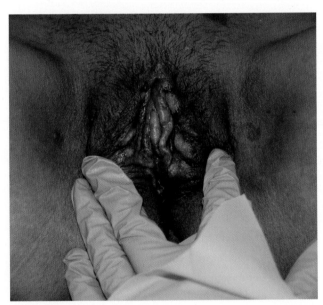

Photograph contributed by Dr. Laura Greer.

a. Rapid plasma reagin

b. Wright-Giemsa stain

c. Herpes simplex 2 antibody assay

d. Positive skin punch biopsy staining for *Candida*

3-25. Your patient is a 24-year-old woman who presents with recent painless vulvar nodules that have now developed into red ulcers that bleed easily. Inguinal lymphadenopathy is minimal on examination. She has been in a mutually monogamous, heterosexual relationship for a year. Wright-Giemsa stain of a swab from one of the lesions shows Donovan bodies (shown here). What is her diagnosis?

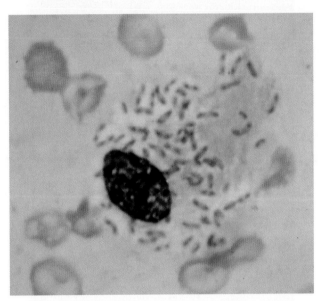

Reproduced, with permission, from Hart G: Donovanosis. In Fauci AS, Braunwald E, Kasper DL, et al (eds): Harrison's Principles of Internal Medicine, 17th ed. New York, McGraw-Hill, 2008, Figure 154-2.

a. Chancroid

b. Primary syphilis

c. Granuloma inguinale

d. Lymphogranuloma venereum

3–26. Risk factors for the vaginal pathogen seen here on potassium hydroxide (KOH) preparation include which of the following?

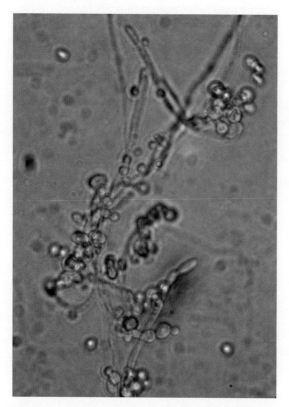

Reproduced, with permission, from Brooks GF, Carroll KC, Butel JS, et al (eds): Medical mycology. In Jawetz, Melnick, & Adelberg's Medical Microbiology, 25th ed. New York, McGraw-Hill, 2010, Figure 45-20.

a. Obesity

b. Orogenital sex

c. Broad-spectrum antibiotic use

d. All of the above

3–27. Your 32-year-old patient has no complaints when presenting for a routine health maintenance visit, but is found to have a clinically abnormal vaginal discharge during speculum examination of the vagina. A saline preparation of vaginal secretions demonstrates the motile pathogens shown here and marked by arrows. Your patient is at highest concurrent risk for which of the following?

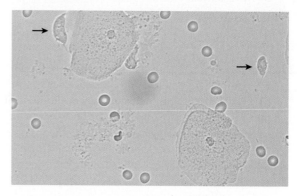

Photograph contributed by Dr. Lauri Campagna and Rebecca Winn, WHNP.

a. Infertility

b. Cervical neoplasia

c. Acute pelvic inflammatory disease

d. Coinfection with other sexually transmitted pathogens

3–28. Treatment of uncomplicated gonorrhea of the cervix recommended by 2011 Centers for Disease Control and Prevention (CDC) guidelines takes into account recent development of antibiotic resistance. Recommended treatment includes which of the following?

a. Erythromycin

b. Ciprofloxacin

c. Ceftriaxone plus azithromycin

d. Ciprofloxacin plus azithromycin

3–29. 2010 Centers for Disease Control and Prevention (CDC) guidelines include annual screening of all sexually active women aged 25 years and younger, regardless of risk factors, for all **EXCEPT** which of the following sexually transmitted infections?

a. Syphilis

b. Gonorrhea

c. *Chlamydia* infection

d. Human immunodeficiency virus

3-30. Your patient presents with vulvar lesions similar to those shown here. Approximately 8 weeks ago, she acquired a new sexual partner. Which of the following patient-applied topical therapies for this infection has shown superiority over the others in clinical trials with nearly 100-percent initial clearance rates?

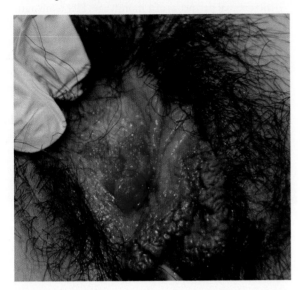

Reproduced, with permission, from Hemsell DL: Gynecologic infection. In Schorge JO, Schaffer JI, Halvorson LM, et al (eds): Williams Gynecology, 1st ed. New York, McGraw-Hill, 2008, Figure 3-17.

   a. Imiquimod

   b. Sinecatechins

   c. Podophyllotoxin

   d. None of the above

3-31. Your patient is a 20-year-old college student with acute onset of urinary frequency and dysuria 2 days ago. She is otherwise healthy and is afebrile. She had one similar episode 15 months ago that resolved quickly with oral antibiotics. Studies have shown that the minimum evaluation required before antibiotics are prescribed for uncomplicated cystitis includes which of the following?

   a. Urinalysis

   b. Physical examination

   c. Urine culture with bacterial sensitivities

   d. None of the above are required

3-32. Which of the following can cause a falsely positive leukocyte esterase testing of a urine specimen?

   a. *Trichomonas* vaginitis

   b. Contamination with colonic or vaginal bacteria

   c. Delayed testing or a poorly preserved specimen

   d. All of the above

3-33. Your patient is a 20-year-old nulligravida with generalized abdominal pain (worse in both lower quadrants), vaginal discharge, anorexia, fever, and chills. She rates her pain as a "9" on a scale of 10. She became sexually active for the first time 1 year ago and has had three sexual partners since. She uses condoms for contraception. Her oral temperature is 39.1°C. Abdominal examination shows diffuse tenderness with bilateral lower quadrant guarding. Her cervix has the appearance shown. Lateral movement of the cervix during bimanual examination elicits increased pain. There are sheets of leukocytes on her vaginal saline wet prep. Her urine pregnancy test result is negative. Which of the following tests would be **LEAST** likely to aid the diagnosis and management of this patient?

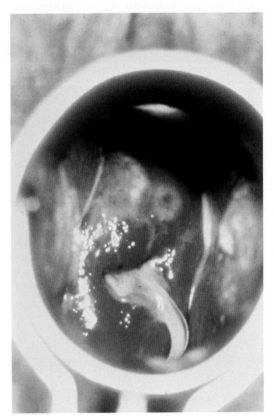

Reproduced, with permission, from Buckley RG, Knoop KJ: Gynecologic and obstetric conditions. In Knoop KJ, Stack LB, Storrow AB, et al (eds): The Atlas of Emergency Medicine, 3rd ed. New York, 2010, Figure 10-4.

   a. Urinalysis

   b. Pelvic sonography

   c. Complete blood count

   d. Endometrial biopsy for bacterial culture

SECTION 1

3-34. The patient in Question 3–31 is admitted to the hospital inpatient gynecology service. Which of the following parenteral antibiotic regimens would **NOT** be appropriate for initial therapy?

a. Cefotetan plus doxycycline

b. Clindamycin plus gentamicin

c. Ciprofloxacin plus metronidazole

d. Ampicillin/sulbactam plus doxycycline

3-35. Your 42-year-old patient underwent an uneventful vaginal hysterectomy for adenomyosis 10 days ago. She received perioperative prophylactic antibiotics. She presents to your office today complaining of diffuse lower abdominal pain. This began several days ago as left-sided lower abdominal pain, but has worsened and become more generalized. She developed subjective fever and anorexia yesterday. On examination, she appears ill. Her temperature is 39.5°C, pulse 110, blood pressure 90/55. Her abdominal and pelvic examinations suggest peritonitis with extreme tenderness and a possible mass in the left adnexal region. Which of the following true gynecologic emergencies does this likely represent?

a. Ovarian abscess

b. Pelvic cellulitis

c. Vaginal cuff cellulitis

d. Infected pelvic hematoma

3-36. You are called to the emergency department to consult on a 26-year-old patient presenting with 36 hours of progressive malaise, fever, muscle aches, anorexia, diarrhea, and confusion. Her last menstrual period began 2 to 3 days ago as expected. She has had an intrauterine device in place for 1 year without problems. She has a new sexual partner as of 1 month ago. Her temperature is elevated, she is hypotensive, and she has erythema of her oropharynx and vaginal mucosa. Her skin demonstrates a diffuse macular rash. Abdominal and bimanual pelvic examinations are mildly tender, but no specific or localized findings are present. After obtaining appropriate laboratory tests and bacterial cultures, you quickly start parenteral antibiotics effective against which of the following pathogens?

a. *Neisseria gonorrhoeae*

b. *Staphylococcus aureus*

c. *Streptococcus pyogenes*

d. *Clostridium perfringens*

References

Amsel R, Totten PA, Spiegel CA, et al: Nonspecific vaginitis. Diagnostic criteria and microbial and epidemiologic associations. Am J Med 74:14, 1983

Centers for Disease Control and Prevention: Cephalosporin susceptibility among Neisseria gonorrhoeae isolates—United States, 2000–2010. MMWR 60(26):873, 2011

Centers for Disease Control and Prevention: Sexually transmitted diseases treatment guidelines, 2010. MMWR 59(12):1, 2010

Chapter 3 ANSWER KEY

Question number	Letter answer	Page cited	Header cited	Question number	Letter answer	Page cited	Header cited
3–1	b	p. 64	Normal Vaginal Flora	3–20	c	p. 75	Tetracyclines
3–2	a	p. 64	Normal Vaginal Flora	3–21	a	p. 75	Tetracyclines
3–3	d	p. 64	Normal Vaginal Flora	3–22	a	p. 76	Pathogens Causing Genital Ulcer Infections
3–4	b	p. 65	Vaginal pH				
3–5	d	p. 65	Vaginal pH	3–23	a	p. 80	Table 3-12
3–6	b	p. 66	Diagnosis	3–24	a	p. 79	Diagnosis
3–7	d	p. 66	Diagnosis	3–25	c	p. 81	Granuloma Inguinale
3–8	a	p. 67	Table 3-3	3–26	d	p. 83	Fungal Infection
3–9	d	p. 67	Treatment	3–27	d	p. 84	Epidemiology
3–10	b	p. 67	Structure	3–28	c	p. 87	Treatment
3–11	d	p. 70	Table 3-5	3–29	a	p. 87	*Chlamydia trachomatis*
3–12	d	p. 67	Penicillins	3–30	d	p. 88	Treatment
3–13	c	p. 69	Cephalosporins	3–31	d	p. 92	Diagnosis
3–14	c	p. 70	Aminoglycosides	3–32	d	p. 92	Leukocyte Esterase
3–15	a	p. 74	Carbapenems	3–33	d	p. 96	Laboratory Testing
3–16	b	p. 74	Clindamycin	3–34	c	p. 99	Table 3-28
3–17	d	p. 74	Vancomycin	3–35	a	p. 103	Ovarian Abscess
3–18	a	p. 75	Metronidazole	3–36	b	p. 105	Toxic Shock Syndrome
3–19	c	p. 75	Fluoroquinolones				

CHAPTER 4

Benign Disorders of the Lower Reproductive Tract

4-1. Pathology involving the vulva is common, and lesions may result from which of the following?

    a. Trauma

    b. Neoplasia

    c. Immune responses

    d. All of the above

4-2. Which of the following agents is commonly implicated in allergic contact dermatitis?

    a. Lanolin

    b. Cosmetic ingredients

    c. Clobetasol propionate

    d. All of the above

4-3. Vulvar hygiene is a cornerstone of lichen sclerosus management and includes all **EXCEPT** which of the following?

    a. Wearing preferably nylon or synthetic underwear

    b. Avoiding use of scented bath products and soaps

    c. Avoiding use of a harsh washcloth to clean the vulva

    d. Avoiding commercial washing detergents for undergarments

4-4. Which of the following vulvar disorders is characterized by a chronic inflammatory skin condition mainly of the anogenital skin as shown in this image?

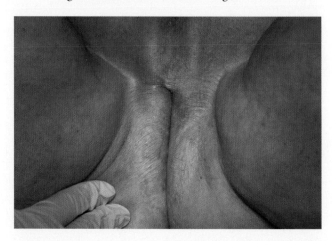

Reproduced, with permission, from Gala RB: Benign disorders of the lower reproductive tract. In Schorge JO, Schaffer JI, Halvorson LM, et al (eds): Williams Gynecology, 1st ed. New York, McGraw-Hill, 2008, Figure 4-1.

    a. Lichen planus

    b. Lichen sclerosus

    c. Contact dermatitis

    d. Hidradenitis suppurativa

4-5. Which of the following autoimmune disorders have been reported to show a consistent relationship with lichen sclerosus?

    a. Graves disease

    b. Diabetes mellitus

    c. Systemic lupus erythematosus

    d. All of the above

4-6. Which of the following preparations provide first-line therapy for lichen sclerosus?

    a. Estrogen cream

    b. Testosterone cream

    c. Ultrapotent topical corticosteroid ointment

    d. All of the above

4–7. Although several treatments are available for psoriasis (shown here), the most widely used, rapid, and effective agent is which of the following?

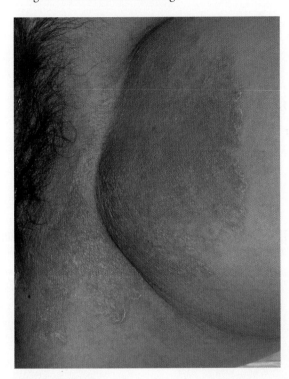

   a. Alefacept

   b. Infliximab

   c. Vitamin D analog

   d. Topical corticosteroid

4–8. Which of the following vulvar dermatoses commonly presents with oral lesions, such as the one shown here?

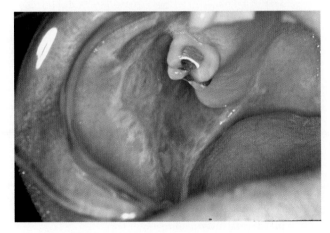

Photograph contributed by Dr. Edward Ellis.

   a. Lichen planus

   b. Lichen sclerosus

   c. Pemphigus vulgaris

   d. Fox-Fordyce disease

4–9. Treatment of vaginal lichen planus is challenging, and symptomatic relief has been reported using which of the following?

   a. Minocycline

   b. Estrogen cream

   c. Sequential vaginal dilators

   d. Vaginal corticosteroid suppositories

4–10. Which of the following vulvar disorders is characterized by this image?

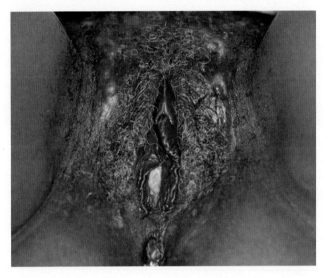

Reproduced, with permission, from Gala RB: Benign disorders of the lower reproductive tract. In Schorge JO, Schaffer JI, Halvorson LM, et al (eds): Williams Gynecology, 1st ed. New York, McGraw-Hill, 2008, Figure 4-10.

   a. Vitiligo

   b. Lichen planus

   c. Lichen sclerosus

   d. Hidradenitis suppurativa

4–11. Which of the following vulvar disorders can be disfiguring and involves apocrine gland-bearing follicular epithelium?

   a. Crohn disease

   b. Lichen planus

   c. Hidradenitis suppurativa

   d. Erythema multiforme major

4–12. Early treatment of hidradenitis suppurativa involves which of the following?

   a. Topical corticosteroid ointment

   b. Infliximab, a monoclonal antibody

   c. Surgical excision of apocrine gland sinus tracts

   d. Warm compresses, topical antiseptics, and systemic antibiotics

4–13. Which of the following is a painful, self-limited mucosal lesion?

   a. Vitiligo

   b. Aphthous ulcer

   c. Pemphigus vulgaris

   d. All of the above

4–14. Epithelium pigmentation changes may include which of the following?

   a. Vitiligo

   b. Melanoma

   c. Acanthosis nigricans

   d. All of the above

4–15. Which of the following is the second most common vulvar malignancy and accounts for up to 10 percent of all vulvar cancers?

   a. Melanoma

   b. Basal cell carcinoma

   c. Squamous cell carcinoma

   d. Bartholin gland adenocarcinoma

4–16. The loss of epidermal melanocytes in areas of depigmented vulvar skin is shown in this image and is termed which of the following?

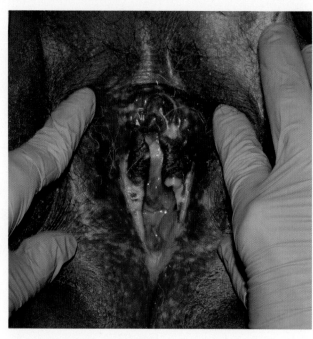

Image contributed by Sharon Irvin, WHNP.

   a. Vitiligo

   b. Acanthosis

   c. Fox-Fordyce disease

   d. Nigricans acrochordon

4–17. The most common cause of vitiligo involves genetic factors. What percent of patients have at least one affected first-degree relative?

   a. 10

   b. 20

   c. 40

   d. 50

4–18. Bartholin gland duct cysts form in direct response to which of the following?

   a. Vulvar irritation

   b. Cervical gonorrhea

   c. Gland duct obstruction

   d. Chronic lichen sclerosus

4–19. The image below best represents which of the following vulvar disorders?

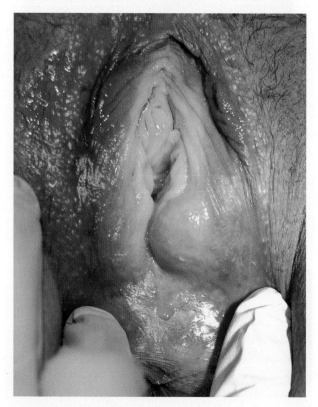

Reproduced with permission from Hoffman BL, Horsager R, Roberts SW: Williams Obstetrics 23rd Edition Study Guide. New York, McGraw-Hill, 2011, Figure 40-13.

   a. Skene gland abscess

   b. Urethral diverticulum

   c. Epidermal inclusion cyst

   d. Bartholin gland duct cyst

4–20. Which of the following is generally the treatment of choice for recurrent Bartholin gland duct abscess?

   a. Systemic antibiotics

   b. 5-percent lidocaine ointment

   c. Bartholin gland duct marsupialization

   d. Warm compresses and frequent sitz baths

4–21. This midline cystic mass best represents which of the following vulvar disorders?

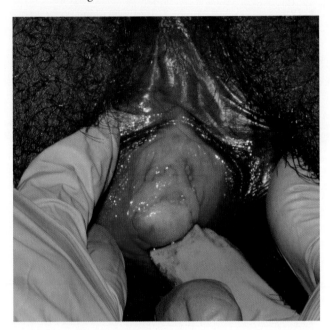

Image contributed by Dr. Sasha Andrews.

   a. Gartner duct cyst

   b. Bartholin gland cyst

   c. Urethral diverticulum

   d. Nabothian cyst

4–22. According to the October 2003 ISSVD World Congress, which of the following terms most often describes burning vulvar pain occurring in the absence of relevant visible findings or specific, clinically identifiable disorders?

   a. Dermatitis

   b. Vulvodynia

   c. Hidradenitis

   d. Vestibulitis

4–23. The pain of vulvodynia is described as which of the following?

   a. Provoked

   b. Unprovoked

   c. Generalized

   d. All of the above

4–24. Although no specific laboratory test can diagnose vulvodynia, which of the following tests may help exclude an underlying vaginitis?

   a. Cervical Pap test

   b. Keyes punch biopsy

   c. Human papillomavirus (HPV) serology

   d. Wet prep, vaginal pH evaluation, and herpes viral serology

4–25. In general, which of the following forms of therapy may be initially recommended to stabilize and improve vulvodynia symptoms?

   a. Surgical excision

   b. Intralesional injections

   c. Oral antidepressants and anticonvulsants

   d. Vulvar care and 5-percent lidocaine ointment

Chapter 4   ANSWER KEY

Question number	Letter answer	Page cited	Header cited	Question number	Letter answer	Page cited	Header cited
4–1	d	p. 110	Vulvar Lesions	4–14	d	p. 120	Disorders of Pigmentation
4–2	d	p. 111	Table 4-1	4–15	a	p. 120	Disorders of Pigmentation
4–3	a	p. 114	Table 4-3	4–16	a	p. 121	Vitiligo
4–4	b	p. 113	Lichen Sclerosus	4–17	b	p. 121	Vitiligo
4–5	d	p. 113	Lichen Sclerosus	4–18	c	p. 123	Bartholin Gland Duct Cyst and Abscess
4–6	c	p. 114	Corticosteroids	4–19	d	p. 123	Bartholin Gland Duct Cyst and Abscess
4–7	d	p. 117	Psoriasis	4–20	c	p. 123	Bartholin Gland Duct Cyst and Abscess
4–8	a	p. 117	Lichen Planus	4–21	c	p. 123	Urethral Diverticulum
4–9	d	p. 118	Treatment of Vaginal Lichen Planus	4–22	b	p. 124	Vulvodynia
4–10	d	p. 118	Hidradenitis Suppurativa	4–23	d	p. 124	Vulvodynia
4–11	c	p. 118	Hidradenitis Suppurativa	4–24	d	p. 126	Laboratory Testing
4–12	d	p. 118	Hidradenitis Suppurativa	4–25	d	p. 126	Treatment
4–13	b	p. 119	Aphthous Ulcers				

CHAPTER 5

Contraception and Sterilization

5-1. Which of the following poses the highest risk of death in fertile women aged 35 to 44 years?

    a. Pregnancy

    b. Oral contraceptive use

    c. Intrauterine device (IUD) use

    d. Surgical tubal sterilization procedure

5-2. Which of the following is a second-tier contraceptive method with an expected failure rate of 3 to 9 percent per 100 users during the first year?

    a. Spermicide

    b. Withdrawal

    c. Intrauterine device

    d. Oral contraceptive pills

5-3. Your patient delivered a healthy infant 2 weeks ago and wishes to initiate use of a contraceptive method during the next few weeks. She is breastfeeding exclusively. For which of the following is there strong evidence that use decreases the quantity and quality of breast milk?

    a. Progestin-only pills

    b. Depot medroxyprogesterone acetate

    c. Combination hormonal contraceptives

    d. None of the above

5-4. A 16-year-old nulligravida is requesting a contraceptive method. She plans to become sexually active with her boyfriend soon. Which of the following is legally required in most states prior to prescribing hormonal contraception for adolescents below the age of consent?

    a. Parental consent

    b. Pelvic examination

    c. Cervical cancer screening

    d. None of the above

5-5. Which of the following conditions is **NOT** listed by the manufacturer as a contraindication of this contraceptive method?

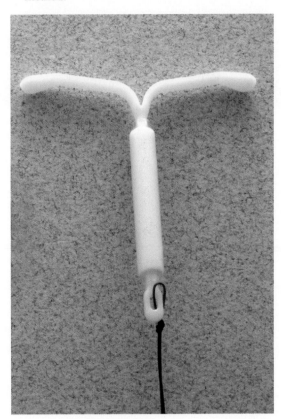

    a. Acute liver disease

    b. Heavy menses due to coagulation disorder

    c. Increased susceptibility to pelvic infection

    d. Uterine anomaly with distortion of the uterine cavity

5–6. Your patient is a 26-year-old multipara who presents for a well-woman examination. She has no complaints. She is satisfied with her current method of contraception (shown here). It was inserted 2 years ago, and she wishes to continue with this contraceptive method. Her pelvic exam is normal. Cervical cytology (Pap test) is obtained and is negative for malignancy, but *Actinomyces* is identified on the smear. Which of the following is **NOT** a reasonable treatment option for managing this incidental finding according to current recommendations from the American College of Obstetricians and Gynecologists (2005)?

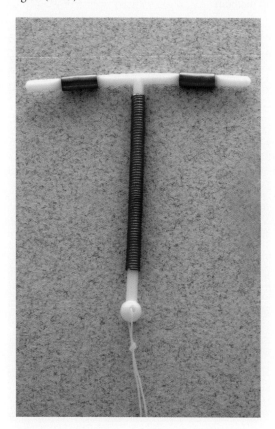

a. Hysterectomy

b. Expectant management (no intervention)

c. Extended course of antibiotics with intrauterine device (IUD) left in place

d. IUD removal and initiation of an alternative contraceptive method

5–7. For which of the following is the use of an intrauterine device associated with an increased complication rate?

a. Adolescence

b. Human immunodeficiency infection

c. Insertion immediately after spontaneous or induced abortion

d. None of the above

5–8. What is the spontaneous expulsion rate for the intrauterine device during the first year after placement?

a. 1 percent

b. 5 percent

c. 10 percent

d. 15 percent

5–9. What is the approximate risk of the complication shown here per intrauterine device insertion?

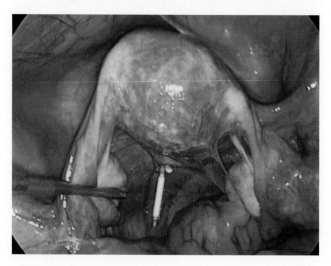

Photograph contributed by Dr. Kimberly Kho.

a. 1 in 100

b. 1 in 1000

c. 1 in 10,000

d. 1 in 100,000

5–10. A 34-year-old multipara with a copper-containing IUD in place presents for intrauterine device (IUD) removal because she plans to become pregnant soon. Her last menstrual period was 8 weeks ago. Her urine pregnancy test is positive, and sonography confirms an eight-week intrauterine gestation. She wishes to continue this pregnancy, if possible. She feels well, is afebrile, and has no cervical discharge or pelvic tenderness. You visualize the IUD tail strings protruding from the external cervical os. Which of the following management strategies is recommended to optimize the outcome for your patient?

a. Perform IUD removal and evacuation of uterine contents

b. Perform IUD removal and plan expectant pregnancy management

c. Leave the IUD in place and plan expectant pregnancy management

d. Leave the IUD in place and administer broad-spectrum antibiotics for the next 4 weeks

5–11. For which of the following contraceptive methods is a history of previous ectopic pregnancy considered by its manufacturer to be a contraindication to its use?

   a. Copper-containing intrauterine device

   b. Progestin-containing subdermal implant

   c. Depot medroxyprogesterone acetate (DMPA)

   d. Levonorgestrel-releasing intrauterine system (LNG-IUS)

5–12. Which of the following is thought to be a mechanism of action by which this device provides contraception?

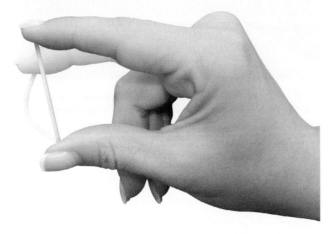

   a. Ovulation suppression

   b. Endometrial atrophic changes

   c. Increased cervical mucus viscosity

   d. All of the above

5–13. Which of the following statements is true regarding the effects of female tubal sterilization?

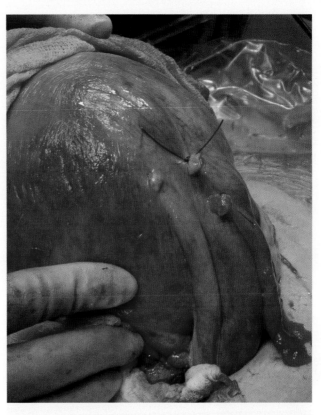

Reproduced, with permission, by Hoffman BL, Horsager R, Roberts SW, et al: Williams Obstetrics 23rd Edition Study Guide. New York, McGraw-Hill, 2011, Figure 33-6B.

   a. Ovarian cancer risk is increased.

   b. The incidence of menorrhagia and dysmenorrhea are increased.

   c. At least 10 percent of pregnancies occurring after the procedure are ectopic.

   d. By 5 years postprocedure, 50 percent of women aged 30 years or younger at the time of sterilization express regret.

5–14. Which of the following statements regarding vasectomy is true?

   a. Semen analysis should be performed 3 months after vasectomy to confirm azoospermia.

   b. The postoperative complication rate is 20 times less than that of female tubal sterilization.

   c. The failure rate is 30 times less than that of female tubal sterilization.

   d. All of the above

5-15. Which of the following is **NOT** a physiologic effect exerted by the progestin component of combination hormonal contraceptives?

   a. Lowered serum free testosterone levels

   b. Suppressed serum levels of luteinizing hormone

   c. Elevated serum levels of follicle-stimulating hormone

   d. All are physiologic effects

5-16. Which of the following is **NOT** an absolute contraindication to use of this contraceptive method?

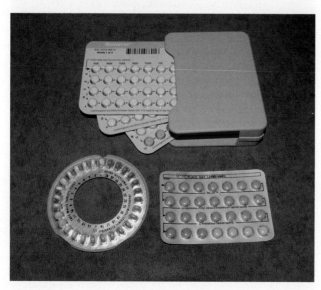

Reproduced, with permission, from Stuart GS: Contraception and sterilization. In Hoffman BL, Schorge JO, Schaffer JI, et al (eds): Williams Gynecology, 2nd ed. New York, McGraw-Hill, 2012, Figure 5-10.

   a. Thrombotic disorders

   b. Cholestatic jaundice

   c. Migraines with focal neurologic deficits

   d. Uncomplicated systemic lupus erythematosus (including negative testing for antiphospholipid antibodies)

5-17. Which of the following statements regarding this method of contraception compared with combination oral contraceptive pills (COCs) is true?

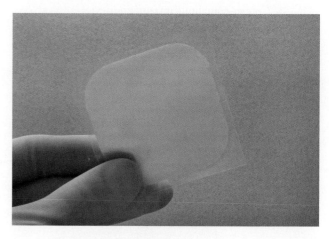

Reproduced, with permission, by Hoffman BL, Horsager R, Roberts SW, et al: Williams Obstetrics 23rd Edition Study Guide. New York, McGraw-Hill, 2011, Figure 32-12.

   a. Total estrogen exposure is greater with this method.

   b. This method is less likely to cause breast tenderness.

   c. This method controls dysmenorrhea in a greater percentage of women.

   d. The pregnancy rate with this method is slightly higher than with COCs.

5-18. Rates of which of the following are increased with use of extended cycle hormonal contraception compared with traditional cyclic hormonal contraception use?

   a. Headaches

   b. Escape ovulation

   c. Endometrial cancer

   d. Unpredictable bleeding

5-19. Use of which of the following drugs most clearly decreases combined hormonal contraceptive efficacy?

   a. Rifampin

   b. Penicillin

   c. Doxycycline

   d. Ciprofloxacin

5-20. Low-dose combination hormonal contraceptives most clearly increase the risk of developing which of the following?

   a. Obesity

   b. Clinically significant hypertension

   c. Overt diabetes in women with prior gestational diabetes

   d. None of the above

5–21. With combination hormonal contraceptive use, stroke risk is elevated by which of the following being coexistent?

a. Tobacco use

b. Hypertension

c. Migraine headaches with aura

d. All of the above

5–22. Your patient is concerned after reading that the risk of deep-vein thrombosis and pulmonary embolism is tripled or quadrupled in current users of combination hormonal contraceptives (CHCs) compared with that of the general population. You explain that this is true, but that the risk is still lower than the risk of venous thrombosis related to pregnancy. What is the approximate rate of thromboembolic events per 10,000 woman years with CHC use?

a. 4 events

b. 24 events

c. 44 events

d. 64 events

5–23. Your patient is an 18-year-old nulligravida who is not sexually active, but takes combination oral contraceptive pills (COCs) to achieve good control of her irregular menses and dysmenorrhea. She has grand mal epilepsy. Her seizures are well controlled on medication. Serum levels of which anticonvulsant medication are decreased significantly by concurrent COC use?

a. Phenytoin

b. Lamotrigine

c. Carbamazepine

d. Phenobarbital

5–24. Contemporary low-dose combination oral contraceptives are most strongly implicated as a risk factor for the development of which of the following neoplasms?

a. Breast cancer

b. Cervical cancer

c. Benign hepatic adenomas

d. Lymphoma, if human immunodeficiency virus (HIV) infection is coexistent

5–25. Your patient has diabetes and hypertension but prefers to use "pills" for contraception. She declines an intrauterine device and barrier methods. She is considering a progestin-only contraceptive and favors progestin-only pills. You counsel her regarding the advantages as well as which of the following disadvantages of progestin-only pills compared with combination oral contraceptives?

a. Higher failure rate

b. High rate of irregular bleeding

c. Higher relative ectopic pregnancy rate

d. All of the above

5–26. Which of the following is generally increased by the use of depot medroxyprogesterone acetate compared with other contraceptive methods?

a. Acne

b. Bone fractures

c. Hepatic neoplasms

d. Interval to resumption of ovulation after method cessation

5–27. Which of the following is an advantage of lambskin condoms compared with latex rubber condoms?

a. Fewer allergic reactions

b. Lower breakage and slippage rates

c. Better protection against sexually transmitted infections

d. All of the above

5–28. Which of the following is an advantage of progestin-only emergency contraception (EC) regimens compared with estrogen-progestin combinations for this purpose?

a. More effective in preventing pregnancy

b. Effective if taken beyond 5 days after exposure

c. Provides better protection against sexually transmitted infections

d. None of the above

References

American College of Obstetricians and Gynecologists: Clinical management guidelines for obstetrician-gynecologists. Practice Bulletin No. 59, January 2005

Chapter 5 ANSWER KEY

Question number	Letter answer	Page cited	Header cited	Question number	Letter answer	Page cited	Header cited
5–1	a	p. 133	Table 5-1	5–15	c	p. 148	Mechanism of Action
5–2	d	p. 132	Chapter 5: Contraception and Sterilization	5–16	d	p. 149	Table 5-7
5–3	d	p. 136	Table 5-4	5–17	a	p. 152	Transdermal System
5–4	d	p. 135	Adolescence and Perimenopause	5–18	d	p. 153	Extended Cycle Contraception
5–5	b	p. 138	Table 5-5	5–19	a	p. 155	Table 5-11
5–6	a	p. 138	Infection	5–20	d	p. 153	Weight Gain; CHC & Medical Disorders
5–7	d	p. 139	Low Parity and Adolescents	5–21	d	p. 155	Cerebrovascular Disorders
5–8	b	p. 139	Expulsion	5–22	a	p. 155	Venous Thromboembolism
5–9	b	p. 139	Uterine Perforation	5–23	b	p. 156	Seizure Disorders
5–10	b	p. 140	Management	5–24	b	p. 156	Neoplastic Diseases
5–11	d	p. 141	Ectopic Pregnancy	5–25	d	p. 158	Counseling
5–12	d	p. 143	Mechanism of Action	5–26	d	p. 158	Delayed Return of Fertility Following Cessation
5–13	c	p. 145	Regret	5–27	a	p. 159	Latex Sensitivity
5–14	d	p. 147	Male Sterilization	5–28	a	p. 163	Progestin-Only Regimens

CHAPTER 6

First-Trimester Abortion

6-1. More than 80 percent of spontaneous abortions occur in the first 12 weeks of pregnancy. What percent of these result from chromosomal anomalies?

a. 25

b. 35

c. 50

d. 75

6-2. Although most early pregnancy losses are clinically silent, approximately what percentage of all pregnancies are reportedly lost after implantation?

a. 11

b. 21

c. 31

d. 41

6-3. Which of the following chromosomal anomalies is most frequently identified with first-trimester abortion?

a. Triploidy

b. Monosomy X (45,X)

c. Autosomal trisomy

d. Balanced Robertsonian translocation

6-4. Maternal factors that contribute to euploid abortion include all **EXCEPT** which of the following?

a. Frequent alcohol use

b. Daily tobacco smoking

c. Dietary nutrient deficiency

d. Poorly controlled diabetes mellitus

6-5. Although moderate caffeine consumption is unlikely to cause spontaneous abortion, studies consistently warn that use above what daily amount of caffeine increases the risk for miscarriage?

a. 200 mg (2 cups of coffee)

b. 300 mg (3 cups of coffee)

c. 400 mg (4 cups of coffee)

d. 500 mg (5 cups of coffee)

6-6. Up to what percentage of women experience vaginal spotting or bleeding during early gestation?

a. 15

b. 25

c. 35

d. 45

6-7. Approximately what percentage of pregnancies abort in women experiencing early gestational bleeding?

a. 5

b. 20

c. 50

d. 60

6-8. A proven, effective therapy for threatened abortion includes which of the following?

a. Bed rest

b. Daily morning acetaminophen (Tylenol)

c. Increased oral fluid intake

d. None of the above

6-9. Which of the following should always be considered in the differential diagnosis of threatened abortion?

a. Paternal factors

b. Ectopic pregnancy

c. Minor maternal trauma

d. Oral contraceptive use

6-10. Your patient presents with complaints of vaginal spotting and a last menstrual period 6 weeks ago. Transvaginal sonography reveals the following, and fetal heart motion is seen. Your diagnosis is which of the following?

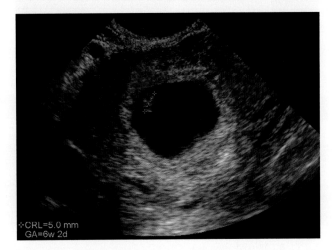

a. Missed abortion

b. Incomplete abortion

c. Threatened abortion

d. All of the above

6–11. The same patient in Question 6–10 represents 2 weeks later with light bleeding and strong cramps. Her blood pressure is 132/78, pulse is 72, and she is afebrile. Her hematocrit is 40. Transvaginal sonography reveals the following. Appropriate management includes which of the following?

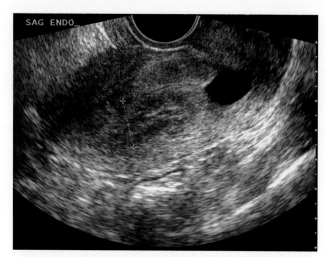

a. Await spontaneous miscarriage

b. Excise cesarean scar pregnancy

c. Perform emergent cerclage placement

d. Administer intramuscular injection of methotrexate

6–12. While in your emergency department, the patient in Question 6–11 passes the tissue shown here. Her bleeding and pain have now subsided significantly. Your diagnosis is which of the following?

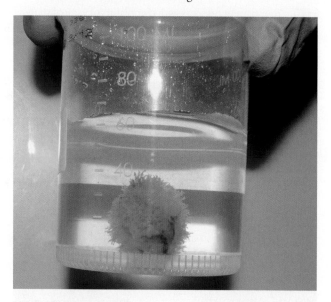

a. Missed abortion

b. Complete abortion

c. Threatened abortion

d. None of the above

6–13. Appropriate management of this patient now includes which of the following?

a. Transvaginal sonography

b. Dilatation and curettage

c. Administration of Rho [D] immunoglobulin, if the patient is Rh negative

d. All of the above

6–14. To correctly define an incomplete abortion, which of the following must be present?

a. Abdominal cramping

b. Heavy vaginal bleeding

c. Dilated external cervical os

d. Dilated internal cervical os

6–15. The transvaginal sonogram shown below displays which of the following?

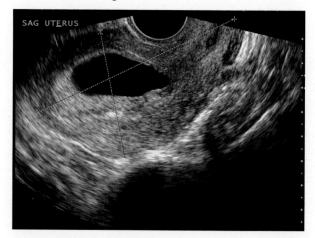

a. Cervical pregnancy

b. Cesarean scar pregnancy

c. Intrauterine anembryonic gestation

d. None of the above

6–16. In 2005, the Centers for Disease Control and Prevention reported four septic abortion deaths following medical abortion. The deaths were all caused by toxic shock syndrome from which of the following bacterial infections?

a. Gonorrhea

b. *Clostridium sordellii*

c. *Staphylococcus aureus*

d. *Streptococcus pyogenes*

6–17. In women experiencing a spontaneous incomplete abortion without dangerous hemorrhage or infection, expectant management results in spontaneous completion in what percent?

a. 10

b. 30

c. 50

d. 80

6-18. Recurrent spontaneous abortion or recurrent miscarriage is formally defined by which of the following?

  a. Two pregnancy losses in 10 years at 20 weeks' gestation or less

  b. Two consecutive pregnancy losses at 20 weeks' gestation or less

  c. Three or more consecutive pregnancy losses at 20 weeks' gestation or less

  d. Two consecutive pregnancy losses with fetal weights more than 500 grams

6-19. Which of the following is more likely to result in recurrent second-trimester losses?

  a. Genetic factors

  b. Infection

  c. Autoimmune or anatomic factors

  d. All of the above

6-20. Acquired defects that may lead to recurrent miscarriage include which of the following?

  a. Leiomyoma

  b. Asherman syndrome

  c. Cervical incompetence

  d. All of the above

6-21. Of müllerian defects, which has the lowest associated risk of recurrent miscarriage and is shown here in this three-dimensional sonographic image?

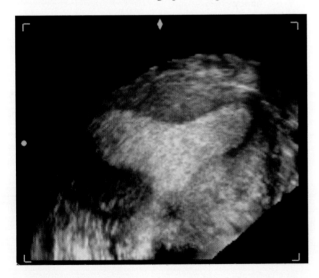

  a. Septate uterus

  b. Arcuate uterus

  c. Uterus didelphys

  d. Unicornuate uterus

6-22. What percent of women with recurrent miscarriage have recognized autoimmune factors?

  a. 5

  b. 15

  c. 30

  d. 45

6-23. Early pregnancy loss is more common in women with which of the following?

  a. Well-controlled type 2 diabetes mellitus

  b. Human immunodeficiency virus (HIV) infection

  c. Systemic lupus erythematosus with antiphospholipid antibodies

  d. Marfan syndrome

6-24. Antiphospholipid antibodies can be correlated with adverse pregnancy outcome. Clinical and laboratory criteria include which of the following?

  a. Serial detection of lupus anticoagulant

  b. Three or more consecutive spontaneous abortion before 10 weeks' gestation

  c. Moderate to high levels of immunoglobulin G (IgG) or immunoglobulin M (IgM) anticardiolipin antibodies

  d. All of the above

6-25. There are treatment regimens for antiphospholipid syndrome that increase live birth rates. A regimen proposed by the American College of Obstetricians and Gynecologists includes which of the following?

  a. Low-dose aspirin daily

  b. 5000 units vitamin D daily

  c. Unfractionated heparin twice daily

  d. Both low-dose aspirin daily along with unfractionated heparin twice daily

6-26. In asymptomatic women with recurrent miscarriage, screening for which of the following infections is indicated to find an underlying etiology?

  a. Gonorrhea

  b. Human immunodeficiency virus (HIV) infection

  c. *Chlamydia trachomatis* infection

  d. None of the above

6-27. An initial scheme for the evaluation of women with recurrent miscarriage includes all **EXCEPT** which of the following?

  a. Partner karyotyping

  b. Diagnostic laparoscopy

  c. Uterine cavity evaluation

  d. Antiphospholipid antibody syndrome testing

6-28. In the United States, how many pregnancies are electively (voluntary) terminated for every four live births?

   a. 1

   b. 2

   c. 3

   d. 4

6-29. Common complications of this method of first-trimester pregnancy termination include all **EXCEPT** which of the following?

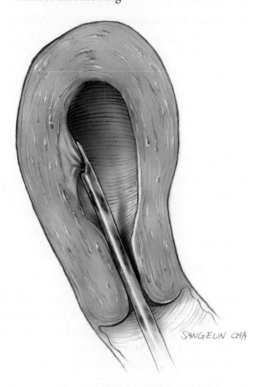

Reproduced, with permission, from Word L: Surgeries for benign gynecologic conditions. In Hoffman BL, Schorge JO, Schaffer JI, et al (eds): Williams Gynecology, 2nd ed. New York, McGraw-Hill, 2012, Figure 41-16.8.

   a. Infection

   b. Hemorrhage

   c. Asherman syndrome

   d. Incomplete abortion

6-30. Prior to surgical pregnancy termination, the device shown here is placed in preparation for pregnancy termination at 14 weeks' gestation. The next day your patient chooses **NOT** to proceed with the abortion. You remove the laminaria and counsel her on which of the following?

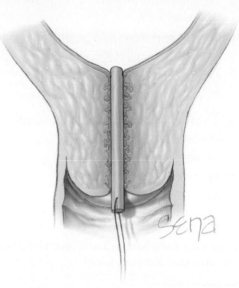

Reproduced, with permission, from Cunningham FG, Leveno KL, Bloom SL, et al: Abortion. In Williams Obstetrics, 23rd ed. New York, McGraw-Hill, 2010, Figure 9-6A.

   a. Observation is recommended.

   b. Abortion will spontaneously occur in most cases.

   c. Oral antimicrobials are required to prevent infection.

   d. Cerclage placement is required to sustain the pregnancy.

Reference

Centers for Disease Control and Prevention: *Clostridium sordellii* toxic shock syndrome after medical abortion with mifepristone and intravaginal misoprostol—United States and Canada, 2001–2005. MMWR 54(29):724, 2005

Chapter 6 ANSWER KEY

Question number	Letter answer	Page cited	Header cited
6–1	c	p. 170	Spontaneous Abortion
6–2	c	p. 171	Incidence
6–3	c	p. 171	Aneuploid Abortion
6–4	c	p. 172	Maternal Factors
6–5	d	p. 174	Caffeine
6–6	b	p. 175	Threatened Abortion
6–7	c	p. 175	Threatened Abortion
6–8	d	p. 175	Threatened Abortion
6–9	b	p. 175	Threatened Abortion
6–10	c	p. 175	Threatened Abortion
6–11	a	p. 176	Incomplete Abortion
6–12	b	p. 177	Complete Abortion
6–13	c	p. 177	Complete Abortion
6–14	d	p. 176	Incomplete Abortion
6–15	c	p. 177	Missed Abortion
6–16	b	p. 177	Septic Abortion

Question number	Letter answer	Page cited	Header cited
6–17	d	p. 178	Management of Spontaneous Abortion
6–18	c	p. 178	Recurrent Miscarriage
6–19	c	p. 178	Recurrent Miscarriage
6–20	d	p. 181	Anatomic Factors
6–21	b	p. 182	Table 6-6
6–22	b	p. 182	Immunologic Factors
6–23	c	p. 182	Autoimmune Factors
6–24	d	p. 182	Antiphospholipid Antibody Syndrome
6–25	d	p. 182	Antiphospholipid Antibody Syndrome
6–26	d	p. 186	Infections
6–27	b	p. 186	Evaluation and Treatment
6–28	a	p. 187	Elective Abortion
6–29	c	p. 189	Techniques for Surgical Abortion
6–30	a	p. 189	Hygroscopic Dilators

CHAPTER 7

Ectopic Pregnancy

7-1. An ectopic or extrauterine pregnancy is one in which the blastocyst implants anywhere other than the endometrial lining of the uterine cavity. Such pregnancies account for what percentage of reported pregnancies in the United States?

  a. 2

  b. 4

  c. 5

  d. 6

7-2. Most ectopic pregnancies implant in the fallopian tube. Where is the **LEAST** common fallopian tube implantation site?

  a. Fimbria

  b. Isthmus

  c. Ampulla

  d. None of the above

7-3. Which of the following carries the highest risk of subsequent ectopic pregnancy?

  a. Smoking

  b. Prior ectopic pregnancy

  c. More than five lifelong sexual partners

  d. Positive test result for cervical *Chlamydia trachomatis*

7-4. Smoking more than one pack of cigarettes daily increases the risk of ectopic pregnancy by what amount?

  a. Twofold

  b. Fourfold

  c. Sixfold

  d. Eightfold

7-5. The levonorgestrel-releasing intrauterine system (Mirena) has a 5-year cumulative pregnancy rate of 0.5 per 100 users. What percentage of these pregnancies are ectopic?

  a. 20

  b. 30

  c. 50

  d. 70

7-6. In a woman with known risk factors for an extrauterine pregnancy who presents with amenorrhea, which of the following symptoms may suggest an ectopic pregnancy?

  a. Breast tenderness

  b. Pain with defecation

  c. Vaginal bleeding and abdominal pain

  d. All of the above

7-7. Inappropriately rising serum β-human chorionic gonadotropin (hCG) levels only indicate a dying pregnancy, not its location. With a robust uterine pregnancy, serum β-hCG levels should increase by which of the following percentage ranges every 48 hours?

  a. 23 to 46 percent

  b. 53 to 66 percent

  c. 63 to 76 percent

  d. 73 to 86 percent

7-8. Using transvaginal sonography, this gestational structure is usually first visible between which of the following weeks of gestation?

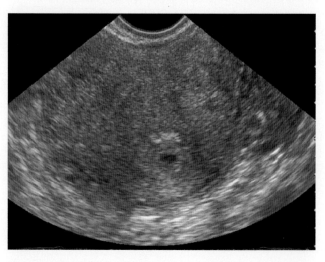

Reproduced, with permission, from Dashe J, Moschos, E, Hoffman BL: Sonographic findings of early intrauterine pregnancy (update). In Cunningham FG, Leveno KL, Bloom SL, et al (eds): Williams Obstetrics, 22nd ed. Online. Accessmedicine.com. New York, McGraw-Hill, 2007, Figure 3.

  a. 4.5 and 5 weeks

  b. 5 and 6 weeks

  c. 5.5 and 6 weeks

  d. After 6 weeks

7–9. A lower-limit serum β-human chorionic gonadotropin (β-hCG) concentration is selected to represent the discriminatory value at which transvaginal sonography can reliably visualize pregnancy? This value may vary by institution but is usually one of which number pairs listed below?

a. 1500 or 2000 IU/L

b. 2500 or 3000 IU/L

c. 4500 or 5000 IU/L

d. 5500 or 6000 IU/L

7–10. The absence of an uterine pregnancy by sonography and a serum β-hCG levels **ABOVE** the discriminatory value may signify which of the following?

a. An ectopic pregnancy

b. An incomplete abortion

c. A resolving completed abortion

d. All of the above

7–11. In this image, a yolk sac is seen within a gestational sac that is adjacent to an ovary. This image most likely represents which of the following?

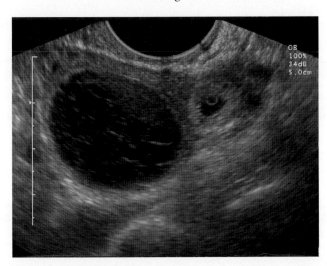

a. An intracervical pregnancy

b. A normal intrauterine pregnancy

c. A pregnancy within the fallopian tube

d. An intraligamentous pregnancy

7–12. In Question 7-11, the cystic mass seen within this ovary most likely represents which of the following?

a. Endometrioma

b. Theca lutein cyst

c. Serous cystadenoma

d. Corpus luteum cyst

7–13. A woman presents with a serum β-hCG level exceeding 2500 IU/L, vaginal bleeding, and abdominal pain. This laparoscopic photograph illustrates which of the following?

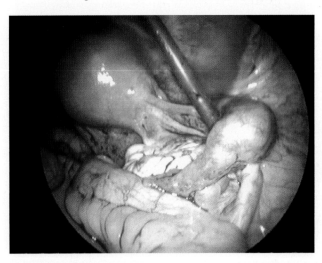

Photograph contributed by Dr. Kevin Doody.

a. A right ovarian mass

b. An intrauterine pregnancy

c. A right interstitial pregnancy

d. A distended right tubal ampulla

7–14. In women presenting with a positive urine pregnancy test result plus abdominal pain with or without vaginal bleeding, use of which of the following strategies helps diagnose a pregnancy of unknown location?

a. Transvaginal sonography

b. Dilatation and curettage

c. Quantitative serum β-hCG measurement

d. All of the above

7–15. Without intervention, an ectopic tubal pregnancy can lead to which of the following?

a. Tubal rupture

b. Spontaneous resolution

c. Expulsion of products of conception through the tubal fimbria

d. All of the above

7–16. In the medical management of ectopic pregnancy, a predictor of success for the use of single-dose methotrexate includes which of the following?

a. Fetal cardiac activity

b. Concomitant use of folinic acid

c. An ectopic mass greater than 3.5 cm

d. An initial serum β-hCG value <5000 IU/L

7–17. Methotrexate is often used in the medical management of selected ectopic pregnancies. The agent methotrexate is which of the following?

a. A protease inhibitor

b. A monoclonal antibody

c. A folic acid antagonist

d. A vascular endothelial growth factor antagonist

7–18. The use of methotrexate to medically treat ectopic pregnancy is contraindicated in which of the following settings?

a. Renal dysfunction

b. Breastfeeding

c. Hemodynamic instability

d. All of the above

7–19. One of the most common side effects of methotrexate includes which of the following?

a. Myelosuppression

b. Pulmonary damage

c. Anaphylactoid reaction

d. Transient liver dysfunction

7–20. For carefully selected patients, medical management of ectopic pregnancy using methotrexate is associated with what overall resolution rate?

a. 30 percent

b. 50 percent

c. 80 percent

d. 90 percent

7–21. Close monitoring of the patient receiving single-dose intramuscular methotrexate for the management of an ectopic pregnancy includes the comparison of serum β-hCG levels on which of the following schedules?

a. Day 1, 2, and 3

b. Day 1, 4, and 7

c. Day 4, 7, and 10

d. None of the above

7–22. During the first few days following methotrexate administration for ectopic pregnancy, which of the following symptoms can be expected in up to half of all patients?

a. Syncope

b. Polyuria

c. Abdominal pain

d. Increased vaginal bleeding

7–23. Contraception is recommended after successful medical therapy with methotrexate, as this drug has been shown to persist in human tissue for up to how many months after a single intramuscular dose?

a. 2 months

b. 4 months

c. 8 months

d. 16 months

7–24. In a number of randomized trials, single-dose intramuscular methotrexate compared with laparoscopic salpingostomy found similar outcomes with regard to which of the following?

a. Treatment complication rates

b. Health-related quality of life

c. Tubal patency and subsequent uterine pregnancy

d. None of the above

7–25. One of the criteria that should be met to diagnose an ovarian ectopic pregnancy includes which of the following?

a. The ipsilateral tube is incorporated into the pregnancy mass.

b. The ectopic pregnancy is connected by the mesoteres to the uterus.

c. Histologically, ovarian tissue is identified in the gestational sac wall.

d. All of the above

7-26. Although this location for an ectopic pregnancy is rare, risk factors compared with other ectopic pregnancy sites are similar. Of the following, what is a specific risk factor for this type of ectopic pregnancy?

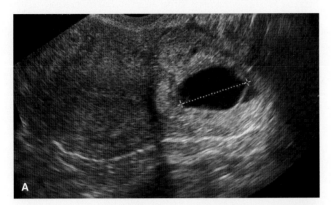

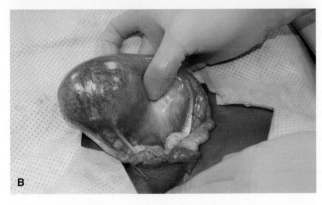

Figure B: Photograph contributed by Dr. Jennifer Muller. Reproduced with permission from Hoffman BL, Horsager R, Roberts SW, et al: Williams Obstetrics 23rd Edition Study Guide. New York, McGraw-Hill, 2011, Figure 10-4.

a. Prior intrauterine device use

b. Prior medical abortion

c. Prior cesarean delivery

d. Prior ipsilateral salpingectomy

7-27. Sonographic criteria that support the diagnosis of a cervical ectopic pregnancy include all **EXCEPT** which of the following?

a. A comma-shaped uterine contour

b. Absent intrauterine gestational tissue

c. Gestational tissue at the level of the cervix

d. A portion of the endocervical canal seen interposed between the gestation and the endometrial canal

7-28. Cesarean scar pregnancy can often be sonographically diagnosed if four criteria are satisfied. These include all **EXCEPT** which of the following?

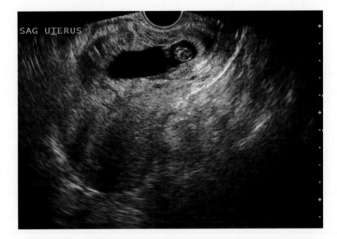

a. An empty uterine cavity

b. An empty cervical canal

c. A gestational sac in the anterior part of the uterine isthmus

d. Normal myometrium between the bladder and gestational sac

Chapter 7   ANSWER KEY

Question number	Letter answer	Page cited	Header cited	Question number	Letter answer	Page cited	Header cited
7–1	a	p. 198	Introduction	7–15	d	p. 207	Management
7–2	a	p. 199	Figure 7-1	7–16	d	p. 207	Medical Management
7–3	b	p. 200	Risk Factors	7–17	c	p. 209	Methotrexate
7–4	b	p. 200	Risk Factors	7–18	d	p. 209	Table 7-3
7–5	c	p. 200	Risk Factors	7–19	d	p. 209	Methotrexate
7–6	d	p. 201	Symptoms	7–20	d	p. 209	Methotrexate
7–7	b	p. 203	Serum β-hCG Measurements	7–21	b	p. 209	Methotrexate
7–8	a	p. 204	Sonography	7–22	c	p. 209	Methotrexate
7–9	a	p. 204	Sonography	7–23	c	p. 210	Surveillance
7–10	d	p. 204	Sonography	7–24	c	p. 211	Medical versus Surgical
7–11	c	p. 204	Sonography	7–25	c	p. 212	Ovarian Pregnancy
7–12	d	p. 204	Sonography	7–26	d	p. 212	Interstitial Pregnancy
7–13	d	p. 206	Summary of Diagnostic Evaluation	7–27	a	p. 213	Cervical Pregnancy
7–14	d	p. 206	Summary of Diagnostic Evaluation	7–28	d	p. 214	Cesarean Scar Pregnancy

CHAPTER 8

Abnormal Uterine Bleeding

8-1. All **EXCEPT** which of the following definitions of abnormal uterine bleeding are true?

   a. Metrorrhagia describes intermenstrual bleeding.

   b. Oligomenorrhea refers to cycles with intervals shorter than 35 days.

   c. Hypomenorrhea refers to menses with diminished flow or shortened interval.

   d. Menorrhagia is defined as prolonged or heavy cyclic menstruation, with menses lasting longer than 7 days or exceeding 80 mL of blood loss.

8-2. All **EXCEPT** which of the following tools are clinically useful to estimate menstrual blood loss?

   a. Pad counts

   b. Hemoglobin and hematocrit

   c. Pictorial blood assessment chart

   d. Sodium hydroxide extraction of hemoglobin

8-3. The most common etiologies of bleeding have been correctly paired with their age demographic in all **EXCEPT** which of the following?

   a. Adolescence—anovulation

   b. Childhood—vulvovaginitis

   c. Perimenopause—anovulation

   d. Menopause—endometrial carcinoma

8-4. Which of the following mechanisms are responsible for control of blood loss during menses?

   a. Thrombi

   b. Platelet aggregation

   c. Vasoconstriction of endometrial arteries

   d. All of the above

8-5. Which of the following may be reasonably considered in the evaluation of postcoital vaginal bleeding?

   a. Conization

   b. Cystoscopy

   c. Colposcopy

   d. Proctoscopy

8-6. Which of the following clinical findings may be associated with abnormal uterine bleeding?

   a. Obesity

   b. Bruising

   c. Acanthosis nigricans

   d. All of the above

8-7. Which laboratory criteria listed below is consistent with iron-deficiency anemia?

   a. Low serum ferritin level

   b. Normal hemoglobin and hematocrit

   c. Low total iron-binding capacity (TIBC)

   d. Increase in mean corpuscular hemoglobin (MCV)

8-8. A patient seeing you for menorrhagia reveals that she has a personal history of gingival bleeding and that during a recent tooth extraction, she bled excessively. You decide to screen her for a coagulation disorder. You order all **EXCEPT** which of the following laboratory tests?

   a. Bleeding time

   b. Prothrombin time (PT)

   c. Partial thromboplastin time (PTT)

   d. Complete blood count (CBC) with platelets

8-9. Which of the following is a limitation of flexible plastic samplers (i.e., Pipelle) used for endometrial biopsy (EMB) in the evaluation of abnormal uterine bleeding?

   a. Low rate of inadequate sampling

   b. Ability to be performed in an office setting

   c. Less patient discomfort compared to stiff metal curette

   d. Low sensitivity and high false-negative rate for focal endometrial pathology

8-10. Which of the following are advantages of transvaginal sonography in the evaluation of abnormal uterine bleeding?

   a. Ability to reduce use of endometrial biopsy

   b. Simultaneous assessment of myometrium and endometrium

   c. Greater patient comfort compared with endometrial biopsy or hysteroscopy

   d. All of the above

8–11. What is the primary advantage of saline infusion sonography compared with transvaginal sonography?

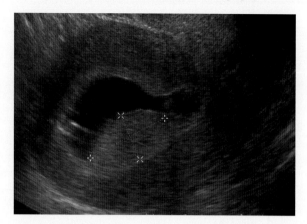

    a. Less patient discomfort

    b. Superior detection of intracavitary masses

    c. Ability to perform at any time of the cycle

    d. Simultaneous assessment of myometrium and endometrium

8–12. A 60-year-old postmenopausal woman presents for evaluation of bleeding, which you have determined from your physical examination to be uterine in origin. Which of the following diagnostic procedures is a logical first step in her evaluation?

    a. Colposcopy

    b. Diagnostic hysteroscopy

    c. Transvaginal sonography

    d. Saline-infusion sonography

8–13. Characteristics of the soft, fleshy intrauterine growth, shown here exhibiting a single feeder vessel, include which of the following?

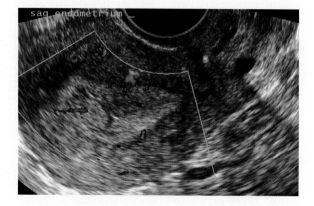

    a. The main diagnostic tool is the Pap smear.

    b. It is an uncommon cause of abnormal uterine bleeding.

    c. Infertility has been linked directly with this growth.

    d. Use of oral contraceptive pills appears to be protective.

8–14. Which characteristics are risk factors for malignant transformation of the structural lesion shown here?

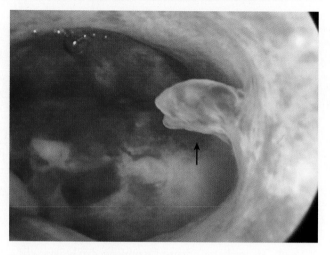

Photograph contributed by Dr. Mayra Thompson.

    a. Tamoxifen use

    b. Postmenopausal status

    c. Size greater than 1.5 cm

    d. All of the above

8–15. Your 27-year-old patient who recently underwent dilatation and curettage for an incomplete abortion presents to the office with new-onset menorrhagia. Transvaginal sonography reveals this hypoechoic tubular structure within the myometrium, with large-caliber vessels and blood flow reversal, as displayed here. What is the next most appropriate step in her evaluation?

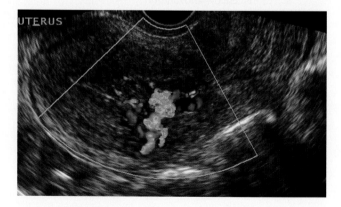

    a. Angiography

    b. Hysteroscopy

    c. Saline-infusion sonography

    d. Computed tomography (CT) of pelvis with contrast

8-16. Which of the following explanations have been suggested as the etiology for abnormal uterine bleeding with use of the device shown below in this three-dimensional sonogram?

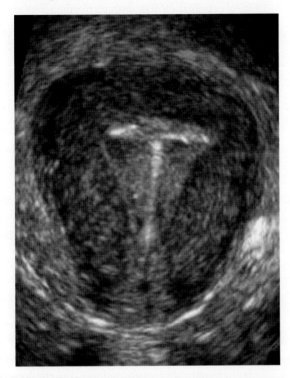

   a. Malposition of the device

   b. Unbalanced ratio of prostaglandins and thromboxane

   c. Increased endometrial vascularity, congestion, and degeneration

   d. All of the above

8-17. A patient for whom you initiated combination oral contraceptive pills (COCs) 3 months ago returns to the office for a routine COC reevaluation. She complains of light but irregular bleeding during this time, but states that it is improving. What is your diagnosis and plan of care?

   a. COC intolerance requiring method discontinuation

   b. Breakthrough bleeding requiring counseling and reassurance

   c. Endometrial pathology necessitating transvaginal sonography

   d. Hormonal imbalance requiring selection of a different COC formulation

8-18. In which situation should irregular spotting or bleeding be evaluated in a postmenopausal patient on hormone replacement therapy (HRT)?

   a. History of endometrial polyps

   b. Continued bleeding after 6 months of HRT use

   c. Abnormal bleeding that develops after initial amenorrhea

   d. All of the above

8-19. Which of the following statements regarding tamoxifen is true?

   a. It acts as an estrogen agonist in the breast and uterus.

   b. Tamoxifen use has been linked to endometrial polyps, hyperplasia, and carcinoma but not to uterine sarcomas.

   c. Women using tamoxifen should undergo evaluation for endometrial cancer only if symptoms of bleeding develop.

   d. It is a selective estrogen-receptor modulator (SERM) used as an adjunct for treatment of estrogen-receptor-negative breast cancer.

8-20. Systemic causes of abnormal uterine bleeding include which of the following?

   a. Liver disease

   b. Severe renal dysfunction

   c. Hypo- and hyperthyroidism

   d. All of the above

8-21. Which is an effective first-line treatment for women with menorrhagia and von Willebrand disease?

   a. Endometrial ablation

   b. Dilatation and curettage (D&C)

   c. Combination oral contraceptive pills (COCs)

   d. Nonsteroidal anti-inflammatory drugs (NSAIDs)

8-22. Which of the following statements regarding dysfunctional uterine bleeding (DUB) is true?

   a. Eighty to 90 percent of DUB is associated with ovulation.

   b. Up to half of women with abnormal uterine bleeding will have DUB.

   c. If structural causes of abnormal uterine bleeding cannot be excluded, the term *DUB* is used.

   d. Bleeding associated with anovulation is thought to stem predominantly from vascular dilatation alone.

8-23. Which of the following medications used to treat dysfunction uterine bleeding (DUB) is correctly paired with its mechanism of action?

   a. Tranexamic acid—increased plasmin levels

   b. Nonsteroidal anti-inflammatory drugs (NSAIDs)—stimulation of cyclooxygenase (COX-1 and 2)

   c. Oral progestins—inhibition of endometrial growth with organized sloughing following their withdrawal

   d. Combination oral contraceptive pills (COCs)—endometrial atrophy with diminished prostaglandin synthesis and increased endometrial fibrinolysis

8-24. Which of the following statements is true regarding the efficacy of the option shown here in this three-dimensional sonogram for the treatment of dysfunctional uterine bleeding (DUB)?

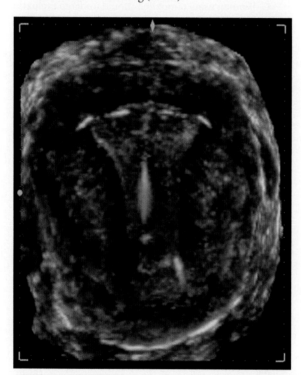

   a. It has been shown to reduce menstrual loss by more than 75 percent after 3 months' use.

   b. It has been shown to be more effective than mefenamic acid or oral progestins in decreasing uterine blood loss.

   c. Compared with endometrial ablation, this method appears to have similar therapeutic effects up to 2 years after treatment.

   d. All of the above

8-25. A patient presents to the emergency department with complaints of a 1-day history of heavy vaginal bleeding. She is tachycardic but not hypotensive, and vital signs do not change with positional changes from lying to sitting. Physical examination demonstrates bleeding from above the cervical os and continued pooling of blood in the vagina. Laboratory studies reveal she is anemic. Which of the following choices is the most appropriate first-line agent in attempting to control her active uterine bleeding?

   a. Tranexamic acid

   b. Intravenous estrogen

   c. Gonadotropin-releasing hormone (GnRH) agonist

   d. Combination oral contraceptive pill (COC) taper

8-26. Which of the following statements regarding tranexamic acid is true?

   a. To be most effective, it requires administration before and during menses.

   b. Contraindications to its usage include a history or intrinsic risk of thromboembolic disease.

   c. It does affect other blood coagulation parameters, such as platelet count, prothrombin time (PT), and partial thromboplastin time (PTT).

   d. It is an antifibrinolytic drug that permanently blocks lysine binding sites on plasminogen, thereby decreasing plasmin levels and fibrinolytic activity.

8-27. When counseling a patient for endometrial ablation, which of the following points is important to discuss with her?

   a. Three fourths of women after ablation experience significantly decreased flow.

   b. Approximately 10 to 15 percent of women will need subsequent hysterectomy by 5 years after the ablation.

   c. Following ablation, later evaluation of the endometrium for recurrent abnormal bleeding can be difficult due to resultant distortion of the endometrial cavity.

   d. All of the above

8-28. All **EXCEPT** which of the following are contraindications for endometrial ablation?

   a. Postmenopausal status

   b. Prior classical cesarean delivery

   c. Anatomically normal endometrial cavity

   d. Women wishing to preserve their fertility

Chapter 8 ANSWER KEY

Question number	Letter answer	Page cited	Header cited
8–1	b	p. 219	Definitions
8–2	d	p. 219	Definitions
8–3	d	p. 220	Incidence
8–4	d	p. 222	Pathophysiology
8–5	c	p. 223	Postcoital Bleeding
8–6	d	p. 225	Table 8-2
8–7	a	p. 223	β-hCG and Hematologic Testing
8–8	a	p. 223	β-hCG and Hematologic Testing; Coagulopathy
8–9	d	p. 226	Sampling methods
8–10	d	p. 227	Sonography; Transvaginal Sonography
8–11	b	p. 228	Saline-Infusion Sonography
8–12	c	p. 229	Summary of Diagnostic Procedures
8–13	d	p. 230	Endometrial Polyp
8–14	d	p. 230	Endometrial Polyp
8–15	a	p. 232	Arteriovenous Malformation (AVM)

Question number	Letter answer	Page cited	Header cited
8–16	d	p. 232	Intrauterine Device (IUD); Copper-Containing Intrauterine Device
8–17	b	p. 233	Combination Hormonal Contraception
8–18	d	p. 233	Hormone Replacement Therapy (HRT)
8–19	c	p. 233	Tamoxifen
8–20	d	p. 234	Systemic Causes
8–21	c	p. 235	Von Willebrand Disease (vWD)
8–22	b	p. 236	Dysfunctional Uterine Bleeding (DUB)
8–23	c	p. 237	Treatment
8–24	d	p. 238	Levonorgestrel-Releasing Intrauterine System (LNG-IUS)
8–25	b	p. 237	Table 8-4
8-26	b	p. 239	Tranexamic Acid
8-27	d	p. 239	Endometrial Destructive Procedures
8-28	c	p. 240	Table 8-5

CHAPTER 8

CHAPTER 9

Pelvic Mass

9-1. Age has the greatest influence in the evaluation of a pelvic mass. Which of the following statements regarding demographic factors and pelvic masses is true?

   a. Malignant ovarian tumors in children and adolescents are common.

   b. Most gynecologic pelvic masses in prepubertal and adolescent girls involve the ovary.

   c. Malignancy is a more frequent cause of pelvic masses in reproductive-aged women than in postmenopausal women.

   d. None of the above

9-2. Which of the following statements regarding the pathology of leiomyomas is true as shown in part by these low- and high-power histologic images?

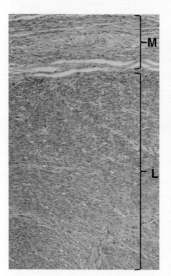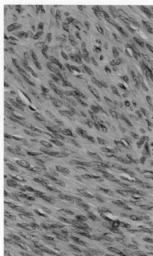

L = leiomyoma; M = myometrium. Photographs contributed by Dr. Kelley Carrick.

   a. Each leiomyoma is derived from multiple progenitor myocytes.

   b. Mitotic activity in their elongated smooth muscle bundles is common.

   c. Leiomyomas possess a distinct autonomy from their surrounding myometrium.

   d. Necrosis and degeneration develop infrequently in leiomyomas because of their abundant and well-organized blood supply.

9-3. Which of the following factors decreases the risk for development of leiomyomas?

   a. Early menarche

   b. Cigarette smoking

   c. Elevated body mass index (BMI)

   d. Polycystic ovarian syndrome (PCOS)

9-4. Mechanisms by which leiomyomas create a hyperestrogenic environment requisite for their growth and maintenance include which of the following?

   a. Leiomyomas convert estradiol to estrone.

   b. Leiomyoma cells contain a greater density of estrogen receptors compared with normal myometrium.

   c. Leiomyomas contain higher levels of cytochrome P450 aromatase, which allows for conversion of androgens to estrogen.

   d. All of the above

9-5. What type of leiomyoma is shown in this sonographic image?

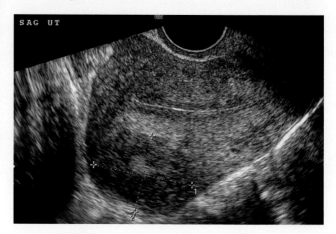

   a. Intramural

   b. Subserosal

   c. Submucosal, type 0

   d. Submucosal, type I

9-6. Symptoms of leiomyomas have been correctly partnered with the appropriate pathophysiology in all **EXCEPT** which of the following pairs?

  a. Asymptomatic—prolapsing fibroid

  b. Menorrhagia—dilatation of endometrial venules

  c. Pelvic pressure—mechanical compression

  d. Acute pelvic pain—leiomyoma degeneration

9-7. Leiomyomas account for 2 to 3 percent of infertility cases. Which of the following describes the mechanisms by which leiomyomas may disrupt fertility?

  a. Occlusion of tubal ostia

  b. Distortion of normal uterine contractions

  c. Disruption of implantation secondary to distortion of the endometrial cavity

  d. All of the above

9-8. Rare complications of leiomyomas include all **EXCEPT** which of the following?

  a. Leiomyomatosis

  b. Cystic degeneration

  c. Pseudo-Meigs syndrome

  d. Myomatous erythrocytosis syndrome

9-9. As shown here, leiomyomas may commonly show which of the following sonographic features?

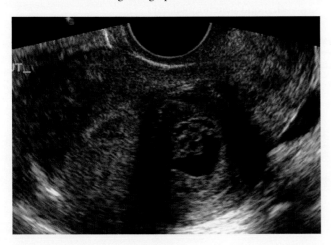

  a. Cystic degeneration

  b. Discrete borders with shadowing

  c. Round hypoechoic myometrial mass

  d. All of the above

9-10. Your 48-year-old patient presents with complaints of worsening menorrhagia. She has no other medical problems. Three-dimensional sonographic evaluation reveals the findings as shown below. All **EXCEPT** which of the following are suitable choices for medical treatment in this patient?

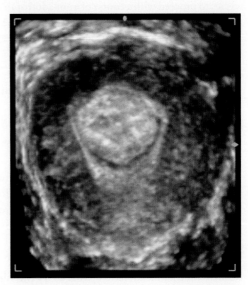

  a. Combination oral contraceptives (COC)

  b. Depot medroxyprogesterone acetate (DMPA)

  c. Gonadotropin-releasing hormone (GnRH) agonist

  d. Levonorgestrel-releasing intrauterine system (LNG-IUS)

9-11. Which of the following are proposed mechanisms of action of gonadotropin-releasing hormone (GnRH) agonists on leiomyomas?

  a. GnRH agonists downregulate estrogen and progesterone receptors on the leiomyomas themselves.

  b. GnRH agonists downregulate receptors on hypothalamic gonadotropes, thereby suppressing estrogen and progesterone levels.

  c. GnRH agonists downregulate receptors on pituitary gonadotropes, thereby suppressing estrogen and progesterone levels.

  d. None of the above

9–12. A 47-year-old woman presents to you with complaints of heavy menstrual bleeding and dysmenorrhea. She also is anemic, which you have determined from your evaluation to be secondary to leiomyoma-related bleeding. After thorough discussion of the various medical and surgical options, she wishes to proceed with a course of a gonadotropin-releasing hormone (GnRH) agonist. Which of the following statements is important to include in your counseling on this treatment?

    a. Treatment can result in loss of trabecular bone, which may not be recouped following therapy discontinuation.

    b. Side effects of GnRH agonists include vasomotor symptoms, libido changes, and vaginal dryness with accompanying dyspareunia.

    c. Anticipated clinical benefits are reduced leiomyoma volume with diminished bleeding and pain. However, once therapy is stopped, leiomyomas regrow and regain pretreatment sizes within 3 to 4 months.

    d. All of the above

9–13. Relative contraindications to uterine artery embolization (UAE) include all **EXCEPT** which of the following?

    a. Desire for future fertility

    b. Pedunculated subserosal or submucosal leiomyomas

    c. Concurrent gonadotropin-releasing hormone (GnRH) agonist use

    d. History of prior *Neisseria gonorrhoeae* or *Chlamydia trachomatis* infection

9–14. Compared with hysterectomy, uterine artery embolization (UAE) is associated with which of the following?

    a. Longer hospitalization

    b. Postembolization syndrome

    c. Higher 24-hour postprocedural pain scores

    d. Equivalent time frame for return to work

9–15. Your 35-year-old nulligravid patient comes to the office for counseling regarding uterine artery embolization (UAE) for treatment of her medically refractory menorrhagia secondary to leiomyomas. She desires future fertility. Which of the following complications of pregnancy is she at increased risk for after UAE?

    a. Miscarriage

    b. Cesarean delivery

    c. Postpartum hemorrhage

    d. All of the above

9–16. Frequent complications associated with uterine artery embolization include which of the following?

    a. Groin hematoma

    b. Leiomyoma tissue passage

    c. Prolonged vaginal discharge

    d. All of the above

9–17. All **EXCEPT** which of the following statements regarding magnetic resonance imaging-guided focused ultrasound therapy (MRgFUS) are true?

    a. Long-term data regarding the duration of symptom relief are limited.

    b. Less than 10 percent of women seek alternative treatments for their symptoms by 12 months following MRgFUS.

    c. This technique focuses ultrasound energy to a degree that heats targeted leiomyomas to incite necrosis.

    d. Contraindications include abdominal wall scars, contraindications to MR imaging, uterine size greater than 24 weeks, and desire for future fertility.

9–18. Advantages of laparoscopic versus open myomectomy include which of the following?

    a. Equivalent febrile morbidity rates

    b. Less adhesion formation

    c. Improved pregnancy rates

    d. Equivalent hospital stays

9–19. Which of the following surgical therapies does not have documented long-term effectiveness in the treatment of menorrhagia?

    a. Myomectomy

    b. Hysterectomy

    c. Dilatation and curettage (D&C)

    d. Hysteroscopic resection of submucous leiomyomas

9–20. A 32-year-old woman presents to the emergency department with complaints of progressively worsening midline lower pelvic pain during the last few months. She denies fever or vaginal discharge. Her last menstrual period (LMP) was 2 years ago. She states that she had a procedure done for heavy uterine bleeding, and after that, she "never had a period again." Physical examination demonstrates a normal sized but tender uterus, her β-human chorionic gonadotropin (β-hCG) test is negative for pregnancy, and sonographic evaluation reveals the findings shown below. What is the most likely etiology for her condition?

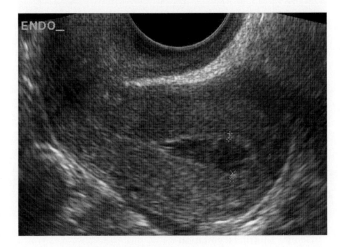

a. Radiation treatment

b. Endometrial ablation

c. Congenital uterine anomaly

d. Prolonged hypoestrogenism with atrophy

9–21. Theories regarding the pathogenesis of adenomyosis include which of the following?

a. Metaplasia of pluripotent müllerian tissue

b. Invagination of the endometrial basalis layer into the myometrium

c. Myometrial weakness caused by pregnancy, uterine surgery, or compromised immunological activity at the endometrial–myometrial junction

d. All of the above

9–22. Which of the following symptoms of adenomyosis is correctly paired with its etiology?

a. Dysmenorrhea—increased prostaglandin production

b. Dysmenorrhea—hemorrhage within the ectopic glandular foci

c. Menorrhagia—increased and abnormal vascularization of the adenomyotic tissue

d. None of the above

9–23. Sonographic characteristics of diffuse adenomyosis may include which of the following?

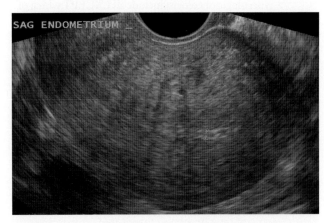

a. Small myometrial hypoechoic cysts

b. Myometrial wall thickening with heterogeneous texture

c. Ill-defined endometrial echo with striated projections extending into the myometrium

d. All of the above

9–24. All **EXCEPT** which of the following are appropriate medical treatments for adenomyosis?

a. Copper intrauterine device

b. Combination oral contraceptives (COCs)

c. Nonsteroidal anti-inflammatory drugs (NSAIDS)

d. Levonorgestrel-releasing intrauterine system (LNG-IUS)

9–25. Which of the following tumor antigens is correctly paired with its ovarian tumor or malignancy?

a. Alpha-fetoprotein (AFP)—dysgerminoma

b. β-hCG—granulosa cell tumor

c. Cancer antigen 19-9 (CA19-9)—mucinous epithelial ovarian carcinoma

d. Lactate dehydrogenase (LDH)—yolk sac tumor and embryonal cell carcinoma

9–26. During the annual visit of a 56-year-old postmenopausal patient, you detect a right adnexal fullness during bimanual examination. Transvaginal sonography reveals a 3-cm thin-walled, unilocular cyst of the right ovary. She is asymptomatic. Which of the following is the most appropriate initial course of treatment?

a. Gynecologic oncology referral

b. Diagnostic laparoscopy with cystectomy

c. Expectant management with periodic surveillance if her CA125 level is normal

d. Prescription of combination oral contraceptive pills to hasten cyst resolution

9-27. Clinical criteria of a newly diagnosed pelvic mass in a premenopausal woman that should prompt referral to a gynecologic oncologist include all **EXCEPT** which of the following?

   a. Ascites

   b. CA125 level of 460 U/mL

   c. Evidence of abdominal or distant metastasis

   d. Family history of breast or ovarian cancer in a first-degree relative

9-28. All **EXCEPT** which of the following are risks factors for development of the ovarian lesion shown here?

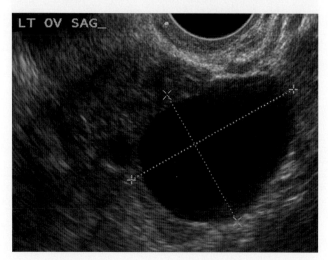

   a. Smoking

   b. Tamoxifen

   c. Combination oral contraceptives (COCs)

   d. Levonorgestrel-releasing intrauterine device (LNG-IUS)

9-29. A 25-year-old patient at 14 weeks' gestation by last menstrual period presents to the emergency department with complaints of bilateral pelvic pain. Transabdominal sonography reveals these bilateral multilocular cystic ovarian masses. Which of the following commonly associated conditions must be excluded in pregnancies with this finding?

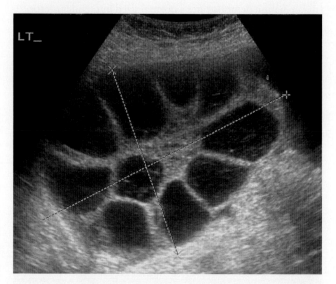

   a. Fetal hydrops

   b. Multifetal gestation

   c. Gestational trophoblastic disease

   d. All of the above

9–30. The sonographic "tip of the iceberg" sign corresponds to the site within a mature cystic teratoma where the most varied tissue types, such as hair and fatty secretions, are found. Pathologically, what is the name of this area?

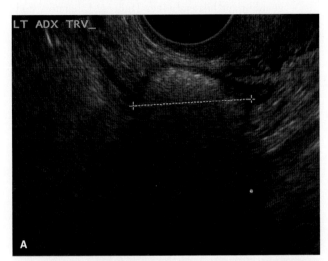

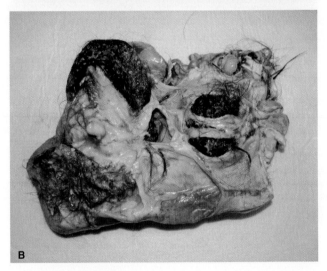

a. Homunculus

b. Struma ovarii

c. Hydatid of Morgagni

d. Rokitansky protuberance

9–31. A 29-year-old G2P2 with a last menstrual period 3 weeks ago presents to the emergency department with complaints of worsening right pelvic pain. She states that she had the sudden onset of sharp pain after bending over to pick up one of her children. She experienced intense nausea with the pain. The pain did not respond to acetaminophen and has intermittently worsened during the past several hours. No adnexal masses were detected on physical examination, but the patient was guarding. Transvaginal sonography demonstrates an 8-cm enlarged right ovary without a dominant mass or cyst, high impedance arterial flow of the ovary on color Doppler interrogation, and no free fluid. These findings are most consistent with which of the following clinical diagnoses?

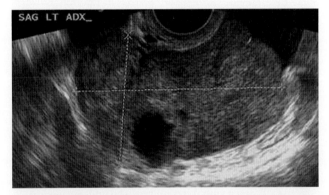

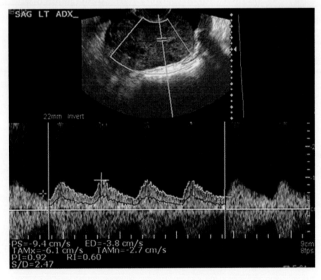

a. Appendicitis

b. Ovarian torsion

c. Hemorrhagic cyst

d. Ruptured corpus luteum cyst

SECTION 1

9–32. Which of the following management plans is most appropriate for the patient in Question 9-31?

　　a. General surgery consultation

　　b. Laparoscopy with adnexectomy

　　c. Laparoscopy with detorsion of the ovary

　　d. Close observation with serial examinations

9–33. Which of the following statements regarding the pathology depicted here are true?

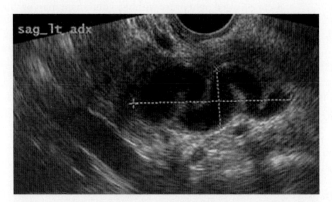

　　a. It can be associated with chronic pelvic pain.

　　b. It is the result of chronic swelling of the fallopian tube.

　　c. Women with this condition who undergo in vitro fertilization (IVF) have approximately half the pregnancy rate of other women.

　　d. All of the above

9–34. A 20-year-old nulligravida with a last menstrual period 5 days ago presents to the emergency department with generalized lower abdominal pain and fever. She reports a new sexual partner. Physical examination demonstrates guarding and bilateral adnexal fullness. Laboratory studies show leukocytosis, and transvaginal sonography reveals no visible ovaries but bilateral adnexal masses as shown here. The diagnosis most consistent with these findings is which of the following?

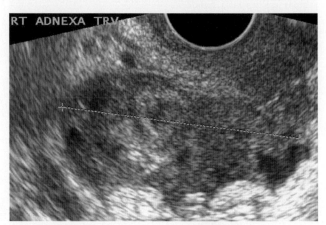

　　a. Endometriosis

　　b. Ovarian torsion

　　c. Tuboovarian abscess

　　d. Malignant ovarian neoplasm

Chapter 9 ANSWER KEY

Question number	Letter answer	Page cited	Header cited
9–1	b	p. 246	Demographic Factors
9–2	c	p. 247	Pathology
9–3	b	p. 249	Table 9-1
9–4	d	p. 247	Estrogen Effects
9–5	b	p. 250	Classification of Uterine Leiomyoma
9–6	a	p. 250	Symptoms
9–7	d	p. 251	Infertility and Pregnancy Wastage
9–8	b	p. 252	Other Clinical Manifestations
9–9	d	p. 253	Imaging
9–10	d	p. 254	Table 9-2
9–11	c	p. 254	GnRH Agonists
9–12	d	p. 254	GnRH Agonists
9–13	d	p. 257	Table 9-3
9–14	b	p. 256	Uterine Artery Embolization
9–15	d	p. 256	Uterine Artery Embolization
9–16	d	p. 256	Uterine Artery Embolization
9–17	b	p. 258	Magnetic Resonance Imaging-Guided Focused Ultrasound

Question number	Letter answer	Page cited	Header cited
9–18	b	p. 258	Laparoscopic Myomectomy
9–19	c	p. 258	Endometrial Ablation
9–20	b	p. 259	Hematometra
9–21	d	p. 259	Pathophysiology
9–22	a	p. 260	Symptoms
9–23	d	p. 260	Sonography
9–24	a	p. 261	Management
9–25	c	p. 262	Tumor Markers
9–26	c	p. 264	Table 9-4
9–27	d	p. 265	Table 9-5
9–28	c	p. 265	Risk Factors
9–29	d	p. 266	Theca Lutein Cysts
9–30	d	p. 267	Pathology
9–31	b	p. 270	Symptoms and Physical Findings
9–32	c	p. 271	Management
9–33	d	p. 273	Hydrosalpinx
9–34	c	p. 274	Tubo-ovarian Abscess (TOA)

CHAPTER 9

CHAPTER 10

Endometriosis

10-1. With endometriosis, as shown here, which of the following is ectopically located?

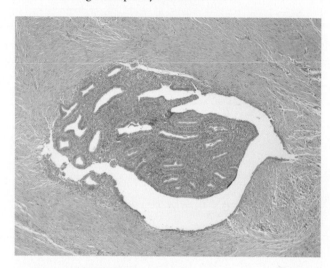

Reproduced, with permission, from Carr BR, Beshay VE: Endometriosis. In Hoffman BL, Schorge JO, Schaffer JI, et al (eds): Williams Gynecology, 2nd ed. New York, McGraw-Hill, 2012, Figure 10-10.

    a. Myometrial cells

    b. Ectocervical cells

    c. Endometrial glands and stroma

    d. Endocervical glands and stroma

10-2. The prevalence of endometriosis is higher in women with which of the following characteristic?

    a. Pelvic pain

    b. Infertility

    c. Affected family member

    d. All of the above

10-3. Which of the following theories is the most widely accepted as the cause of endometriosis?

    a. Lymphatic spread

    b. Hormonal induction

    c. Coelomic metaplasia

    d. Retrograde menstruation

10-4. Persistence of endometriosis is directly dependent on which of the following hormones?

    a. Estrogen

    b. Testosterone

    c. Progesterone

    d. Androstenedione

10-5. An enzyme important in creating a unique hormonal environment within endometriotic implants includes which of the following?

    a. Aromatase

    b. Cyclooxygenase type 2

    c. 17β-Hydroxysteroid dehydrogenase type 1

    d. All of the above

10-6. Which of the following conditions is a risk factor for developing endometriosis?

    a. Multiparity

    b. Transverse vaginal septum

    c. Prior chemotherapy exposure

    d. Autoimmune connective tissue disorders

10-7. Which of the following environmental toxins has been implicated in the development of endometriosis?

    a. Arsenic

    b. Asbestos

    c. DEHP—bis(2-ethylhexyl)phthalate

    d. TCDD—tetrachlorodibenzo-*p*-dioxin

10-8. Which of the following is the focus of the classification system developed by the American Society for Reproductive Medicine (ASRM)?

    a. Degree of pelvic pain

    b. Degree of infertility

    c. Anatomic extent of endometriosis

    d. All of the above

10-9. In the ASRM classification system, mild endometriosis found during laparoscopy is described as which of the following?

    a. Stage 1

    b. Grade 1

    c. Stage A

    d. Grade A

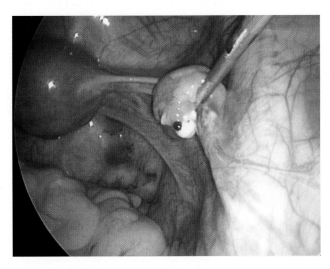

Photograph contributed by Dr. Karen Bradshaw.

10-10. At the time of laparoscopy, this patient was noted to have endometriotic surface lesions limited to the locations shown below. According to the ASRM classification, which of the following stages is assigned?

a. Stage 1

b. Stage 2

c. Stage 3

d. Stage 4

10-11. At the time of laparoscopy, your patient was noted to have bilateral adnexal cysts. Incision of one of the surgical specimens is seen here. Prior to laparoscopy, the ovarian cysts were measured by sonography and found to be 4 cm (right), 7 cm (left). According to the ASRM classification, this degree of endometriosis would be assigned which stage?

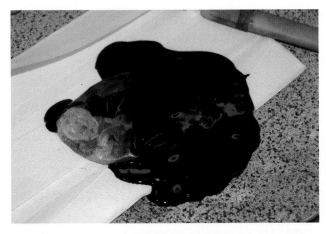

Reproduced, with permission, from Carr BR, Beshay VE: Endometriosis. In Hoffman BL, Schorge JO, Schaffer JI, et al (eds): Williams Gynecology, 2nd ed. New York, McGraw-Hill, 2012, Figure 10-4B.

a. Stage 1

b. Stage 2

c. Stage 3

d. Stage 4

10-12. In which of the following locations is endometriosis **LEAST** likely to be found?

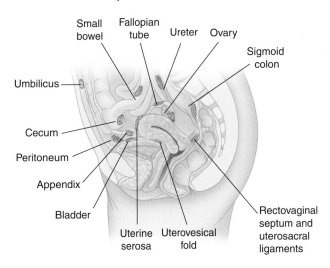

Reproduced, with permission, from Carr BR: Endometriosis. In Schorge JO, Schaffer JI, Halvorson LM, et al (eds): Williams Gynecology, 1st ed. New York, McGraw-Hill, 2008, Figure 10-3.

a. Ovary

b. Bladder

c. Posterior cul-de sac

d. Uterosacral ligaments

10-13. Which of the following locations is endometriosis **MOST** likely to be found?

a. Bladder

b. Small bowel

c. Large bowel

d. Posterior cul-de sac

10-14. Which of the following patient complaints is **LEAST** likely to be encountered in women with endometriosis?

a. Dysuria

b. Dyschezia

c. Dyspareunia

d. Dysmenorrhea

10-15. Which of the following statements is true regarding endometriosis?

a. Depth of disease invasion correlates with degree of pain

b. Severity of disease correlates with degree of infertility

c. Severity of disease correlates with degree of dyspareunia

d. All of the above

10–16. In women presenting with chronic pelvic pain, what percentage of women are expected to have endometriosis at the time of laparoscopy?

   a. 1–5

   b. 10–30

   c. 40–60

   d. 80–90

10–17. Which of the following is the most likely etiology for infertility in women with endometriosis?

   a. Tubal obstruction

   b. Implantation defect

   c. Ovulatory dysfunction

   d. Abnormalities of the endocervical mucus

10–18. Compared with women without endometriosis, women with endometriosis undergoing in vitro fertilization (IVF) treatment for infertility will have which of the following?

   a. Higher pregnancy rates

   b. Fewer blastomeres per embryo

   c. Higher oocyte yields at oocyte retrieval

   d. Lower embryonic developmental arrest rates

10–19. When considering the diagnosis of endometriosis, which of the following gynecologic conditions should be considered in the differential diagnosis?

   a. Tubo-ovarian abscess

   b. Interstitial cystitis

   c. Degenerating leiomyoma

   d. All of the above

10–20. Which of the following manifestations is most likely encountered during the physical examination of a patient with endometriosis?

   a. Tenderness to lower abdominal palpation

   b. Endocervical polyp during speculum examination

   c. Powder burn lesions on the cervix during speculum examination

   d. Uterosacral ligament nodularity during bimanual examination

10–21. Which of the following is true regarding laboratory testing during evaluation of suspected endometriosis?

   a. It should rarely be performed.

   b. It identifies most cases of endometriosis.

   c. It is used mainly to exclude other conditions.

   d. Reference ranges vary widely among laboratories that perform endometriosis-specific assays.

10–22. Which of the following methods can reliably assist in making the diagnosis of endometriosis?

   a. Sonography

   b. Laparoscopy

   c. Computed tomography

   d. Magnetic resonance imaging

10–23. Sonographically, endometriomas are typically described as which of the following?

   a. Solid with intracystic blood flow

   b. Cystic with hyperechoic internal echoes

   c. Solid with diffuse internal low level echoes

   d. Cystic with diffuse internal low level echoes

10–24. The following pelvic sonogram image signifies which of the following conditions?

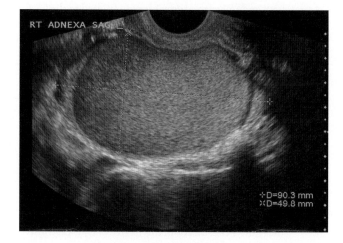

   a. Ovarian torsion

   b. Mature teratoma

   c. Tubo-ovarian abscess

   d. Ovarian endometrioma

10–25. Which of the following peritoneal implant colorings most commonly correlates with histologic findings of endometriosis?

   a. Red

   b. Blue

   c. Black

   d. Clear

10–26. Medical treatment for endometriosis may include all **EXCEPT** which of the following?

   a. Progestins

   b. Oral contraceptives

   c. Aromatase inhibitors

   d. Androgen-receptor blockers

10-27. Which of the following combination oral contraceptive formulations is most effective in the management of endometriosis?

 a. Monophasic

 b. Multiphasic

 c. Low dose (20 μg ethinyl estradiol)

 d. All are equally effective

10-28. The treatment effect of progestins on endometriosis is secondary to which of the following?

 a. Estrogen antagonism

 b. Androgen antagonism

 c. Aromatase inhibition

 d. Glucocorticoid stimulation

10-29. Women seeking immediate fertility and who suffer from endometriosis would most likely benefit from which of the following treatments?

 a. Danazol

 b. Aromatase inhibitors

 c. Laparoscopic ablation of lesions

 d. Gonadotropin-releasing hormone (GnRH) agonists

10-30. All **EXCEPT** which of the following are danazol side effects?

 a. Hirsutism

 b. Hot flashes

 c. Voice deepening

 d. Breast hypertrophy

10-31. The most troublesome side effects of GnRH agonist use stem from which of the following?

 a. Hypoestrogenism

 b. Hypoandrogenism

 c. Hyperestrogenism

 d. Hyperandrogenism

10-32. When should add-back therapy be considered during the course of GnRH agonist treatment?

 a. At 1 month

 b. At 6 months

 c. Not necessary

 d. At initiation of therapy

10-33. With deeply infiltrating endometriosis, which of the following surgical approaches may most likely benefit the patient?

 a. Laser ablation

 b. Radical excision

 c. Bipolar electrosurgical ablation

 d. Monopolar electrosurgical ablation

10-34. For surgical treatment of endometriomas, which of the following approaches is superior?

 a. Drainage

 b. Cystectomy

 c. Cyst wall ablation

 d. None of the above

10-35. Which of the following statements is most likely true regarding presacral neurectomy?

 a. It may be performed laparoscopically.

 b. It effectively treats lateral adnexal pain.

 c. It is a procedure that excises the uterosacral ligaments.

 d. It should commonly be used for most women with endometriosis.

10-36. Which of the following is a concern with the use of estrogen replacement therapy following bilateral salpingo-oophorectomy for endometriosis?

 a. Recurrence of endometriotic lesions

 b. Persistence of endometriotic lesions

 c. Cancer development within endometriotic lesions

 d. All of the above

Chapter 10 ANSWER KEY

Question number	Letter answer	Page cited	Header cited	Question number	Letter answer	Page cited	Header cited
10–1	c	p. 281	Introduction	10–20	d	p. 289	Physical Examination
10–2	d	p. 281	Incidence	10–21	c	p. 289	Laboratory Testing
10–3	d	p. 282	Pathophysiology	10–22	b	p. 290	Diagnostic Imaging
10–4	a	p. 282	Hormonal Dependence	10–23	d	p. 290	Sonography
10–5	d	p. 282	Hormonal Dependence	10–24	d	p. 290	Sonography
10–6	b	p. 284	Anatomic Defects	10–25	a	p. 291	Diagnostic Laparoscopy
10–7	d	p. 284	Environmental Toxins	10–26	d	p. 292	Medical Treatment of Pain
10–8	c	p. 285	Classification System	10–27	d	p. 292	Combination Oral Contraceptives
10–9	a	p. 285	Classification System				
10–10	a	p. 285	Classification System	10–28	a	p. 292	Progestins
10–11	c	p. 285	Classification System	10–29	c	p. 298	Treatment of Endometriosis-Related Infertility
10–12	b	p. 285	Anatomic Sites				
10–13	d	p. 285	Anatomic Sites	10–30	d	p. 294	Androgens
10–14	b	p. 286	Patient Symptoms	10–31	a	p. 295	GnRH Agonists
10–15	d	p. 286	Patient Symptoms	10–32	b	p. 295	Add-Back Therapy
10–16	c	p. 287	Noncyclic Pain	10–33	b	p. 296	Lesion Removal and Adhesiolysis
10–17	a	p. 287	Infertility				
10–18	b	p. 288	Folliculogenesis and Embryogenesis Effects	10–34	b	p. 297	Endometrioma Resection
				10–35	a	p. 297	Presacral Neurectomy
10–19	d	p. 289	Table 10-1	10–36	d	p. 298	Postoperative Hormone Replacement

CHAPTER 11

Pelvic Pain

11-1. Depending on the type of afferent nerve fibers involved, pain may be categorized as visceral or somatic. Somatic pain stems from nerve afferents of the somatic nervous system, which innervates which of the following?

a. Muscle

b. Parietal peritoneum

c. Subcutaneous tissue and skin

d. All of the above

11-2. The following illustration describes which of the following?

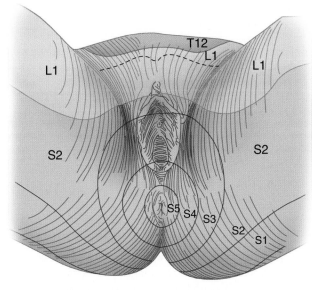

Reproduced, with permission, from Rogers DE, Hoffman BL: Pelvic pain. In Hoffman BL, Schorge JO, Schaffer JI, et al (eds): Williams Gynecology, 2nd ed. New York, McGraw-Hill, 2012, Figure 11-1B.

a. Dermatome map

b. Central sensitization

c. Peripheral sensitization

d. Viscerosomatic convergence

11-3. Visceral pain stems from afferent fibers of the autonomic nervous system that transmit information from the viscera and visceral peritoneum, resulting in pain described as which of the following?

a. Sharp

b. Stabbing

c. Localized

d. Generalized, dull ache

11-4. Sustained noxious stimuli can lead to persistent central sensitization and to a permanent loss of neuronal inhibition. As a result, a decreased threshold to painful stimuli remains despite resolution of the inciting stimuli. This persistence characterizes which type of pain?

a. Acute

b. Neuropathic

c. Inflammatory

d. All of the above

11-5. Acute lower abdominal pain and acute pelvic pain are common complaints. By definition, these present in general for which of the following durations?

a. <7 days

b. 1 month

c. 2 months

d. 3 consecutive months

11-6. Etiologies of acute lower abdominal and acute pelvic pain are extensive. Common etiologies of right lower quadrant pain include all **EXCEPT** which of the following?

a. Hepatitis

b. Urolithiasis

c. Ovarian torsion

d. Ectopic pregnancy

11–7. In addition to a thorough medical and surgical history, a verbal description of the pain experienced and its associated factors is essential. As an example, pain without diarrhea, constipation, or gastrointestinal bleeding lowers the probability of which of the following sources?

   a. Urinary

   b. Neurologic

   c. Gynecologic

   d. Gastrointestinal

11–8. The initial examination of a patient experiencing pain includes the assessment of vital signs. If intravascular hypovolemia is suspected, pulse and blood pressure assessment for orthostatic changes is required. Between lying and standing after 1 minute, which of the following values often reflect hypovolemia?

   a. An unchanged pulse, systolic blood pressure decrease of 10 mm Hg

   b. A pulse increase of 15 beats per minute, systolic blood pressure unchanged

   c. A pulse increase of 30 beats per minute, systolic blood pressure decline of 20 mm Hg

   d. A pulse decrease of 15 beats per minute, systolic blood pressure decline of 10 mm Hg

11–9. Which of the following is suggested by abdominal rebound tenderness and involuntary guarding?

   a. Bowel obstruction

   b. Uterine leiomyomata

   c. Peritoneal irritation

   d. None of the above

11–10. Cervical motion tenderness is associated with peritoneal irritation and is commonly found with which of the following?

   a. Appendicitis

   b. Liver disease

   c. Pyelonephritis

   d. Unruptured ectopic pregnancy

11–11. Your patient presents with acute lower abdominal pain, 8 weeks of amenorrhea, and vaginal spotting. She has a history of gonorrhea, and her pregnancy test result is positive. A transvaginal sonographic sagittal view of her uterus and cul-de-sac is shown here. These findings are most suggestive of which of the following?

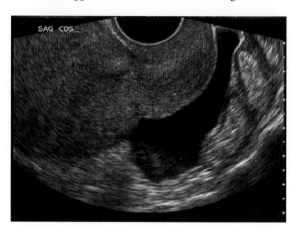

Reproduced, with permission, from Gala RB: Ectopic pregnancy. In Hoffman BL, Schorge JO, Schaffer JI, et al (eds): Williams Gynecology, 2nd ed. New York, McGraw-Hill, 2012, Figure 7-8B.

   a. Hydrosalpinx

   b. Hemoperitoneum

   c. Corpus luteum cyst

   d. Abdominal pregnancy

11–12. Chronic pelvic pain is a common gynecologic problem, and its prevalence in reproductive-aged women has been estimated at which of the following?

   a. 5

   b. 10

   c. 15

   d. 20

11–13. Many investigators, as well as the American College of Obstetricians and Gynecologists, define chronic pelvic pain. It is pain that is localized to the pelvis, infraumbilical anterior abdominal wall, or lumbosacral back or buttocks in addition to which of the following?

   a. Dyspareunia

   b. Cyclic pain

   c. Dysmenorrhea

   d. Pain leading to degrees of functional disability

11–14. Although causes of chronic pelvic pain fall within a broad spectrum, which of the following is commonly diagnosed?

   a. Endometriosis

   b. Interstitial cystitis

   c. Irritable bowel syndrome

   d. All of the above

11–15. A detailed history and physical examination are integral to diagnosing the etiology of chronic pelvic pain. A brief historical survey generally includes all **EXCEPT** which of the following questions?

   a. Are you taking any drugs?

   b. Do you believe you are imagining this pain?

   c. What do you believe or fear is the cause of your pain?

   d. Are you now or have you been abused physically or sexually?

11–16. Abdominal pain elicited with elevation of the head and shoulders while tensing the abdominal wall muscles is typical of anterior abdominal wall pathology and is termed which of the following?

   a. Carnett sign

   b. Iliopsoas test

   c. Straight leg test

   d. Trendelenburg test

11–17. During the physical examination for chronic pelvic pain, the technique shown here should be included. Nodularity may be found most commonly with which of the following?

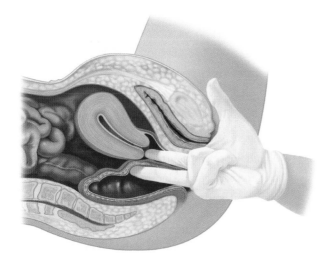

Reproduced, with permission, from Pearson MJ, Hoffman BL: Well woman care. In Hoffman BL, Schorge JO, Schaffer JI, et al (eds): Williams Gynecology, 2nd ed. New York, McGraw-Hill, 2012, Figure 1-9.

   a. Chronic ectopic pregnancy

   b. Endometriosis or neoplasia

   c. Pelvic inflammatory disease

   d. Uterine or cervical leiomyomas

11–18. In patients with combined urinary and chronic pelvic pain symptoms, which of the following tests is typically advised?

   a. Cystoscopy

   b. Cystometrics

   c. Retrograde cystourethrography

   d. Computed tomography scanning of the abdomen and pelvis

11–19. During laparoscopy for chronic pelvic pain, the following are identified in the upper abdomen and pelvis, respectively. These are most consistent with which of the following?

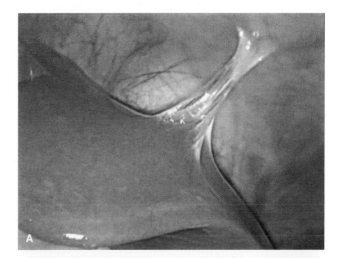

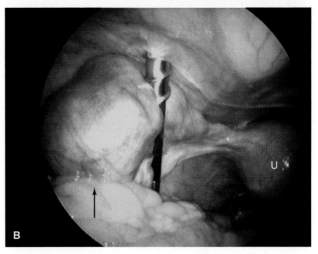

Figure A: Photograph contributed by Dr. David Rogers. Figure B: Photograph contributed by Dr. Kevin Doody. Reproduced, with permission, from Hoffman BL: Pelvic mass. In Schorge JO, Schaffer JI, Halvorson LM, et al (eds): Williams Gynecology, 1st ed. New York, McGraw-Hill, 2008, Figure 9-17.

   a. Endometriosis

   b. Chronic appendicitis

   c. Salpingitis isthmic nodosum

   d. Prior pelvic inflammatory disease

11–20. Medical management of chronic pelvic pain in patients in whom pathology is not identifiable may be directed toward dominant symptoms using which of the following?

   a. Hormonal suppression

   b. Antidepressants and anticonvulsants

   c. Analgesics such as nonsteroidal anti-inflammatory drugs

   d. All of the above

11–21. Surgical hysterectomy may serve as a treatment of chronic pelvic pain. In patients with no identified pelvic pathology, surgery fails to resolve pain in what percentage of these women?

   a. 10

   b. 20

   c. 30

   d. 40

11–22. Which of the following terms describes cyclic menstrual pain without identifiable associated pathology?

   a. Adenomyosis

   b. Primary dysmenorrhea

   c. Secondary dysmenorrhea

   d. Menstrual outlet obstruction

11–23. Primary dysmenorrhea is positively associated with which of the following?

   a. Smoking

   b. Early age at menarche

   c. Increased body mass index

   d. All of the above

11–24. The pathophysiology of primary dysmenorrhea is initiated by endometrial sloughing, during which endometrial cells release what substance that stimulates myometrial contractions and ischemia?

   a. Estrogen

   b. Follicle-stimulating hormone (FSH) and luteinizing hormone (LH)

   c. Progesterone

   d. Prostaglandins

11–25. Dyspareunia is a frequent gynecologic complaint noted in up to 20 percent of U.S. women and can be subclassified as insertional or deep. Which of the following is commonly associated with deep dyspareunia?

   a. Vulvodynia

   b. Endometriosis

   c. Poor vaginal lubrication

   d. All of the above

11–26. Patient complaints suggestive of interstitial cystitis commonly include all **EXCEPT** which of the following?

   a. Hematuria

   b. Urinary urgency

   c. Urinary frequency

   d. Stress urinary incontinence

11–27. Direct hernias commonly bulge through Hesselbach triangle, whose boundaries shown here include all **EXCEPT** which of the following?

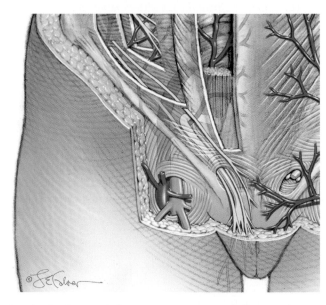

Reproduced, with permission, from Corton MM: Anatomy. In Hoffman BL, Schorge JO, Schaffer JI, et al (eds): Williams Gynecology, 2nd ed. New York, McGraw-Hill, 2012, Figure 38-4.

   a. Inguinal ligament

   b. Inferior epigastric artery

   c. Superficial epigastric artery

   d. Lateral border of rectus abdominis muscle

11–28. Treatment options for pelvic muscle trigger points include all **EXCEPT** which of the following?

   a. Biofeedback

   b. Hysterectomy

   c. Muscle relaxants

   d. Trigger point needling

11–29. Chronic lower anterior abdominal wall pain may follow this incision and may be linked to nerve entrapment of all **EXCEPT** which of the following nerves?

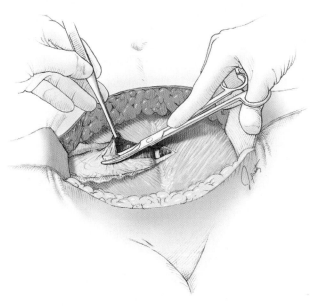

Reproduced, with permission, from Hoffman BL: Surgeries for benign gynecologic conditions. In Schorge JO, Schaffer JI, Halvorson LM, et al (eds) Williams Gynecology, 1st ed. New York, McGraw-Hill, 2008, Figure 41-2.1.

    a. Femoral

    b. Ilioinguinal

    c. Genitofemoral

    d. Iliohypogastric

Chapter 11   ANSWER KEY

Question number	Letter answer	Page cited	Header cited	Question number	Letter answer	Page cited	Header cited
11–1	d	p. 304	Somatic Pain	11–17	b	p. 313	Lithotomy
11–2	a	p. 304	Somatic Pain	11–18	a	p. 313	Radiologic Imaging and Endoscopy
11–3	d	p. 304	Visceral Pain	11–19	d	p. 313	Radiologic Imaging and Endoscopy
11–4	b	p. 306	Neuropathic Pain				
11–5	a	p. 306	Acute Pain	11–20	d	p. 314	Treatment
11–6	a	p. 306	Table 11-1	11–21	d	p. 316	Hysterectomy
11–7	d	p. 306	History	11–22	b	p. 318	Dysmenorrhea
11–8	c	p. 307	Vital Signs	11–23	d	p. 318	Risks for Primary Dysmenorrhea
11–9	c	p. 307	Abdominal Examination				
11–10	a	p. 307	Pelvic Examination	11–24	d	p. 318	Pathophysiology
11–11	b	p. 308	Sonography	11–25	b	p. 319	Dyspareunia
11–12	c	p. 310	Chronic Pelvic Pain	11–26	d	p. 320	Interstitial Cystitis/Painful Bladder Syndrome
11–13	d	p. 310	Chronic Pelvic Pain				
11–14	d	p. 310	Etiology	11–27	c	p. 323	Abdominal Wall Hernia
11–15	b	p. 310	Table 11-3	11–28	b	p. 326	Treatment
11–16	a	p. 312	Supine	11–29	a	p. 326	Anterior Abdominal Wall Nerve Entrapment Syndromes

CHAPTER 12

Breast Disease

12-1. Which of the following is **NOT** a common presentation of breast disease in women?

    a. Breast pain

    b. Palpable mass

    c. Nipple discharge

    d. Skin pigmentation abnormalities

12-2. The areola contains numerous lubricating sebaceous glands referred to as which of the following?

    a. Mallory glands

    b. Montgomery glands

    c. Mammosebaceous units

    d. Mammolactiferous glands

12-3. Which group of lymph nodes receives most of the lymphatic drainage from the breasts and are therefore most often involved by breast cancer metastases?

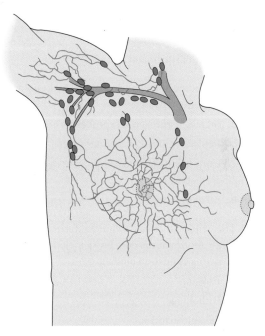

Reproduced, with permission, from Poggi MM, Harney K: The breast. In DeCherney AH, Nathan L (eds): CURRENT Diagnosis & Treatment Obstetrics & Gynecology, 10th ed. New York, McGraw-Hill, 2007, Figure 63-3.

    a. Axillary

    b. Supraclavicular

    c. External mammary

    d. Internal mammary

12-4. The primordial breast develops from which of the following tissues?

    a. Mesoderm

    b. Primitive fat lobules

    c. Basal layer of the epidermis

    d. Multipotent cells within the dermis

12–5. Final histologic differentiation of breast tissue is not completed until which of the following occurs?

   a. Menarche

   b. Onset of puberty

   c. First full-term pregnancy

   d. Breastfeeding for several months

12–6. Most benign and malignant breast disease occurs within the breast structures that are the most sensitive to ovarian hormones and prolactin. Which structures are these?

   a. Lobular fat

   b. Collecting ducts

   c. Collagenous stroma

   d. Terminal ducts and acini

12–7. Which of the following describes the physiology of the breast in menopause?

   a. Increased estrogen-receptor expression

   b. Replacement of collagenous stroma with fat

   c. Conversion of adrenal androgens to estrogen by aromatase

   d. All of the above

12–8. The "triple test" that best guides the management of breast abnormalities does **NOT** include which of the following evaluation modalities?

   a. Imaging

   b. Pathology

   c. Genetic markers

   d. Clinical examination

12–9. Frequently mistaken for a breast mass, the axillary extension of normal breast tissue is referred to as the tail of which of the following?

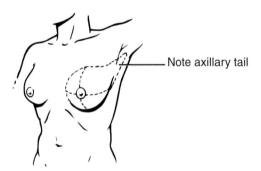

Note axillary tail

Reproduced, with permission, from LeBlond RF, Brown DD, DeGowin RL: The chest: chest wall, pulmonary, and cardiovascular Systems; the breasts. In DeGowin's Diagnostic Examination, 9th ed. New York, McGraw-Hill, 2009, Figure 8-55.

   a. Rahn

   b. Spence

   c. Pearson

   d. Griffith

12–10. Which of the listed mammographic features of solid breast masses suggests malignancy?

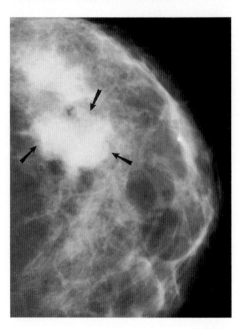

Reproduced, with permission, from Hunt KK, Newman LA, Copeland EM III: The breast. In Brunicardi FC, Andersen DK, Billiar TR, et al (eds): Schwartz's Principles of Surgery, 9th ed. New York, McGraw-Hill, 2010, Figure 17-28.

   a. Irregular margins

   b. Absent internal echoes

   c. Width-to-height ratio of 3 or greater

   d. None of the above

12–11. The reporting system for mammographic results in general use is referred to as which of the following acronyms?

   a. BI-RADS

   b. MAM-IMGS

   c. RISK-OPS

   d. GAIL-MODS

12–12. Which of the following initial diagnostic techniques is currently favored because of its minimal invasiveness, its lower insufficient-sample rate, and its ability to provide superior diagnostic tissue samples?

   a. Core-needle biopsy

   b. Fine-needle aspiration

   c. Open excisional biopsy

   d. Intraductal washings for cytology

12–13. What is the accuracy of a concordant benign triple test for correctly predicting that a breast mass is benign?

   a. 60%

   b. 70%

   c. 80%

   d. >99%

12-14. A 40-year-old woman is evaluated for a self-discovered breast mass. Clinical examination shows a left breast mass that is smooth, mobile, 1.5 cm in greatest diameter, and located at 4 o'clock and 3 cm from the nipple. Diagnostic mammography shows the mass with smooth borders, no calcifications, presence of internal echoes, and a width-to-height ration of 1. Core needle biopsy shows benign ductal and lobular structures. Which of the following is the most appropriate clinical management of this mass?

a. Excision

b. Breast sonography

c. Repeat core biopsy in 3 months

d. Clinical examination at 6-month intervals

12-15. A 50-year-old woman without any family history of breast or related cancers is found to have a palpable, 2-cm breast cyst with complex sonographic features. The mass is asymptomatic. What is the most reasonable management of this complex mass?

a. Excision

b. Fine-needle biopsy

c. Aspiration with cytology

d. Aspiration and if sonographic abnormality persists, then excision

12-16. A 17-year-old presents with a 0.5-cm breast mass with a triple test classification of benign concordant. The diagnosis of fibroadenoma is strongly suspected. The mass is asymptomatic. Repeat examinations 6 months and 1 year later show the mass to be unchanged in size and character. What is the best option for further management of this mass?

a. Excision

b. Core needle biopsy

c. Magnetic resonance imaging

d. Continued clinical monitoring

12-17. Which statement regarding phyllodes tumors of the breast is **FALSE**?

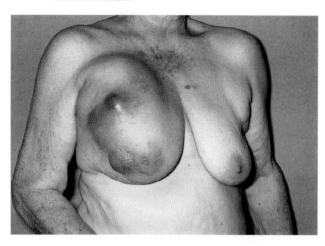

Reproduced, with permission, from Hunt KK, Newman LA, Copeland EM III: The breast. In Brunicardi FC, Andersen DK, Billiar TR, et al (eds): Schwartz's Principles of Surgery, 9th ed. New York, McGraw-Hill, 2010, Figure 17-40A.

a. Lymph node metastasis is rare.

b. The lung is the most common site of metastasis.

c. Local recurrence is common (>30%) for malignant tumors.

d. Primary treatment consists of chemotherapy and radiation.

12-18. Which of the following scenarios involving breast nipple discharge is most concerning for an underlying malignancy?

a. Spontaneous, bloody, multiduct discharge in a 36-year-old pregnant patient

b. Spontaneous, single-duct serous discharge in a 28-year-old on oral contraceptive pills

c. Greenish multiduct discharge expressed during routine clinical examination of a 50-year-old woman

d. Milky white discharge expressed from several ducts during clinical examination of a 40-year-old multipara

12–19. Which of the following is **NOT** part of the therapeutic approach to puerperal mastitis?

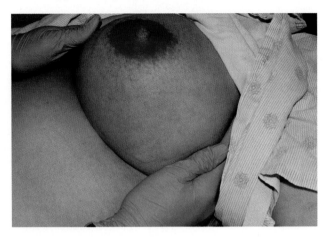

Photograph contributed by Dr. La'Keisha Demerson.

a. Antibiotics

b. Breastfeeding cessation

c. Sonography if abscess suspected

d. Topical treatment of any nipple cracks

12–20. Which of the following is an infrequent presentation of cancer in the nonpuerperal breast?

a. Abscess

b. Mastalgia

c. Cellulitis

d. All of the above

12–21. The presence of atypical epithelial hyperplasia carries what increased relative risk of breast cancer?

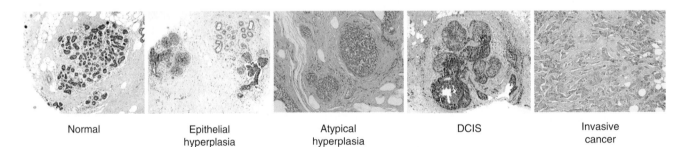

| Normal | Epithelial hyperplasia | Atypical hyperplasia | DCIS | Invasive cancer |

Reproduced, with permission, from Euhus D: Breast disease. In Schorge JO, Schaffer JI, Halvorson LM, et al (eds): Williams Gynecology, 1st ed. New York, McGraw-Hill, 2008, Figure 12-9.

a. 1.5

b. 2.5

c. 3.5

d. 4.5

12–22. Lobular carcinoma of the breast is a marker of increased cancer risk rather than a direct cancer precursor. Which of the following interventions is **NOT** a reasonable strategy for reducing that risk?

a. Chemoprevention

b. Prophylactic unilateral mastectomy

c. Twice-yearly clinical examinations

d. Alternating mammography and magnetic resonance imaging

12–23. Which histologic feature of ductal carcinoma in situ is the most predictive of the presence of invasive cancer, the extent of disease, and the recurrence risk after treatment?

a. Nuclear grade

b. Morphologic type

c. Mammographic features

d. Presence or absence of comedonecrosis

12–24. Paget disease of the nipple is a type of which of the following breast neoplasias?

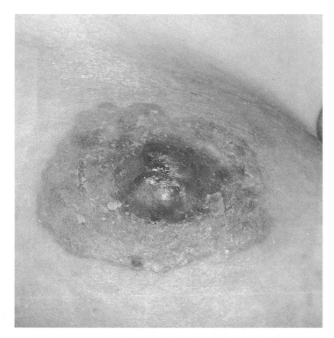

Reproduced, with permission, from Neuhaus IM, Grekin RC: Mammary and extramammary Paget disease. In Wolff K, Goldsmith LA, Katz SI, et al (eds): Fitzpatrick's Dermatology in General Medicine, 7th ed. New York, McGraw-Hill, 2008, Figure 121-1.

    a. Fibrocystic change

    b. Ductal carcinoma in situ

    c. Lobular carcinoma in situ

    d. Atypical epithelial hyperplasia

12–25. Which of the following has the strongest association with increased breast cancer risk?

    a. Increasing parity

    b. Earlier age of first live birth

    c. Increasing lifetime number of menstrual cycles

    d. Use of estrogen-only hormone replacement therapy

12–26. Which of the following breast cancer risk evaluation tools has been independently validated and is widely used?

    a. Gail model

    b. Richardson model

    c. Tryer-Cuzick model

    d. Bloom-Schwarz model

12–27. What percentage of breast cancers are caused by inherited gene mutations such as BRCA1 and BRCA2?

    a. Fewer than 10

    b. Approximately 25

    c. Approximately 50

    d. Greater than 75

12–28. Up to 40 percent of male breast cancers are related to which genetic syndrome?

    a. BRCA1

    b. BRCA2

    c. $p16^{INK4a}$

    d. Li-Fraumeni

12–29. Carriers of *BRCA* gene mutations, in addition to breast cancer, are at increased risk for which of the following?

    a. Melanoma

    b. Ovarian cancer

    c. Pancreatic cancer

    d. All of the above

12–30. Approximately what percentage of abnormalities detected by screening mammography represent a malignancy?

    a. 5

    b. 15

    c. 35

    d. 55

12–31. Up to what percentage of women diagnosed with breast cancer will have had a normal mammogram during the preceding 12 to 24 months?

    a. 5

    b. 10

    c. 15

    d. 25

12–32. An advantage of breast screening with magnetic resonance imaging compared with screening using mammography includes which of the following?

    a. Lower cost per procedure

    b. Lower false positive rate

    c. Increased ease of test performance

    d. Better performance in dense breast tissue

12–33. Breast cancers positive for estrogen and progesterone receptors generally demonstrate a better prognosis and allow more treatment options. What proportion of breast cancers are estrogen- and progesterone-receptor positive?

    a. One third

    b. Two thirds

    c. One fourth

    d. Three fourths

12–34. What is the most common site of distant breast cancer metastasis?

   a. Bone

   b. Liver

   c. Lungs

   d. Ovaries

12–35. At present, what is standard treatment following lumpectomy for apparently localized breast cancer?

   a. Bilateral axillary radiation

   b. Ipsilateral axillary radiation

   c. Whole breast radiation of affected breast

   d. Whole breast radiation of both affected and contralateral breasts

12–36. Which of the following therapeutic agents used to treat breast cancer in postmenopausal women increases the risk of bone fractures?

   a. Tamoxifen

   b. Bisphosphonates

   c. Aromatase inhibitors

   d. None of the above

12–37. Which of the following characteristics is **NOT** typical of inflammatory breast cancer?

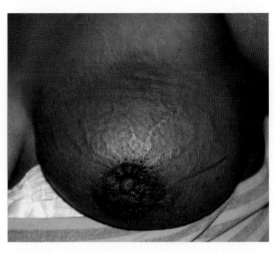

Reproduced, with permission, from Euhus D: Breast disease. In Schorge JO, Schaffer JI, Halvorson LM, et al (eds): Williams Gynecology, 1st ed., New York, McGraw-Hill, 2008, Figure 12-16B.

   a. Slow onset

   b. Breast induration

   c. Breast enlargement

   d. Erythematous skin changes

12–38. Which of the following are known to be effective breast cancer prevention strategies?

   a. Regular physical activity in average risk women

   b. Tamoxifen for 5 years in women at increased risk

   c. Prophylactic oophorectomy in women at very high risk

   d. All of the above

Chapter 12 ANSWER KEY

Question number	Letter answer	Page cited	Header cited
12–1	d	p. 333	Breast Disease
12–2	b	p. 333	Ductal System
12–3	a	p. 333	Lymphatic Drainage
12–4	c	p. 334	Development and Physiology
12–5	c	p. 334	Development and Physiology
12–6	d	p. 334	Development and Physiology
12–7	d	p. 334	Development and Physiology
12–8	c	p. 334	Evaluation of a Breast Lump
12–9	b	p. 334	Physical Examination
12–10	a	p. 336	Diagnostic Imaging
12–11	a	p. 336	Breast Imaging Reporting and Data System
12–12	a	p. 336	Breast Biopsy
12–13	d	p. 337	Triple Test
12–14	a	p. 337	Triple Test
12–15	a	p. 337	Cysts
12–16	d	p. 337	Fibroadenoma
12–17	d	p. 338	Phyllodes Tumors
12–18	b	p. 338	Nipple Discharge
12–19	b	p. 340	Puerperal Infections

Question number	Letter answer	Page cited	Header cited
12–20	d	p. 340	Nonpuerperal Infections
12–21	d	p. 343	Ductal and Lobular Hyperplasia
12–22	b	p. 343	Lobular Carcinoma in Situ
12–23	a	p. 344	Ductal Carcinoma in Situ
12–24	b	p. 345	Paget Disease of the Nipple
12–25	c	p. 345	Reproductive Factors
12–26	a	p. 346	Gail Model
12–27	a	p. 346	Breast Cancer Genetics
12–28	b	p. 346	Inherited Breast-Ovarian Cancer Syndrome; Table 12-5
12–29	d	p. 347	Table 12-5
12–30	a	p. 347	Screening Mammography
12–31	d	p. 347	Screening Mammography
12–32	d	p. 348	Screening Magnetic Resonance Imaging
12–33	b	p. 349	Tumor Characteristics
12–34	a	p. 349	Breast Cancer Staging
12–35	c	p. 350	Surgery
12–36	c	p. 350	Hormone Therapy and Targeted Therapies
12–37	a	p. 351	Inflammatory Breast Cancer
12–38	d	p. 351	Breast Cancer Prevention

CHAPTER 13

Psychosocial Issues and Female Sexuality

13-1. Which of the following common psychiatric problem frequently accompanies reproductive disorders?

   a. Mood disorder

   b. Anxiety disorder

   c. Alcohol or substance abuse

   d. All of the above

13-2. The diagnostic criteria defining a major depressive episode include nearly daily feelings of depressed mood and/or decreased interest or pleasure in most activities. Diagnostic criteria may also include all **EXCEPT** which of the following?

   a. Insomnia

   b. Poor concentration

   c. Compulsive, repetitive behaviors

   d. Inappropriate guilt or feelings of worthlessness

13-3. Anxiety disorders are more common in women and of the mood disorders, have the highest prevalence rates in the United States. What is the approximate lifetime prevalence rate (percent)?

   a. 10

   b. 20

   c. 30

   d. 40

13-4. Which of the following is more commonly diagnosed in men than in women at the present time?

   a. Anxiety

   b. Depression

   c. Eating disorders

   d. Substance misuse

13-5. The etiology of anorexia nervosa may be multifactorial with both biologic and psychosocial factors at play. What is the approximate concordance rate (percent) of the restricting type of anorexia among monozygotic twins?

   a. 11

   b. 33

   c. 66

   d. 99

13-6. A characteristic clinical feature of bulimia nervosa includes *Russell sign*. This finding refers to which of the following?

   a. Patchy alopecia

   b. Knuckle calluses

   c. Electrolyte imbalance

   d. Gastric and proximal small bowel dilation

13-7. Nearly 300 symptoms have been reported by women during the luteal phase of the menstrual cycle (premenstrual syndrome). In most women, these symptoms are self-limited and cause no excessive distress or functional impairment. In approximately what percentage of women are such symptoms severe enough to cause functional impairment or require special attention?

   a. 5

   b. 15

   c. 25

   d. 35

13-8. The etiology of premenstrual disorders remains obscure and likely involves a variety of biological factors. Activity of which of the following is **NOT** currently suspected of playing a significant role in these disorders?

   a. Prolactin

   b. Serotonin

   c. Sex steroids

   d. Renin-angiotensin-aldosterone system

13-9. At present, which of the following is considered primary therapy for psychological symptoms of premenstrual syndrome?

   a. Prostaglandin inhibitors

   b. Combination oral contraceptives

   c. Selective serotonin-reuptake inhibitors

   d. None of the above

13-10. Which of the following is the unique progestin in Yaz, an oral contraceptive that has received Food and Drug Administration (FDA) approval for the treatment of premenstrual dysphoric disorder?

  a. Gestodene

  b. Desogestrel

  c. Drospirenone

  d. Etonogestrel

13-11. Which of the following statements regarding pregnancy and depression is **FALSE**?

  a. Suicide is a leading cause of maternal death in developed countries.

  b. Depression in pregnancy has diagnostic criteria and prognosis different from those in nonpregnant women.

  c. During pregnancy, there is an increased risk of relapse of a preexisting psychiatric disorder.

  d. The prevalence of depression is highest in the first trimester with a slight decrease in the second and third trimesters.

13-12. Selective serotonin-reuptake inhibitor use during pregnancy has been associated with a small increased risk of which of the following in the exposed neonate?

  a. Congenital malformations

  b. Irritability and feeding problems

  c. Persistent pulmonary hypertension

  d. All of the above

13-13. Which of the following is a **FALSE** statement regarding postpartum depression?

  a. There is no standardized screening tool available.

  b. DSM-IV diagnostic criteria include diagnosis within 4 weeks of delivery.

  c. Postpartum "blues" place a woman at increased risk of developing frank depression.

  d. Postpartum depression affects approximately 15 percent of women after pregnancy.

13-14. Which of the following statements is true regarding clinician involvement in the grieving process following a perinatal loss?

  a. Couples and family therapy may be helpful.

  b. Clinicians should limit information regarding the loss.

  c. Support efforts should be concentrated on the grieving mother.

  d. There are no clinician interventions that aid the grieving process.

13-15. Which of the following is **FALSE** regarding mood disorders that develop during the menopausal transition?

  a. Thyroid function should be assessed along with other possible new-onset medical conditions.

  b. Depression or anxiety symptoms are a normal and expected feature of menopausal transition.

  c. A short-term trial of estrogen is a reasonable therapeutic option in the absence of contraindications.

  d. Rates of new-onset depression during the menopausal transition are nearly double those before menopause.

13-16. As in the general population, what is the most common psychiatric disorder diagnosed in the elderly?

  a. Anxiety

  b. Depression

  c. Alcohol and substance misuse

  d. Obsessive-compulsive behaviors

13-17. Approximately what percentage of sexual assault cases are reported by victims to authorities?

  a. 10

  b. 30

  c. 50

  d. 70

13-18. What percentage of rape victims show no gross findings during physical examination of having been assaulted?

  a. 10

  b. 30

  c. 50

  d. 70

13-19. Emergency contraception is routinely offered to rape victims who are not pregnant. What is the per rape risk (percent) of pregnancy in women of reproductive age?

  a. 1

  b. 5

  c. 10

  d. 20

13–20. A 24-year-old rape victim understands that she is at increased risk of contracting any sexually transmitted infection, but is especially fearful of human immunodeficiency virus (HIV) infection. Her assailant was not known to her. She is trying to decide whether or not to accept postexposure HIV prophylaxis. What is her approximate risk (percent) of HIV infection with receptive penile–vaginal rape?

   a. 0.1

   b. 1

   c. 3

   d. 5

13–21. Rape may result in long-term psychological symptoms that include which of the following?

   a. Anxiety

   b. Depression

   c. Somatic complaints

   d. All of the above

13–22. A 1-year-old female toddler is brought for evaluation of suspected sexual abuse. The presence of which of the following infections is the strongest indicator that such abuse has indeed occurred?

   a. Gonorrhea

   b. Hepatitis B

   c. Genital warts

   d. Trichomoniasis

13–23. Which of the following demographic characteristics does **NOT** increase a woman's risk of falling victim to intimate partner violence?

   a. Pregnancy

   b. Younger age

   c. Hispanic race

   d. Witness to violence as a child

13–24. What is reported as the leading cause of death during pregnancy?

   a. Suicide

   b. Homicide

   c. Thromboembolic event

   d. Motor vehicle accident

13–25. In women, which of the following is thought to be most involved in feelings of empathy, love, and emotional intimacy?

   a. Dopamine

   b. Oxytocin

   c. Androgens

   d. Estrogens

13–26. Which of the following is **NOT** a component of the normal female sexual response?

   a. Vaginal narrowing

   b. Clitoral engorgement

   c. Elevated heart and respiratory rates

   d. Increased production of vaginal transudate

13–27. Which of the following therapies has been shown to positively affect postmenopausal sexual difficulties related to urogenital atrophy?

   a. Estrogen

   b. Progesterone

   c. Testosterone

   d. Selective serotonin-reuptake inhibitors

Chapter 13   ANSWER KEY

Question number	Letter answer	Page cited	Header cited	Question number	Letter answer	Page cited	Header cited
13-1	d	p. 356	Common Psychiatric Presentations	13-14	a	p. 368	Perinatal loss
				13-15	b	p. 369	Menopausal Transition and Menopause
13-2	c	p. 359	Table 13-3				
13-3	c	p. 357	Anxiety Disorders	13-16	a	p. 369	Mental Disorders in the Elderly
13-4	d	p. 357	Alcohol and Substance Disorders	13-17	c	p. 370	Sexual Assault
13-5	c	p. 358	Pathophysiology	13-18	d	p. 370	Common Physical Findings with Sexual Assault
13-6	b	p. 362	Bulimia Nervosa				
13-7	b	p. 364	Premenstrual Disorders	13-19	b	p. 371	Pregnancy Prevention
13-8	a	p. 364	Pathophysiology of Premenstrual Syndrome	13-20	a	p. 371	Sexually Transmitted Disease Prevention
13-9	c	p. 366	Treatment of Premenstrual Syndrome	13-21	d	p. 372	Psychological Response to Sexual Assault
13-10	c	p. 366	Treatment of Premenstrual Syndrome	13-22	a	p. 373	Table 13-18
				13-23	c	p. 374	Risk Factors
13-11	b	p. 367	Pregnancy and Postpartum Disorders	13-24	b	p. 374	Intimate Partner Violence During Pregnancy
13-12	d	p. 367	Treatment of Depression in Pregnancy	13-25	b	p. 376	Arousal
				13-26	a	p. 376	Clitoral Changes with Arousal
13-13	a	p. 367	Diagnosis of Depression in the Perinatal Period	13-27	a	p. 377	Sexuality During Menopausal Transition

Pediatric Gynecology

14-1. Which of the following statements is **FALSE** regarding development of the hypothalamic-pituitary-ovarian axis in the female fetus and neonate?

    a. The gonadotropin-releasing hormone (GnRH) "pulse generator" remains functionally dormant until shortly after birth.

    b. By 5 months' gestation, 6 to 7 million oocytes have been created from accelerated germ cell division.

    c. At birth, follicle-stimulating hormone (FSH) and luteinizing hormone (LH) concentrations rise and remain high during the first 3 months of life.

    d. Neonatal breast budding, minor uterine bleeding, and transient ovarian cysts may occur as a normal response to initially high gonadotropin levels.

14-2. Which of the following statements is true regarding pelvic anatomy in the female infant and child?

    a. The ovaries have obtained their normal adult size by birth.

    b. At birth, the uterus and cervix are approximately equal in size.

    c. Presence of an endometrial stripe or fluid within the endometrial cavity of the newborn uterus is a normal finding with sonography.

    d. All the above are true statements.

14-3. Which of the following generally occurs first among the major developmental events of female puberty?

    a. Menarche

    b. Pubarche

    c. Thelarche

    d. Growth spurt

14-4. Precocious puberty is defined as initial pubertal changes occurring prior to what age?

    a. 6.5 years

    b. 8 years

    c. 9.5 years

    d. 10 years

14-5. Delayed puberty is characterized by a lack of initial pubertal changes, usually thelarche, by what age?

    a. 13 years

    b. 14 years

    c. 15 years

    d. 16 years

14-6. During the past several decades, the ages at which U.S. girls experience thelarche and menarche have shown which of the following trends?

    a. Later than in past

    b. Earlier than in past

    c. No significant change from past

    d. No clear trend has been observed

14-7. Indications for an internal vaginal examination in a child include which of the following?

    a. Possible tumor

    b. Vaginal bleeding

    c. Suspected foreign body

    d. All of the above

14-8. Management of labial adhesion or agglutination in a child includes which of the following options?

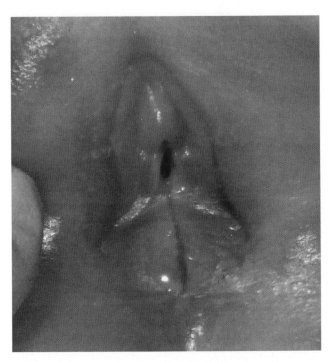

Reproduced, with permission, from Ellen Wilson: Pediatric gynecology. In Hoffman BL, Schorge JO, Schaffer JI, et al (eds): Williams Gynecology, 2nd ed. New York, McGraw-Hill, 2012, Figure 14-7.

a. Emollients

b. Topical estrogen cream

c. Await spontaneous resolution

d. All of the above

14-9. A 14-year-old female presents with increasingly painful, cyclic menses since menarche 9 months ago. Oral analgesics and nonsteroidal antiinflammatory medications no longer adequately control her dysmenorrhea. Which of the following congenital anomalies is most likely present?

a. Obstructed hemivagina and ipsilateral renal anomaly (OHVIRA) syndrome

b. Imperforate hymen

c. Müllerian agenesis

d. Complete transverse vaginal septum

14-10. A 13-year-old female presents with increasing abdominal pain. She has begun appropriate pubertal development, although menarche has not occurred. During examination, a central abdominopelvic mass is appreciated and is shown in Figure A. Physical examination findings prompt sonography and then magnetic resonance (MR) imaging with contrast. The MR imaging results are shown in Figure B. Which of the following congenital anomalies is most likely present?

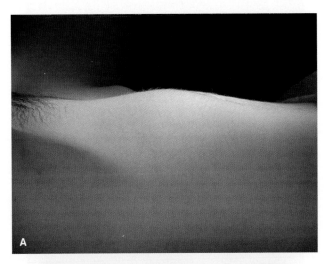

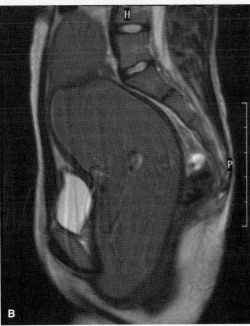

Figure A: Photograph contributed by Dr. Ellen Wilson. Figure B: Reproduced, with permission, from Wilson EE, Bradshaw KD, Hoffman BL: Case report: imperforate hymen (update) In Schorge JO, Schaffer JI, Halvorson LM, et al (eds): Williams Gynecology, 1st ed. Online. New York, McGraw-Hill, 2008, July 29, Figure 3.

a. Müllerian agenesis

b. Cervical agenesis

c. Imperforate hymen

d. Obstructed hemivagina and ipsilateral renal anomaly (OHVIRA) syndrome

14–11. A 7-year-old girl has experienced vulvar irritation with external itching and burning with urination for several months. Symptoms have persisted despite attempts to eliminate potential irritants and contact allergens from the bath and laundry products used by the family. Examination shows symmetrical hypopigmentation and a parchment-like thinning of the vulvar and perianal skin. What is the most likely diagnosis?

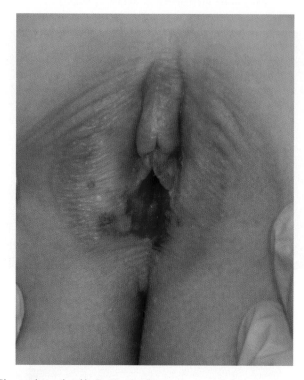

Photograph contributed by Dr. Mary Jane Pearson.

  a. Eczema

  b. Candidiasis

  c. Sexual abuse

  d. Lichen sclerosus

14–12. What approximate percentage of malignant tumors diagnosed in childhood are of ovarian origin?

  a. 1

  b. 5

  c. 10

  d. 15

14–13. What is the preferred imaging modality when a congenital müllerian anomaly is suspected?

  a. Computed tomography

  b. Transabdominal sonography

  c. Magnetic resonance imaging

  d. Abdominopelvic x-ray series

14–14. Which of the following is true regarding isolated premature thelarche?

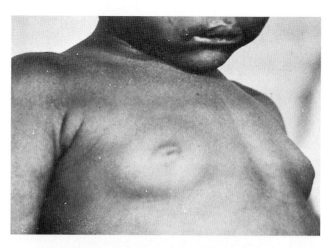

Reproduced, with permission, from Muram D: Pediatric & adolescent gynecology. In DeCherney AH, Nathan L (eds): CURRENT Diagnosis & Treatment Obstetrics & Gynecology, 10th ed. New York, McGraw-Hill, 2007, Figure 34–25.

  a. Bone age is advanced.

  b. Gonadotropin levels are elevated.

  c. It is most common in girls less than 2 years of age.

  d. None of the above.

14–15. A 13-year-old adolescent is brought in for examination due to her left breast being noticeably larger than her right when she is undressed. Thelarche occurred at age 11.5 years. She is left handed and plays softball, tennis, and lacrosse. She cannot think of any specific trauma to the right breast. The breasts are otherwise normal upon examination. Cosmetically, the difference is not obvious when she is clothed. Which of the following is the most common cause of asymmetric breast growth in a female adolescent?

  a. Physical trauma

  b. Surgical trauma

  c. No identifiable cause

  d. Strong right- or left-handedness

14–16. What is the best approach to remedy the case of the breast asymmetry described in Question 14–15?

  a. Initiate combination oral contraceptive pills

  b. Refer now for plastic surgery before asymmetry progresses

  c. Temporarily discourage sports requiring dominant use of one arm or one side of the torso

  d. Reassure that most cases of breast asymmetry resolve by completion of breast development

14–17. Abnormal breast development may be due to either fascial adherence to the underlying muscle layer or high-dose exogenous hormone exposure. In such cases, there is excessive forward and limited lateral development of the breasts, causing an abnormal shape. This condition is referred to as which of the following?

  a. Polythelia

  b. Tuberous breasts

  c. Breast hypertrophy

  d. Asymmetric lactiferous hyperplasia

14–18. A breast mass that is noted in a young adolescent female prompts you to order breast sonography. What is the most likely outcome of the lesion found and shown below?

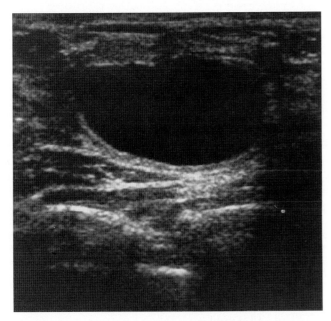

Reproduced, with permission, from Freimanis RI, Ayoub JS: Radiology of the breast. In Chen MYM, Pope TL, Ott DJ (eds): Basic Radiology, 2nd ed. New York, McGraw-Hill, 2011, Figure 5—7.

  a. Spontaneous regression over time

  b. Persistence with little change in size

  c. Gradual increase in size with hormonal stimulation

  d. Development of more generalized fibrocystic changes

14–19. A smooth, firm, mobile, nontender right breast mass is palpable on examination of a 12-year-old girl. It is 1 cm in its greatest dimension and appears solid by sonography. She has had no major health problems to date. What is the most likely diagnosis?

  a. Malignancy

  b. Fibroadenoma

  c. Ductal ectasia

  d. Asymmetric breast budding

14–20. Mastitis is unusual in children and adolescents. What is the most common pathogen isolated from breast abscesses in the pediatric population?

  a. *Escherichia coli*

  b. *Staphylococcus aureus*

  c. *Streptococcus pyogenes*

  d. *Staphylococcus epidermidis*

14–21. An 8-year-old girl is brought in for evaluation of 4 days of intermittent vaginal bleeding. She shows no signs of pubertal development. The cause of the bleeding is not apparent during physical examination, and the decision is made to proceed with examination under anesthesia and saline vaginoscopy. What is the most likely finding?

  a. Foreign object

  b. Atrophic vaginitis

  c. Endocervical polyp

  d. Sarcoma botryoides

14–22. Which of the following is the most common cause of central precocious puberty?

  a. Idiopathic

  b. Head trauma

  c. Hydrocephalus secondary to surgery

  d. Congenital central nervous system anomaly

14–23. Primary therapy for central (gonadotropin dependent) precocious puberty consists of which of the following?

  a. Bromocriptine

  b. Depot medroxyprogesterone acetate

  c. Combination oral contraceptive pills

  d. Gonadotropin-releasing hormone (GnRH) agonist

14–24. A primary goal of therapy for central precocious puberty includes prevention of which of the following consequences?

  a. Short stature

  b. Excessive breast size

  c. Learning disabilities

  d. None of the above

14–25. A 5-year-old girl suffers from precocious puberty. Gonadotropin levels are low, even following gonadotropin-releasing hormone (GnRH) infusion stimulation testing. However, estrogen levels are elevated. Which of the following could be a cause of her disorder?

  a. Primary hypothyroidism

  b. Ovarian granulosa cell tumor

  c. Congenital adrenal hyperplasia

  d. All of the above

14-26. Pubarche, with development of axillary and pubic hair, is stimulated by the androgens derived from which of the following?

   a. Adrenal glands

   b. Ovarian stroma

   c. Peripheral aromatization of estrogens

   d. All of the above

14-27. Delayed puberty in females is defined as lack of secondary sexual characteristics by age 13 or lack of menarche by what age?

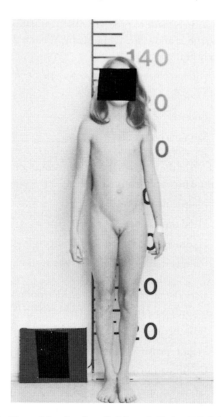

Reproduced, with permission, from Styne D: Puberty. In Gardner DG, Shoback D (eds): Greenspan's Basic & Clinical Endocrinology, 8th ed. New York, McGraw-Hill, 2007, Figure 16—6A.

   a. 14

   b. 15

   c. 16

   d. 18

14-28. Sexually active adolescents are particularly vulnerable to partner violence. In a study by Abma and associates (2010), what percentage of adolescent females who experienced coitarche prior to age 20 years described their first sexual intercourse as nonvoluntary?

   a. 1

   b. 3

   c. 5

   d. 7

14-29. Which of the following contraceptive methods is generally contraindicated in adolescents (age less than 21 years)?

   a. Vaginal ring

   b. Intrauterine devices

   c. Extended-use oral contraceptive pills

   d. None of the above

14-30. Which of the following is required when initiating a contraceptive method for a healthy, sexually active adolescent?

   a. Pap screening

   b. Pelvic examination

   c. Human papillomavirus (HPV) vaccination

   d. None of the above

14-31. In the United States, adolescents can obtain medical care without parental knowledge or consent for which of the following?

   a. Pregnancy

   b. Contraception

   c. Substance abuse

   d. All of the above

References:

Abma JC, Martinez GM, Copen CE: Teenagers in the United States: sexual activity, contraceptive use, and childbearing, National Survey of Family Growth 2006–2008. National Center for Health Statistics. Vital Health Stat 23:30, 2010

Chapter 14 ANSWER KEY

Question number	Letter answer	Page cited	Header cited
14–1	a	p. 382	Hypothalamic-Pituitary-Ovarian (HPO) Axis
14–2	c	p. 383	Anatomy
14–3	c	p. 383	Pubertal Changes
14–4	b	p. 383	Pubertal Changes
14–5	a	p. 383	Pubertal Changes
14–6	b	p. 383	Pubertal Changes
14–7	d	p. 383	Gynecologic Examination
14–8	d	p. 386	Labial Adhesion
14–9	a	p. 387	Congenital Anatomic Anomalies
14–10	c	p. 387	Congenital Anatomic Anomalies
14–11	d	p. 387	Lichen Sclerosus
14–12	a	p. 389	Ovarian Tumors
14–13	c	p. 390	Prepubertal Ovarian Masses
14–14	c	p. 391	Premature Thelarche
14–15	c	p. 391	Breast Asymmetry
14–16	d	p. 391	Breast Asymmetry

Question number	Letter answer	Page cited	Header cited
14–17	b	p. 391	Tuberous Breasts
14–18	a	p. 392	Breast Cysts
14–19	b	p. 392	Breast Masses
14–20	b	p. 392	Breast Masses
14–21	a	p. 393	Vaginal Bleeding
14–22	a	p. 394	Table 14-3
14–23	d	p. 393	Central Precocious Puberty (Gonadotropin Dependent)
14–24	a	p. 393	Central Precocious Puberty (Gonadotropin Dependent)
14–25	d	p. 393	Peripheral Precocious Puberty (Gonadotropin Independent)
14–26	a	p. 394	Variations of Normal Puberty
14–27	b	p. 395	Delayed Puberty
14–28	d	p. 396	Adolescent Perceptions of Sexual Activity
14–29	d	p. 396	Contraception
14–30	d	p. 396	Contraception
14–31	d	p. 396	Contraception

REPRODUCTIVE ENDOCRINOLOGY, INFERTILITY, AND THE MENOPAUSE

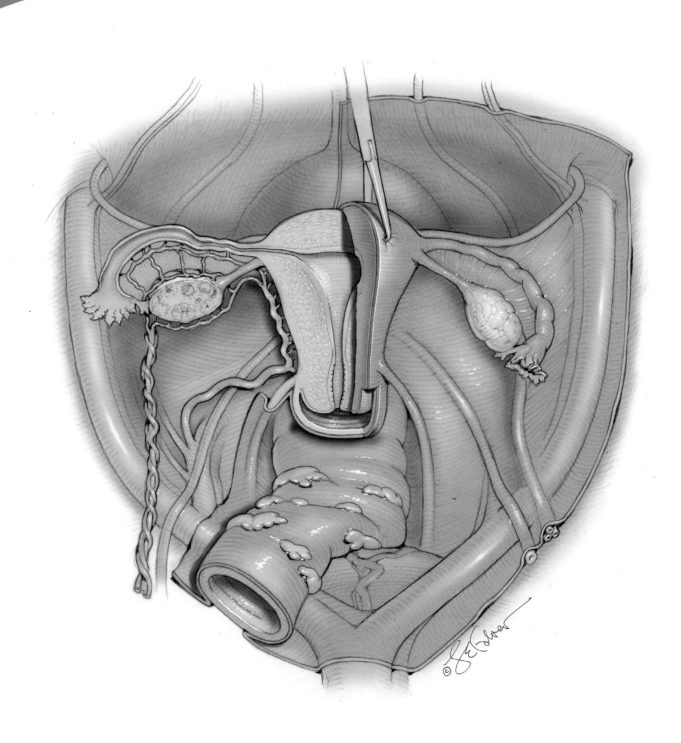

CHAPTER 15

Reproductive Endocrinology

15–1. Which of the following terms most accurately describes autocrine hormone communication?

    a. The hormone produced and secreted acts on its own cell

    b. The hormone produced and secreted acts on distant organs

    c. The hormone produced and secreted acts on neighboring cells

    d. The hormone produced acts intracellularly prior to secretion

15–2. The image below portrays which type of hormone action?

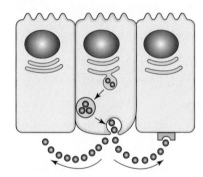

Reproduced, with permission, from Halvorson LM: Reproductive endocrinology. In Schorge JO, Schaffer JI, Halvorson LM, et al (eds): Williams Gynecology, 1st ed. New York, McGraw-Hill, 2008, Figure 15-2B.

    a. Autocrine

    b. Endocrine

    c. Paracrine

    d. Intracrine

15–3. Luteinizing hormone (LH) and human chorionic gonadotropin (hCG) have similar biologic activity for which of the following reasons?

    a. Their β-subunits have 80% homology.

    b. They have nearly homologous α-subunits.

    c. They are produced by the same pituitary cell type.

    d. They are converted to the same amino acid sequence peripherally.

15–4. The last step in estrogen synthesis requires which of the following enzymes?

    a. Aromatase

    b. 5α-Reductase

    c. 21-Hydroxylase

    d. 11β-Hydroxylase

15–5. Based on the diagram below, Enzyme A is which of the following?

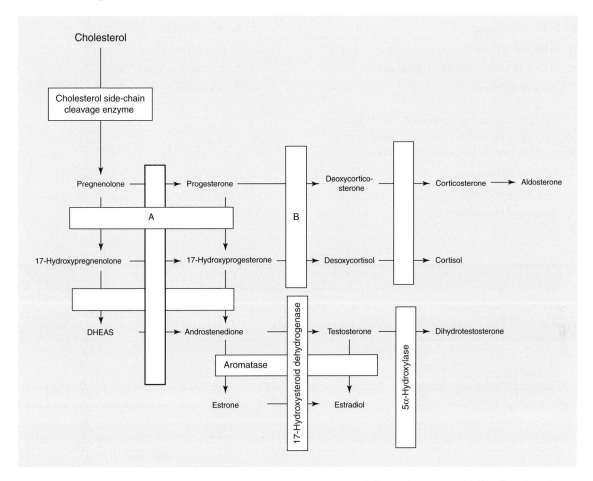

Reproduced, with permission, from Halvorson LM: Reproductive endocrinology. In Schorge JO, Schaffer JI, Halvorson LM, et al (eds): Williams Gynecology, 1st ed. New York, McGraw-Hill, 2008, Figure 15-13.

a. 21-Hydroxylase

b. 11β-Hydroxylase

c. 17α-Hydroxylase

d. 3β-Hydroxysteroid dehydrogenase

15–6. Based on the diagram in Question 15–5, Enzyme B is which of the following?

a. 21-Hydroxylase

b. 11β-Hydroxylase

c. 17α-Hydroxylase

d. 3β-Hydroxysteroid dehydrogenase

15–7. Which of the following hormones is the primary androgen and/or androgen precursor produced by the ovary?

a. Testosterone

b. Androstenedione

c. Dihydrotestosterone

d. Dehydroepiandrosterone sulfate

15–8. Peripheral conversion of androstenedione contributes what percentage to the circulating testosterone concentration in women?

a. 10

b. 25

c. 50

d. 75

15–9. Which of the following will most likely increase circulating sex hormone-binding globulin (SHBG) levels?

a. Insulin

b. Estrogen

c. Androgens

d. Progestins

15–10. Patients with congenital adrenal hyperplasia (CAH) secondary to 21-hydroxylase deficiency will have a deficiency in which of the following hormones?

a. Cortisol

b. Testosterone

c. Androstenedione

d. 17-Hydroxyprogesterone

15–11. Steroid receptors can be found in which of the following locations?

  a. In the cell nucleus

  b. In the cell cytoplasm

  c. In both the cell nucleus and cytoplasm

  d. None of the above

15–12. Gonadotropin-releasing hormone (GnRH) agonists, such as leuprolide acetate, reduce gonadotropin secretion via which of the following mechanisms?

  a. Receptor antagonism

  b. Receptor destruction

  c. Receptor downregulation

  d. None of the above

15–13. As shown here, β-melanocyte stimulating hormone (MSH) is a direct product of which of the following?

  a. β-Endorphin

  b. β-Lipoprotein

  c. Pro-opiomelanocortin

  d. Adrenocorticotropic hormone (ACTH) intermediate

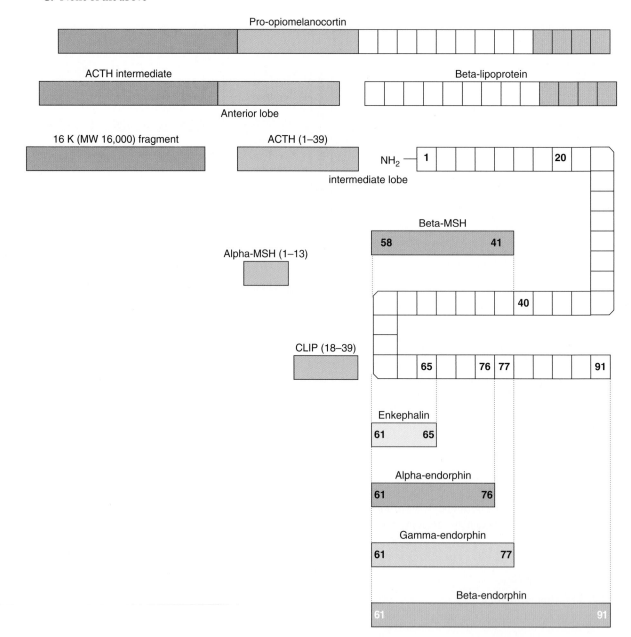

Reproduced, with permission, from Halvorson LM: Reproductive endocrinology. In Schorge JO, Schaffer JI, Halvorson LM, et al (eds): Williams Gynecology, 1st ed. New York, McGraw-Hill, 2008, Figure 15-4.

15–14. Which of the following conditions causes the release of neuropeptide Y?

   a. Obesity

   b. Anorexia

   c. Diabetes mellitus

   d. Hyperprolactinemia

15–15. All **EXCEPT** which of the following are anterior pituitary hormones?

   a. Prolactin

   b. Growth hormone

   c. Thyrotropin-releasing hormone

   d. Follicle-stimulating hormone (FSH)

15–16. Sustained gonadotropin secretion requires which of the following patterns of gonadotropin-releasing hormone (GnRH) secretion?

   a. Pulsatile release of GnRH

   b. Nocturnal release of GnRH

   c. Low doses of GnRH secretion

   d. High doses of GnRH secretion

15–17. Endorphin levels in the brain peak during which of the following menstrual cycle events?

   a. Menses

   b. Ovulation

   c. Luteal phase

   d. Follicular phase

15–18. Which of the following potentiates the release of prolactin from the anterior pituitary gland?

   a. Dopamine

   b. Thyrotropin-releasing hormone

   c. Gonadotropin-releasing hormone

   d. Corticotropin-releasing hormone

15–19. Cells of the anterior pituitary primarily express which of the following dopamine receptors?

   a. D1

   b. D2

   c. D3

   d. None of the above

15–20. Growth hormone effects are mediated through which of the following?

   a. Insulin-like growth factor I

   b. Insulin-like growth factor II

   c. Both, insulin-like growth factors I and II

   d. None of the above

15–21. If affecting the pituitary gland, which of the following can lead to hypogonadotropic hypogonadism?

   a. Brain surgery

   b. Pituitary infarction

   c. Head radiation therapy

   d. All of the above

15–22. A 27-year-old female presents with bilateral nipple discharge. Microscopic evaluation of the discharge reveals galactorrhea. During examination, no breast masses are noted. Patient has a history of schizophrenia. Further laboratory evaluation reveals a mildly elevated prolactin level. Which of the following is most likely the cause of her hyperprolactinemia?

   a. Renal disease

   b. Medication side effect

   c. Prolactin-producing pituitary adenoma

   d. Breast examination performed prior to venipuncture

15–23. The arrow in the diagram shown below is pointing toward which of the following?

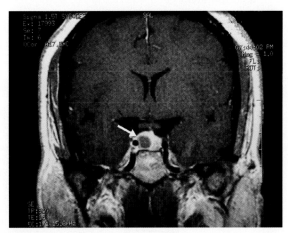

Reproduced, with permission, from Halvorson LM: Reproductive endocrinology. In Schorge JO, Schaffer JI, Halvorson LM, et al (eds): Williams Gynecology, 1st ed. New York, McGraw-Hill, 2008, Figure 15-8A.

   a. The optic chiasm

   b. A pituitary tumor

   c. The third ventricle

   d. A hypothalamic tumor

15–24. A 33-year-old female is being followed for a 5-mm prolactin-producing pituitary adenoma, which is well controlled on bromocriptine 0.5 mg orally daily. She presents with a positive pregnancy test result. How should you manage her treatment at this point?

   a. Discontinue bromocriptine therapy

   b. Increase bromocriptine to 1 mg daily

   c. Check a prolactin level and if it is elevated, continue bromocriptine therapy

   d. Obtain magnetic resonance (MR) imaging of the brain and base decisions on these findings

15-25. What is the first-line of treatment for a pituitary macroadenoma?

   a. Radiation therapy

   b. Dopamine-agonist therapy

   c. Transsphenoidal resection

   d. Somatostatin-agonist therapy

15-26. At what stage of the female life is the highest number of oocytes found in the ovary?

   a. Age 35

   b. At birth

   c. At puberty

   d. In utero at 5 months' gestation

15-27. Meiosis I of the oocytes is completed at which of the following times?

   a. Birth

   b. Puberty

   c. Ovulation

   d. Fertilization

15-30. Which of the following enzymes is absent in the granulosa cell?

   a. Aromatase

   b. 17-Hydroxylase

   c. 3β-Hydroxysteroid dehydrogenase

   d. Cholesterol side chain cleavage enzyme

15-31. Which hormone is the first to rise during female puberty?

   a. Luteinizing hormone

   b. Follicle-stimulating hormone

   c. Estradiol

   d. Progesterone

15-32. Which of the following zona pellucida proteins is responsible for zona hardening after sperm penetration?

   a. ZP1

   b. ZP2

   c. ZP3

   d. None of the above

15-28. In the image below, which line corresponds to luteinizing hormone level changes during the menstrual cycle?

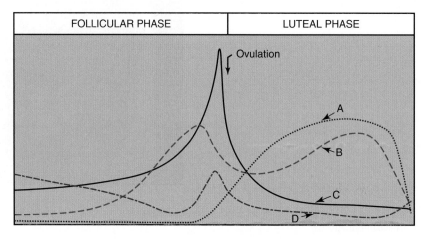

Reproduced, with permission, from Halvorson LM: Reproductive endocrinology. In Schorge JO, Schaffer JI, Halvorson LM, et al (eds): Williams Gynecology, 1st ed. New York, McGraw-Hill, 2008, Figure 15-18.

   a. A

   b. B

   c. C

   d. D

15-29. In the image found in Question 15-28, which line corresponds to estradiol level changes during the menstrual cycle?

   a. A

   b. B

   c. C

   d. D

15-33. An ovarian follicle that is visible on sonography has reached what stage of development?

   a. Primary

   b. Secondary

   c. Preantral

   d. Tertiary

15-34. Which of the following follicle developmental stages requires gonadotropin stimulation for further development?

   a. Primary

   b. Secondary

   c. Preantral

   d. Tertiary

15–35. What is the estradiol concentration and duration needed to initiate a luteinizing hormone surge?

a. 100 pg/mL for 24 hours

b. 100 pg/mL for 50 hours

c. 200 pg/mL for 24 hours

d. 200 pg/mL for 50 hours

15–36. Steroidogenesis in the corpus luteum is mainly under the control of which of the following hormones?

a. Luteinizing hormone

b. Follicle-stimulating hormone

c. Activin

d. Follistatin

15–37. Ovulation can be assumed at which of the following mid-luteal progesterone levels?

a. 0.5 ng/mL

b. 1.0 ng/mL

c. 2.0 ng/mL

d. 3.0 ng/mL

15–38. Images A and B, respectively, correspond to which of the following menstrual cycle phases?

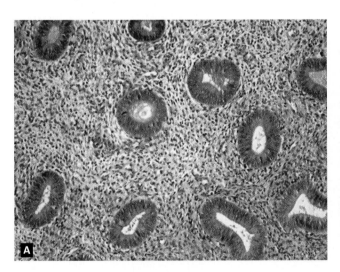 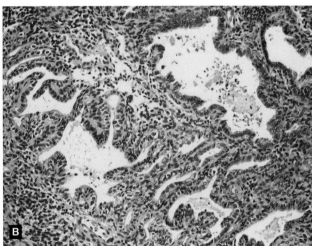

Reproduced, with permission, from Bradshaw KB: Menopausal transition. In Schorge JO, Schaffer JI, Halvorson LM, et al (eds): Williams Gynecology, 1st ed. New York, McGraw-Hill, 2008, Figure 21-4.

a. Secretory, menstrual

b. Menstrual, proliferative

c. Proliferative, secretory

d. Late secretory, proliferative

15–39. Formation of endometrium pinopods, important for embryo implantation, is dependent on which of the following hormones?

a. Estriol

b. Cortisol

c. Estradiol

d. Progesterone

15–40. Which of the following growth factors is involved in embryo implantation?

a. Tumor necrosis factor-β (TNF-β)

b. Leukemia inhibitory factor (LIF)

c. Transforming growth factor-β (TGF-β)

d. Insulin-like growth factors (IGF-II)

Chapter 15   ANSWER KEY

Question number	Letter answer	Page cited	Header cited	Question number	Letter answer	Page cited	Header cited
15–1	a	p. 400	Reproductive Endocrinology	15–20	c	p. 416	Growth Hormone-Releasing Hormone (GHRH)
15–2	c	p. 400	Reproductive Endocrinology	15–21	d	p. 417	The Hypothalamic-Pituitary Axis
15–3	a	p. 401	Luteinizing Hormone, Follicle-Stimulating Hormone, and Human Chorionic Gonadotropin	15–22	b	p. 417	Hyperprolactinemia
				15–23	b	p. 418	Pituitary Adenomas
				15–24	a	p. 420	Pregnancy and Pituitary Adenomas
15–4	a	p. 403	Figure 15-5	15–25	b	p. 420	Treatment of Hyperprolactinemia and Pituitary Adenomas
15–5	c	p. 403	Figure 15-5				
15–6	a	p. 403	Figure 15-5	15–26	d	p. 424	Embryology of the Ovary
15–7	b	p. 404	Figure 15-6	15–27	c	p. 425	Meiotic Division During Oocyte Maturation
15–8	c	p. 404	Figure 15-6				
15–9	b	p. 404	Steroid Hormone Transport in the Circulation	15–28	c	p. 423	Figure 15-19
				15–29	b	p. 423	Figure 15-19
15–10	a	p. 405	Congenital Adrenal Hyperplasia (CAH)	15–30	b	p. 425	Two-Cell Theory of Ovarian Steroidogenesis
15–11	c	p. 406	Estrogen, Progesterone, and Androgen Receptors	15–31	a	p. 427	Puberty
15–12	c	p. 407	Receptor Expression and Desensitization	15–32	b	p. 429	Primary Follicle
				15–33	d	p. 429	Tertiary Follicle
15–13	b	p. 412	Endogenous Opiates	15–34	d	p. 429	Gonadotropins and Follicular Development
15–14	b	p. 413	Neuropeptide Y (NPY) and Galanin				
15–15	c	p. 413	Anterior Pituitary Hormones	15–35	d	p. 430	Ovulation and the Luteinizing Hormone Surge
15–16	a	p. 415	Pulsatile Gonadotropin-Releasing Hormone Secretion	15–36	a	p. 431	Luteal Phase
				15–37	d	p. 431	Luteal Phase
15–17	c	p. 415	Opioid Peptides and Gonadotropin-Releasing Hormone	15–38	c	p. 432	Histology across the Menstrual Cycle
				15–39	d	p. 434	Implantation Window
15–18	b	p. 415	Dopamine and Prolactin	15–40	b	p. 434	Table 15-10
15–19	b	p. 415	Dopamine and Prolactin				

CHAPTER 16

Amenorrhea

16–1. Which of the following clinical scenarios meets the definition of amenorrhea?

    a. 12-year-old with Tanner stage I breast development

    b. 16-year-old with Tanner stage II breast development

    c. 14-year-old with Tanner stage III breast development

    d. 18-year-old with Tanner stage V breast development and cessation of menses for the last two cycles

16–2. Inhibin inhibits synthesis and secretion of which of the following hormones?

    a. Luteinizing hormone (LH)

    b. Follicle-stimulating hormone (FSH)

    c. Corticotropin-releasing hormone (CRH)

    d. Gonadotropin-releasing hormone (GnRH)

16–3. Which of the following hormones can have a negative as well as a positive feedback at the level of the pituitary?

    a. Cortisol

    b. Oxytocin

    c. Estradiol

    d. Progesterone

16–4. Which of the following hormones "rescues" the corpus luteum from luteolysis?

    a. Luteinizing hormone (LH)

    b. Human placental lactogen (hPL)

    c. Follicle-stimulating hormone (FSH)

    d. Human chorionic gonadotropin (hCG)

16–5. Which of the following conditions is considered the most frequent cause of primary amenorrhea?

    a. Turner syndrome

    b. Asherman syndrome

    c. Androgen insensitivity syndrome

    d. Mayer-Rokitansky-Küster-Hauser syndrome

16–6. An 18-year-old nulligravid female presents with primary amenorrhea. During examination, Tanner stage IV breast development and sparse pubic and axillary hair are noted. Also, a blind-ending vagina is identified. What is the likely diagnosis in this patient?

    a. Müllerian agenesis

    b. Premature ovarian failure

    c. Androgen insensitivity syndrome

    d. Congenital adrenal hyperplasia (CAH)

16–7. The patient in question 16–6 undergoes laparoscopy. The white oval structure above the blunt probe represents which of the following?

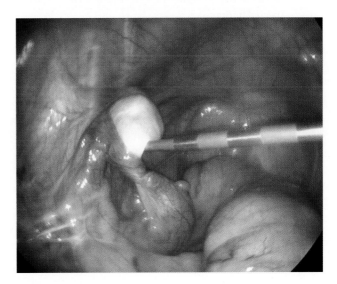

    a. Ovary

    b. Testis

    c. Oophoron

    d. Epoophoron

16–8. What is the expected testosterone level in a patient with müllerian agenesis?

    a. Male level

    b. Female level

    c. Not measurable

    d. Significantly elevated (> 1000 ng/dL)

16–9. What follicle-stimulating hormone (FSH) threshold is needed to diagnose a patient with premature ovarian failure?

    a. 15 mIU/mL with a persistently elevated repeat test result 1 month later

    b. 20 mIU/mL with a persistently elevated repeat test result 1 month later

    c. 30 mIU/mL with a persistently elevated repeat test result 1 month later

    d. 40 mIU/mL with a persistently elevated repeat test result 1 month later

16–10. Findings classic for Turner syndrome include all **EXCEPT** which of the following?

    a. Macrognathia

    b. Neck webbing

    c. Aortic coarctation

    d. Shield-like chest shape

16–11. A 28-year-old nulligravida presents with primary amenorrhea. She is diagnosed with 46,XY gonadal dysgenesis. During pelvic laparoscopy, what is the expected finding?

    a. Streak gonads and male internal genitalia

    b. Streak gonads and female internal genitalia

    c. Empty pelvis (no gonads or internal genitalia)

    d. Bilateral abdominal testes and male internal genitalia

16–12. A 20-year-old female is diagnosed with gonadal dysgenesis, and her karyotype reveals 45,X/46,XY mosaicism. Laparoscopy is performed for which of the following reasons?

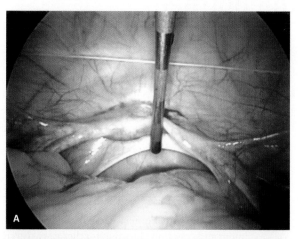

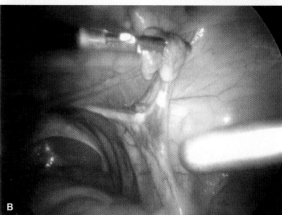

Figure B: Reproduced, with permission, from Halvorson LM: Amenorrhea. In Hoffman BL, Schorge JO, Schaffer JI, et al (eds): Williams Gynecology, 2nd ed. New York, McGraw-Hill, 2012, Figure 16-4.

    a. Gonadectomy due to increased risk of malignant transformation in retained gonads

    b. Oophoropexy due to increased rate of torsion

    c. Endometriosis ablation due to increased rate of endometriosis

    d. None of the above

16–13. An 18-year-old female with primary amenorrhea and sexual infantilism presents for evaluation. During examination, she is noted to be hypertensive, and a patent vagina and a cervix is visualized. Pelvic sonography confirms presence of a uterus, but gonads could not be visualized. Laboratory evaluation is significant for hypokalemia. Which of the following conditions is likely her diagnosis?

    a. 5α-Reductase deficiency

    b. 21-Hydroxylase deficiency

    c. 17-Hydroxylase deficiency

    d. 3β-Hydroxysteroid dehydrogenase deficiency

16–14. Which of the following chemotherapeutic classes is the most damaging to the ovaries?

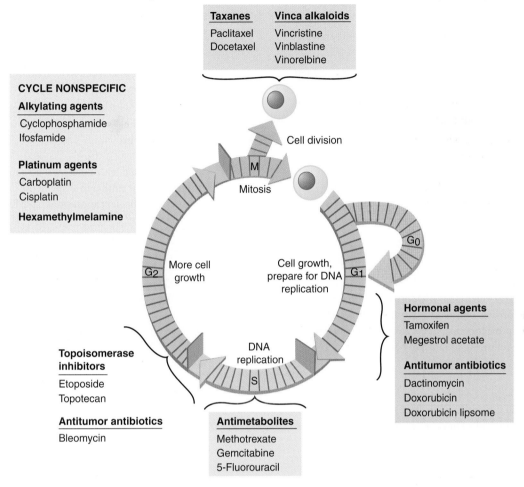

Reproduced, with permission, from Schorge JO: Principles of chemotherapy. In Hoffman BL, Schorge JO, Schaffer JI, et al (eds): Williams Gynecology, 2nd ed. New York, McGraw-Hill, 2012, Figure 27-1.

a. Hormonal agents

b. Antimetabolites

c. Antibiotic agents

d. Alkylating agents

16–15. What radiation dose is high enough to cause permanent ovarian damage?

a. 100 rads

b. 400 rads

c. 600 rads

d. 800 rads

16–16. Which of the following is true of Kallmann syndrome?

a. Gonadotropin-releasing hormone (GnRH) neurons fail to develop.

b. It is a condition that leads to hypergonadotropic hypogonadism.

c. Intact sense of smell differentiates it from other similar conditions.

d. Can be inherited as an autosomal dominant or autosomal recessive disorder.

16–17. What is the lowest body mass index (BMI) that is required to begin menstruation?

a. $15 \, \text{kg/m}^2$

b. $20 \, \text{kg/m}^2$

c. $22 \, \text{kg/m}^2$

d. $24 \, \text{kg/m}^2$

16–18. An 18-year-old with previously regular menses, presents with amenorrhea. She is also diagnosed with anorexia nervosa. Which of the following is likely to be seen in this patient?

a. Elevated luteinizing hormone (LH) level

b. Elevated gonadotropin-releasing hormone (GnRH) level

c. Elevated leptin level

d. Elevated neuropeptide Y level

16–19. Which of the following statements is true regarding polycystic ovarian syndrome?

a. Patients typically present with amenorrhea.

b. It is the most common cause of chronic anovulation.

c. It is characterized by hypogonadotropic hypogonadism.

d. It is characterized by persistently elevated follicle-stimulating hormone (FSH) and estradiol levels.

16–20. Congenital adrenal hyperplasia is most commonly caused by mutations in genes coding for which of the following enzymes?

a. 17-Hydroxylase

b. 21-Hydroxylase

c. 11β-Hydroxylase

d. 3β-Hydroxysteroid dehydrogenase

16–21. A 27-year-old nulligravida presents with 6 months of amenorrhea. During evaluation, she is noted to have hyperprolactinemia. Laboratory tests measuring which of the following should also be obtained?

a. Total testosterone

b. 24-hour urinary free cortisol

c. Thyroid-stimulating hormone (TSH)

d. Insulin-like growth factor II (IGF-II)

16–22. A 15-year-old with primary amenorrhea and Tanner stage V breast development presents for evaluation. Assessing levels for which of the following is the appropriate next step in her evaluation?

a. Luteinizing hormone (LH)

b. Follicle-stimulating hormone (FSH)

c. Human chorionic gonadotropin (hCG)

d. Thyroid-stimulating hormone (TSH)

16–23. An 18-year-old nulligravida presents with primary amenorrhea. She reports vaginal bleeding following a progesterone withdrawal test. Which of the following conditions is most likely excluded?

a. Müllerian agenesis

b. Hypothalamic amenorrhea

c. Premature ovarian failure

d. Polycystic ovarian syndrome (PCOS)

16–24. Measurement of which of the following serum levels is helpful in evaluating patients suspected of having late-onset congenital adrenal hyperplasia (CAH)?

a. Follicle-stimulating hormone (FSH)

b. Testosterone

c. 17-Hydroxyprogesterone

d. Dehydroepiandrosterone sulfate (DHEAS)

16–25. In which of the following patients is a karyotype most likely needed?

a. 22-year-old with amenorrhea and hirsutism

b. 25-year-old with amenorrhea and an elevated prolactin level

c. 20-year-old with amenorrhea and no müllerian structures on sonography

d. 16-year-old with amenorrhea and a persistently elevated follicle-stimulating hormone (FSH) level of 80 mIU/mL

16–26. You are presented with a patient with a unicornuate uterus that is similar in shape to the one shown here. What is the next appropriate step in your management?

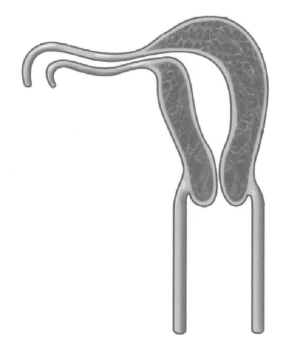

Reproduced, with permission, from Cunningham FG, Leveno KL, Bloom SL, et al (eds): Williams Obstetrics, 23rd ed. New York, McGraw-Hill, 2010, Figure 40-3.

a. Renal scan

b. Diagnostic laparoscopy

c. Diagnostic hysteroscopy

d. Brain magnetic resonance (MR) imaging

16–27. Which of the following medications is used for achieving a pregnancy in a patient with hypogonadotropic hypogonadism?

a. Estradiol

b. Letrozole

c. Gonadotropins

d. Clomiphene citrate (Clomid)

Chapter 16 ANSWER KEY

Question number	Letter answer	Page cited	Header cited
16–1	b	p. 440	Introduction
16–2	b	p. 440	Normal Menstrual Cycle
16–3	c	p. 440	Normal Menstrual Cycle
16–4	d	p. 440	Normal Menstrual Cycle
16–5	a	p. 441	Table 16-1
16–6	c	p. 441	Anatomic Disorders
16–7	b	p. 443	Müllerian Defects
16–8	b	p. 443	Müllerian Defects
16–9	d	p. 444	Hypergonadotropic Hypogonadism (Premature Ovarian Failure)
16–10	a	p. 445	Table 16-6
16–11	b	p. 444	Chromosomal Defects
16–12	a	p. 444	Chromosomal Defects
16–13	c	p. 446	Specific Genetic Defects
16–14	d	p. 446	Acquired Abnormalities
16–15	d	p. 446	Acquired Abnormalities
16–16	d	p. 447	Inherited Abnormalities of the Hypothalamus
16–17	b	p. 448	Exercise-Induced Amenorrhea
16–18	d	p. 449	Pathophysiology of Functional Hypothalamic Amenorrhea
16–19	b	p. 451	Polycystic Ovarian Syndrome (PCOS)
16–20	b	p. 451	Adult-Onset Congenital Adrenal Hyperplasia (CAH)
16–21	c	p. 451	Hyperprolactinemia and Hypothyroidism
16–22	c	p. 454	Exclusion of Pregnancy
16–23	a	p. 454	Progesterone Withdrawal
16–24	c	p. 454	Table 16-7
16–25	d	p. 456	Chromosomal Analysis
16–26	a	p. 456	Anatomic Disorders
16–27	c	p. 457	Infertility

CHAPTER 17

Polycystic Ovarian Syndrome and Hyperandrogenism

17–1. Which of the following criteria for diagnosis of polycystic ovarian syndrome (PCOS) is not part of the Rotterdam criteria?

 a. Oligo-/anovulation

 b. Sonographic polycystic appearance of ovaries

 c. Clinical or biochemical signs of hyperandrogenism

 d. Peripheral distribution of follicles on sonography

17–2. In ovarian hyperthecosis, which of the following is **LEAST** likely to be seen?

 a. Irregular menstrual cycles

 b. Physical signs of hyperandrogenism

 c. Biochemical evidence of hyperandrogenism

 d. More than 12 follicles per ovary during sonography

17–3. First-degree male relatives of women with PCOS have been shown to have higher levels of which of the following circulating hormones?

 a. Testosterone

 b. Androstenedione

 c. Dihydrotestosterone

 d. Dehydroepiandrosterone sulfate

17–4. In PCOS, increased testosterone production from the ovaries is secondary to stimulation by which of the following hormones?

 a. Inhibin

 b. Estradiol

 c. Luteinizing hormone (LH)

 d. Follicle-stimulating hormone (FSH)

17–5. All **EXCEPT** which of the following hormones are increased in women with PCOS?

 a. Luteinizing hormone (LH)

 b. Follicle-stimulating hormone (FSH)

 c. Estradiol

 d. Testosterone

17–6. All **EXCEPT** which of the following are true regarding sex hormone-binding globulin (SHBG)?

 a. It is a product of the liver.

 b. Levels are increased by insulin.

 c. Levels are increased by estradiol.

 d. It binds most of the circulating testosterone.

17–7. Which of the following is **NOT** typical of PCOS?

 a. Acne

 b. Clitoromegaly

 c. Androgenic alopecia

 d. Increased facial hair

17–8. Of the following conditions, which is most likely associated with the following finding?

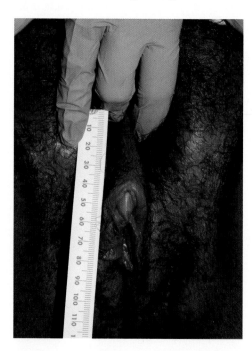

Photograph contributed by Dr. Ben Li. Reproduced, with permission, from Wilson EE: Polycystic ovarian syndrome and hyperandrogenism. In Hoffman BL, Schorge JO, Schaffer JI, et al (eds): Williams Gynecology, 2nd ed. New York, McGraw-Hill, 2012, Figure 17-11.

 a. PCOS

 b. Endometriosis

 c. Hyperprolactinemia

 d. Ovarian androgen-producing tumor

17–9. Which of the following hormones is the most effective in converting vellus hairs to terminal hairs?

   a. Testosterone

   b. Androstenedione

   c. Dihydrotestosterone

   d. Dehydroepiandrosterone (DHEA)

17–10. Which of the following medications is **NOT** a cause of hypertrichosis or hirsutism?

   a. Danazol

   b. Minoxidil

   c. Methyldopa

   d. Ketoconazole

17–11. All **EXCEPT** which of the following is true of acanthosis nigricans?

   a. It is limited to the nape of the neck.

   b. It is a cutaneous sign of insulin resistance.

   c. It is secondary to keratinocyte and skin fibroblast growth.

   d. It is characterized by a thickened, velvety appearance of the skin.

17–12. Of the following laboratory test results, which is most closely associated with the following clinical finding?

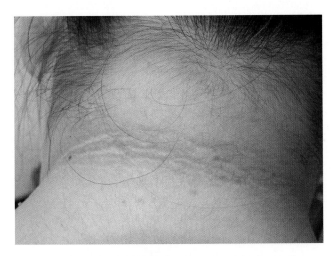

Reproduced, with permission, from Wilson EE: Polycystic ovarian syndrome and hyperandrogenism. In Schorge JO, Schaffer JI, Halvorson LM, et al (eds): Williams Gynecology, 1st ed. New York, McGraw-Hill, 2008, Figure 17-7.

   a. Low progesterone level

   b. Elevated estradiol level

   c. Abnormal glucose tolerance test result

   d. Elevated dehydroepiandrosterone (DHEA) level

17–13. A 22-year-old obese nulligravida presents with a long history of irregular cycles and amenorrhea. After appropriate evaluation, you diagnose her with PCOS. Which of the following findings is **LEAST** likely to be seen in her condition?

   a. Abnormal glucose tolerance test results

   b. Thickened, dark skin on the inner thighs

   c. High serum levels of high density lipoprotein

   d. Male-pattern hair growth on the lower abdomen

17–14. Which of the following is **NOT** characteristic of the metabolic syndrome?

   a. Obesity

   b. Hirsutism

   c. Dyslipidemia

   d. Insulin resistance

17–15. During evaluation for PCOS, a patient is noted to have a total testosterone level of 350 ng/dL. Which of the following endocrine glands most likely harbors the androgen-producing tumor?

   a. Ovary

   b. Adrenal

   c. Pancreas

   d. Pituitary

17–16. During evaluation for PCOS, a serum 17-hydroxyprogesterone level is obtained to exclude which of the following conditions?

   a. Cushing syndrome

   b. Insulin resistance

   c. Congenital adrenal hyperplasia

   d. Androgen-producing adrenal tumor

17–17. Which of the following conditions can result in a false positive elevation in serum 17-hydroxyprogesterone level results?

   a. Obesity

   b. Ovulation

   c. Insulin resistance

   d. Endometrial hyperplasia

17–18. A 23-year-old G1P1 female presents with a recent history of irregular cycles and a desire to conceive. She reports recent weight gain. During examination, she is noted to have facial hirsutism as well as purple stria on the abdomen. Which of the following test is most likely to be helpful in making the diagnosis?

   a. Serum progesterone level

   b. Serum total testosterone level

   c. 24-hour urinary cortisol measurement

   d. Abdominal computed tomography (CT) scanning

17–19. Several patients undergo 2-hour glucose tolerance testing. Which of the following results is specifically equated with the term *impaired glucose tolerance*?

a. 2-hour blood glucose is 80 mg/dL.

b. 2-hour blood glucose is 150 mg/dL.

c. Fasting blood glucose is 80 mg/dL.

d. Fasting blood glucose is 150 mg/dL.

17–20. A 29-year-old female with irregular cycles presents for evaluation. A sonogram of her ovaries reveals the following findings. The ovarian follicles seen are which type?

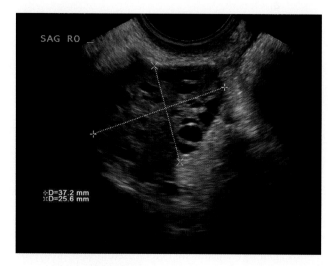

a. Antral follicles

b. Primary follicles

c. Apoptotic follicles

d. Preantral follicles

17–21. According to the Rotterdam criteria, which of the following is **NOT** a criterion for sonographic findings in PCOS?

a. Ovarian volume >10 mL

b. At least 10 follicles per ovary

c. Follicles 2–9 mm in mean diameter

d. Only one ovary with findings is sufficient to define PCOS

17–22. A 25-year-old nulligravida presents for infertility evaluation. She reports monthly cyclic menses. During pelvic sonography, she has 15 follicles measuring 2–9 mm in diameter per ovary. What percentage of young women without PCOS will exhibit polycystic-appearing ovaries during sonographic evaluation?

a. 25

b. 45

c. 65

d. 85

17–23. In treatment of PCOS with combination oral contraceptives, ethinyl estradiol has which of the following effects?

a. Reduces luteinizing hormone (LH) production

b. Increases sex hormone-binding globulin (SHBG) production

c. Reverses endometrial hyperplasia

d. Increases angiotensinogen production

17–24. In treatment of PCOS with combination oral contraceptives, what is one effect of the progesterone component?

a. Reduces follicle-stimulating hormone (FSH) production

b. Increases luteinizing hormone (LH) production

c. Antagonizes androgen receptors

d. Reduces ovarian androgen production

17–25. Which of the following medications can be added to improve the clomiphene citrate (Clomid) response in women with PCOS?

a. Dehydroepiandrosterone (DHEA)

b. Insulin

c. Metformin

d. Progesterone

17–26. Which of the following enzymes necessary for hair follicle division and development is the target of eflornithine hydrochloride (Vaniqa)?

a. Pyrroline carboxylate

b. Pyruvate dehydrogenase

c. Ornithine decarboxylase

d. Glucose-6-phosphate dehydrogenase

17–27. Which of the following statements is **LEAST** likely to be true regarding spironolactone?

a. It reduces luteinizing hormone (LH) production.

b. Is an androgen-receptor blocker.

c. It is a potassium-sparing diuretic.

d. It lowers dihydrotestosterone production.

17–28. Which of the following is true of the procedure shown here?

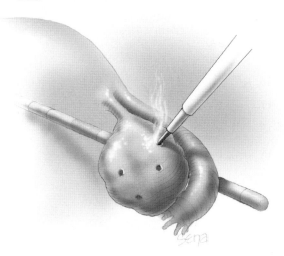

Reproduced, with permission, from Hoffman BL: Surgeries for benign gynecologic conditions. In Schorge JO, Schaffer JI, Halvorson LM, et al (eds): Williams Gynecology, 1st ed. New York, McGraw-Hill, 2008, Figure 41-32.1.

a. Is used now mainly to treat severe hirsutism

b. Is a first-line treatment of women with PCOS seeking fertility

c. Is performed less frequently than ovarian wedge resection in suitable candidates

d. None of the above

Chapter 17   ANSWER KEY

Question number	Letter answer	Page cited	Header cited	Question number	Letter answer	Page cited	Header cited
17–1	d	p. 460	Definition	17–15	a	p. 470	Testosterone
17–2	d	p. 461	Ovarian Hyperthecosis and HAIRAN Syndrome	17–16	c	p. 471	17-alpha Hydroxyprogesterone
				17–17	b	p. 471	17-Hydroxyprogesterone
17–3	d	p. 461	Etiology	17–18	c	p. 471	Cortisol
17–4	c	p. 461	Gonadotropins	17–19	b	p. 472	Table 17-6
17–5	b	p. 461	Pathophysiology	17–20	a	p. 472	Sonography
17–6	b	p. 463	Sex Hormone-Binding Globulin (SHBG)	17–21	b	p. 472	Sonography
				17–22	a	p. 472	Sonography
17–7	b	p. 464	Hyperandrogenism	17–23	b	p. 474	Combination Oral Contraceptive Pills
17–8	d	p. 464	Hyperandrogenism				
17–9	c	p. 464	Pathophysiology of Hirsutism	17–24	d	p. 474	Combination Oral Contraceptive Pills
17–10	d	p. 464	Table 17-3	17–25	c	p. 474	Insulin Sensitizing Agents
17–11	a	p. 466	Acanthosis Nigricans	17–26	c	p. 475	Eflornithine Hydrochloride
17–12	c	p. 466	Acanthosis Nigricans	17–27	a	p. 475	Androgen-Receptor Antagonists
17–13	c	p. 463	Signs and Symptoms				
17–14	b	p. 467	Metabolic Syndrome and Cardiovascular Disease	17–28	d	p. 477	Surgical Therapy

CHAPTER 18

Anatomic Disorders

18-1. Congenital anatomic disorders of the female reproductive tract may result from which of the following mechanisms?

a. Genetic mutation

b. Developmental arrest

c. Abnormal hormonal exposure or exposure to environmental insults

d. All of the above

18-2. Which of the following organs is correctly paired with its embryologic origin?

a. Uterus—mesonephric duct

b. Bladder—mesonephric duct

c. Kidney—paramesonephric duct

d. Testes and ovaries—genital ridge

18-3. What percentage of females with uterovaginal malformations have associated urinary tract anomalies?

a. 5

b. 25

c. 50

d. 75

18-4. Which of the following statements is true regarding sexual differentiation in humans?

a. The SRY acts as a testis-deleting factor (TDF).

b. Without the influence of SRY, gonads develop as testes.

c. The gene is located on the Y chromosome and is named the sex-determining region of the Y (SRY).

d. The presence or absence of gonadal determinant genes is not thought to determine fetal gender.

18-5. Anti-müllerian hormone is involved in all **EXCEPT** which of the following?

a. Regression of the ipsilateral paramesonephric system

b. Peaking of testosterone production as a result of stimulation of the testes

c. Rapid gubernacular growth necessary for the transabdominal descent of testes

d. Prediction of successful ovarian hyperstimulation cycles during assisted reproduction

18-6. In female development, when do germ cells that carry two X chromosomes reach their peak number of 5 to 7 million oocytes?

a. At birth

b. After menarche

c. Just before menarche

d. In utero at 20 weeks' gestation

18-7. The vagina forms partly from both the müllerian ducts and which other structure?

a. genital ridge

b. urogenital sinus

c. mesonephric duct

d. paramesonephric duct

18-8. The hymen is the partition that remains between which structures?

a. Cloacal membrane and genital tubercle

b. Sinovaginal bulb and urogenital sinus

c. Unfused cephalad portions of the two müllerian ducts

d. None of the above

18-9. Which of the following anatomic structures is correctly paired with its embryologic origin?

a. Genital tubercle—clitoris

b. Urethral folds—labia minora

c. Labioscrotal folds—labia majora

d. All of the above

18-10. Which of the following is the most common cause of female pseudohermaphroditism?

a. Maternal exposure to androgen-derivative medications

b. Maternal virilizing ovarian tumors, such as Sertoli-Leydig tumor

c. Fetal congenital adrenal hyperplasia due to deficiency of 21-hydroxylase

d. Fetal congenital adrenal hyperplasia due to deficiency of 11-beta hydroxylase

18–11. Female pseudohermaphroditism (category I) and male pseudohermaphroditism (category II) share which of the following characteristics?

a. Patients have testes.

b. Patients with either disorder are potentially fertile.

c. Both disorders result from excessive androgen exposure.

d. Surgery plays an important role in their respective treatment plans.

18–12. All of the following statements regarding complete androgen insensitivity syndrome (CAIS) are true **EXCEPT** which of the following?

a. On external examination, patients appear as phenotypically normal females.

b. These women develop breasts during puberty due to abundant androgen-to-estrogen conversion.

c. Surgical excision of the testes is recommended prior to puberty to decrease the associated risk of germ cell tumors.

d. Estrogen replacement after puberty is important to maintain bone mass and to provide relief from vasomotor symptoms.

18–13. Which of the following statements are true regarding Turner syndrome?

a. There are classic physical stigmata of the syndrome.

b. They comprise the majority of patients with gonadal dysgenesis.

c. Although the uterus and vagina are normal, patients with the syndrome have streak gonads and subsequently present with primary amenorrhea.

d. All of the above

18–14. What is the male (46,XY) gonadal dysgenesis syndrome called?

a. Swyer syndrome

b. Klinefelter syndrome

c. Mixed gonadal dysgenesis

d. Embryonic testicular regression

18–15. All **EXCEPT** which of the following characteristics of Klinefelter syndrome are true?

a. These patients are tall, overvirilized men.

b. Patients have significantly reduced fertility.

c. The syndrome occurs in 1 to 2 percent of all males.

d. Men with Klinefelter syndrome are at increased risk for germ cell tumors, osteoporosis, and breast cancer.

18–16. When faced with ambiguous external genitalia of a newborn at delivery, the obstetrician should do which of the following?

a. Examine the mother for signs of hyperandrogenism.

b. Refer to the newborn as "your baby" and not as "it."

c. Refrain from gender assignment by explaining that the genitalia are incompletely formed.

d. All of the above

18–17. All **EXCEPT** which of the following statements regarding bladder exstrophy are true?

a. This anomaly displays a predilection for females of 2:1.

b. It is characterized by an exposed bladder lying outside the abdomen.

c. Surgical closure is performed early in life and as a staged procedure.

d. It occurs from failure of the cloacal membrane to be reinforced by an ingrowth of mesoderm.

18–18. Causes of newborn clitoromegaly include which of the following?

a. Prematurity

b. Neurofibromatosis

c. Fetal exposure to excessive androgens

d. All of the above

18–19. A 14-year-old nulligravida presents to the emergency department with complaints of worsening lower abdominal pain over the past few days. She states that she has had a similar pain in the past, usually for a few days each month, but then it subsides. She is afebrile with stable vital signs. Although she has breasts and axillary and pubic hair, she has never had a period. Examination reveals a tender abdominal mass as well as a bluish bulging vaginal mass, shown here. Based on her history and your physical examination, which of the following conditions is your most likely diagnosis?

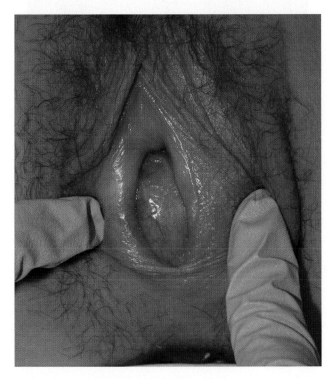

Photograph contributed by Dr. Ellen Wilson. Reproduced, with permission, from Bradshaw KD: Anatomic disorders. In Schorge JO, Schaffer JI, Halvorson LM, et al (eds): Williams Gynecology, 1st ed. New York, McGraw-Hill, 2008, Figure 18-10.

   a. Bartholin cyst

   b. Imperforate hymen

   c. Gartner duct cyst

   d. Longitudinal vaginal septum

18–20. Appropriate techniques for the surgical correction of the condition diagnosed in Question 18–19 involve all **EXCEPT** which of the following?

   a. Hymenectomy

   b. Laparoscopy to exclude endometriosis

   c. Repair in infancy or after thelarche

   d. Needle aspiration of the hematocolpos

18–21. Compared with other müllerian duct defects, transverse vaginal septum is associated with which of the following?

   a. Lower rates of endometriosis

   b. Lower rates of urologic abnormalities

   c. Lower success rates of surgical correction

   d. None of the above

18–22. A 16-year-old nulligravida presents to the emergency department with complaints of abdominal and vaginal pain, worsening during the past several months. She describes the pain as being mostly on her right side and much worse during menstruation. During your physical examination, a patent vagina and cervix are noted, but a unilateral vaginal and pelvic mass is palpated. Transvaginal sonography demonstrates a single uterus and cervix but also a large pelvic mass filled with complex fluid, as shown below, and absence of the right kidney. What is your most likely diagnosis?

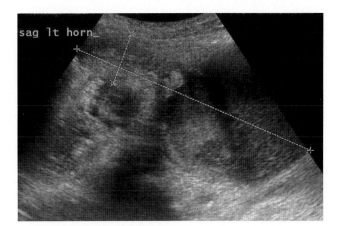

   a. Imperforate hymen

   b. Uterine didelphys

   c. Transverse vaginal septum

   d. Longitudinal vaginal septum

18–23. Why is careful preoperative planning warranted with congenital vaginal cysts?

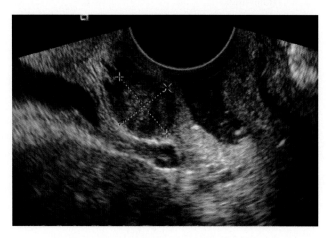

a. The recurrence rate after excision is high.

b. They are frequently large, measuring greater than 8 cm in size.

c. Their typical location is in the posterior-lateral wall of the vagina.

d. Some may extend up into the broad ligament and anatomically approximate the distal course of the ureter.

18–24. Müllerian anomalies are associated with anomalies of all **EXCEPT** which of the following systems?

a. Anal

b. Liver

c. Renal

d. Skeletal

18–25. A 22-year-old G3P0 presents to your office as a new patient for consultation regarding her history of multiple miscarriages. Her gynecologic history is otherwise unremarkable. During physical examination, you note that the uterus is markedly deviated to the left. Transvaginal sonography is performed, and three-dimensional images reveal a single uterus that is deviated and has a banana-shaped cavity, as shown below. What is your diagnosis?

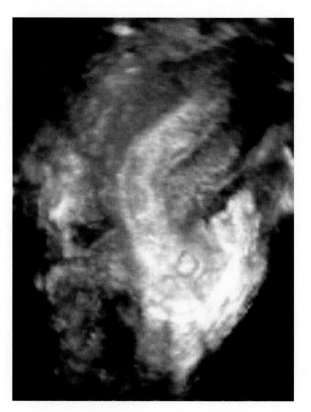

a. Septate uterus

b. Bicornuate uterus

c. Uterine didelphys

d. Unicornuate uterus

18–26. The pathogenesis of poor pregnancy outcomes with a unicornuate uterus is thought to be related to which of the following factors?

a. Cervical incompetence

b. Reduced uterine capacity

c. Anomalous distribution of the uterine artery

d. All of the above

18–27. Which of the müllerian anomalies, as illustrated in this sonogram, has the best reproductive prognosis? A gestational sac is seen on the image's left.

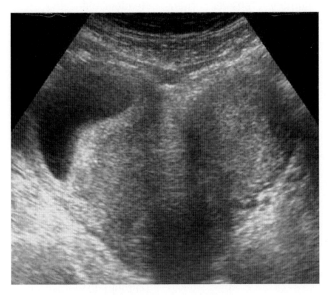

 a. Septate uterus

 b. Bicornuate uterus

 c. Uterine didelphys

 d. Unicornuate uterus

18–28. When should surgical reconstruction of a bicornuate uterus (Strassman metroplasty) be performed?

 a. Only for complete bicornuate anomalies

 b. In all women with the diagnosis of bicornuate uterus

 c. Strassman metroplasty is not performed for repair of bicornuate uterus.

 d. For women in whom recurrent pregnancy loss occurs with no other identifiable cause except their uterine anomaly

18–29. Septate uterus has a significantly higher spontaneous abortion rate and early pregnancy loss rate than bicornuate uterus. As illustrated in the figure below, what is the primary mechanism thought to be responsible for this extraordinarily high pregnancy wastage?

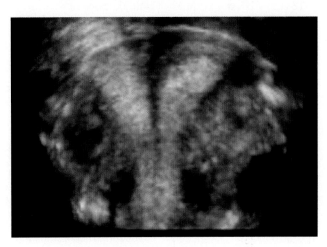

 a. Associated cervical anomalies

 b. Distortion of the uterine cavity

 c. Distortion of the uterine serosal contour

 d. Partial or complete implantation on the largely avascular septum

18–30. Which of the following are seen in offspring of women who took diethylstilbestrol (DES)?

 a. Impaired conception rates in female offspring

 b. Cryptorchidism, testicular hypoplasia, and malformations of the penis in male offspring

 c. T-shaped uterus, "cockscomb" cervix, and increased rates of clear cell adenocarcinoma in female offspring

 d. All of the above

Chapter 18 ANSWER KEY

Question number	Letter answer	Page cited	Header cited
18–1	d	p. 481	Introduction
18–2	d	p. 481	Overview
18–3	c	p. 481	Overview
18–4	c	p. 482	Gonadal Differentiation
18–5	b	p. 482	Gonadal Differentiation
18–6	d	p. 482	Gonadal Differentiation
18–7	b	p. 484	Ductal System Development
18–8	b	p. 484	Ductal System Development
18–9	d	p. 485	External Genitalia
18–10	c	p. 488	Female Pseudohermaphroditism
18–11	d	p. 488	Female Pseudohermaphroditism; Male Pseudohermaphroditism
18–12	c	p. 489	Male Pseudohermaphroditism
18–13	d	p. 489	Gonadal Dysgenesis
18–14	a	p. 489	Gonadal Dysgenesis
18–15	a	p. 490	Embryonic Testicular Regression
18–16	d	p. 491	Gender Assignment

Question number	Letter answer	Page cited	Header cited
18–17	a	p. 491	Defects of the Bladder and Perineum
18–18	d	p. 491	Defects of the Clitoris
18–19	b	p. 492	Hymenal Defects
18–20	d	p. 492	Hymenal Defects
18–21	b	p. 493	Transverse Vaginal Septum
18–22	d	p. 494	Longitudinal Vaginal Septum
18–23	d	p. 495	Congenital Vaginal Cysts
18–24	b	p. 495	Müllerian Anomalies
18–25	d	p. 497	Unicornuate Uterus
18–26	d	p. 497	Unicornuate Uterus
18–27	c	p. 499	Uterine Didelphys
18–28	d	p. 499	Bicornuate Uterus
18–29	d	p. 500	Septate Uterus
18–30	d	p. 502	Diethylstilbestrol-Induced Reproductive Tract Abnormalities

CHAPTER 19

Evaluation of the Infertile Couple

19-1. What is the expected per-cycle fecundability rate (percent)?

    a. 25

    b. 50

    c. 75

    d. 85

19-2. In couples attempting pregnancy, what percentage of women are expected to conceive within 1 year?

    a. 15

    b. 30

    c. 60

    d. 85

19-3. Of the causes of infertility, which of the following is most likely encountered?

    a. Unexplained

    b. Male factors

    c. Tubal disease

    d. Ovulatory dysfunction

19-4. A 30-year-old nulligravida has been trying to conceive for the past 2 years. She has no medical problems. She consumes five alcoholic drinks weekly and smokes one half pack of cigarettes daily. She describes herself as a heavy coffee drinker. She works in a dry cleaning facility. Which of the following exposures is **LEAST** likely to be affecting her fertility?

    a. Alcohol

    b. Caffeine

    c. Cigarettes

    d. Dry cleaning fluid

19-5. How long does the spermatogenesis process take, starting from stem cell to mature sperm?

    a. 10 days

    b. 30 days

    c. 60 days

    d. 90 days

19-6. Which of the following letters points toward the sperm nucleus?

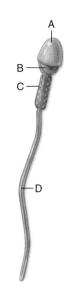

Reproduced, with permission, from McKinley M, O'Loughlin VD (eds): Reproductive system. In Human Anatomy. New York, McGraw-Hill, 2006, Figure 28-13.

    a. A

    b. B

    c. C

    d. D

19-7. In the figure in Question 19-6, which letter indicates the source of kinetic energy generated by mitochondria in the sperm?

    a. A

    b. B

    c. C

    d. D

19-8. With regard to a varicocele, which of the following is most likely true?

    a. It should be repaired once encountered.

    b. It is a frequent cause of male infertility.

    c. Repair of subclinical varicoceles leads to correction of semen abnormalities.

    d. Its negative effect on fertility is secondary to elevated scrotal temperatures.

19–9. Which of the following may lead to permanent damage to sperm production?

a. Spironolactone

b. Anabolic steroids

c. Diabetes mellitus

d. Alcohol consumption

19–10. Gynecomastia in a male patient may suggest the presence of which of the following conditions?

a. Noonan syndrome

b. Klinefelter syndrome

c. Pituitary prolactinoma

d. 17β-Hydroxysteroid dehydrogenase deficiency

19–11. Which of the following is **LEAST** likely true of basal body temperature testing in the adult female?

a. It can be an insensitive test in many women.

b. With ovulation, the temperature rises roughly 0.8°F.

c. It is an inexpensive and easy test for ovulation monitoring.

d. Once the temperature rises, a patient should expect ovulation in the next 12 hours.

19–12. When does ovulation take place in women monitoring with urinary luteinizing hormone (LH) kits?

a. Day of positive results

b. Day after positive results

c. Day prior to positive results

d. Two days after positive results

19–13. Which of the following midluteal progesterone level values signifies ovulation?

a. 0.5 ng/mL

b. 1.0 ng/mL

c. 2.5 ng/mL

d. 5.0 ng/mL

19–14. Which of the following is true of luteal phase deficiency?

a. It affects approximately 50% of menstrual cycles.

b. It is seen when the follicular phase is shorter than 14 days.

c. Fertile women have the same incidence of luteal phase deficiency as infertile women.

d. It is determined by histologic analysis of the endometrium and defined by a greater than 4-day discrepancy between the specimen-derived cycle date and the actual menstrual cycle day.

19–15. At the onset of puberty, what is the estimated number of follicles in a woman's ovaries?

a. 2 million

b. 7 million

c. 1 thousand

d. 300 thousand

19–16. In the evaluation of ovarian function, all **EXCEPT** which of the following laboratory tests are helpful?

a. Cycle day 3 inhibin B level

b. Cycle day 3 estradiol level

c. Random anti-müllerian hormone level

d. Cycle day 3 follicle-stimulating hormone (FSH) level

19–17. Reduction in secretion of which of the following hormones is most likely responsible for the rising serum follicle-stimulating hormone (FSH) level seen as a woman ages?

a. Activin

b. Inhibin B

c. Estradiol

d. Follistatin

19–18. Which of the following is the protocol for a clomiphene citrate (Clomid) challenge test (CCCT)?

a. 50 mg Clomid, cycle days 3–7

b. 50 mg Clomid, cycle days 5–9

c. 100 mg Clomid, cycle days 3–7

d. 100 mg Clomid, cycle days 5–9

19–19. What is the estimated tubal infertility rate after three episodes of pelvic inflammatory disease (PID)?

a. 10%

b. 20%

c. 30%

d. 50%

19–20. What is your interpretation of the following hysterosalpingogram (HSG)?

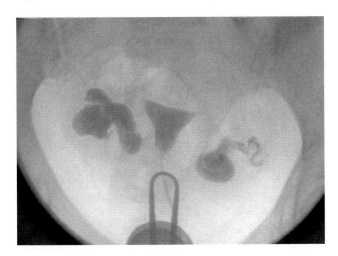

Image contributed by Dr. Kevin Doody. Reproduced, with permission, from Halvorson LM: Evaluation of the infertile couple. In Schorge JO, Schaffer JI, Halvorson LM, et al (eds): Williams Gynecology, 1st ed. New York, McGraw-Hill, 2008, Figure 19-5C.

   a. Normal

   b. Uterine didelphys

   c. Bilateral hydrosalpinges

   d. Unilateral proximal tubal blockage

19–21. What is your interpretation of the following hysterosalpingogram?

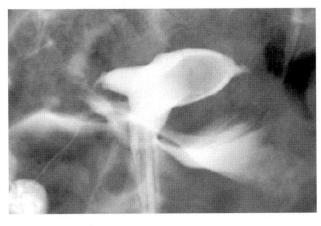

Image contributed by Drs. Kevin Doody. Reproduced, with permission, from Halvorson LM: Evaluation of the infertile couple. In Schorge JO, Schaffer JI, Halvorson LM, et al (eds): Williams Gynecology, 1st ed. New York, McGraw-Hill, 2008, Figure 19-6A.

   a. Normal

   b. Asherman syndrome

   c. Submucous leiomyoma

   d. Bilateral hydrosalpinges

19–22. Which of the following is the gold standard technique for tubal evaluation?

   a. Hysterosalpingography

   b. Laparoscopic evaluation

   c. Saline infusion sonography

   d. Magnetic resonance imaging

19–23. Which of the following is most likely true regarding hysterosalpingography?

   a. It has 98% sensitivity for tubal obstruction.

   b. It has 98% sensitivity for detecting intrauterine pathology.

   c. It is a reliable method to detect peritubal and pelvic adhesions.

   d. The most common cause for proximal tubal obstruction found during HSG is tubal agglutination.

19–24. In this sample of cervical mucus, the effect of which of the following hormones can be seen?

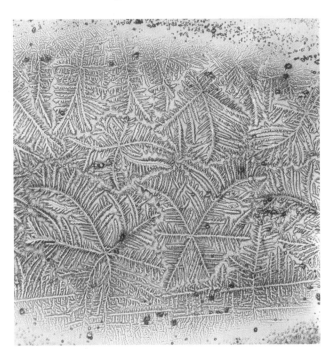

Image contributed by Dr. James C. Glenn. Reproduced, with permission, from Halvorson LM: Evaluation of the infertile couple. In Schorge JO, Schaffer JI, Halvorson LM, et al (eds): Williams Gynecology, 1st ed. New York, McGraw-Hill, 2008, Figure 19-9A.

   a. Estrone

   b. Estradiol

   c. Progesterone

   d. Testosterone

19–25. Liquefaction of the semen specimen after ejaculation is due to secretions from which of the following?

   a. Prostate

   b. Epididymis

   c. Cowper gland

   d. Seminiferous tubules

19–26. In treating hypertension with β-blockers, which of the following semen parameter abnormalities may be seen?

   a. Azoospermia

   b. Oligospermia

   c. Teratospermia

   d. Low semen volume

19–27. Asthenospermia refers to which of the following semen abnormalities?

   a. Sperm count

   b. Semen volume

   c. Sperm motility

   d. Sperm morphology

19–28. Which of the following tests can differentiate between dead and nonmotile sperm?

   a. Zona penetration assay

   b. DNA fragmentation index

   c. Hypoosmotic swelling test

   d. Mannose fluorescence assay

19–29. Genetic testing should be performed in which of the following male patients?

   a. Those with semen volume <2.0 mL

   b. Those with sperm concentration <5 million/mL

   c. Those with fructose present in semen sample

   d. Those with normal sperm morphology <8% by Kruger criteria

19–30. Which of the following Y-chromosome deletions carries the best prognosis for recovering sperm from the testes in an azoospermic patient?

   a. AZFa

   b. AZFb

   c. AZFc

   d. AZFd

Chapter 19 ANSWER KEY

Question number	Letter answer	Page cited	Header cited
19–1	a	p. 506	Introduction
19–2	d	p. 506	Introduction
19–3	d	p. 507	Table 19-1
19–4	d	p. 508	Social
19–5	d	p. 508	The Male History
19–6	b	p. 510	Figure 19-4
19–7	c	p. 510	Figure 19-4
19–8	d	p. 508	The Male History
19–9	b	p. 508	The Male History
19–10	b	p. 511	Examination of the Male Patient
19–11	d	p. 512	Basal Body Temperature
19–12	b	p. 513	Ovulation Predictor Kits
19–13	d	p. 513	Serum Progesterone
19–14	c	p. 513	Endometrial Biopsy
19–15	d	p. 514	Physiology
19–16	a	p. 514	Female Aging and Ovulatory Dysfunction

Question number	Letter answer	Page cited	Header cited
19–17	b	p. 514	Inhibin B
19–18	d	p. 515	Clomiphene Citrate Challenge Test
19–19	d	p. 515	Tubal and Pelvic Factors
19–20	c	p. 515	Tubal and Pelvic Factors; Uterine Abnormalities
19–21	c	p. 515	Tubal and Pelvic Factors; Uterine Abnormalities
19–22	b	p. 516	Radiologic and Surgical Approaches for Evaluation of Pelvic Structures
19–23	b	p. 516	Hysterosalpingography
19–24	b	p. 520	Cervical Factors
19–25	a	p. 522	Semen Analysis
19–26	d	p. 522	Semen Volume
19–27	c	p. 523	Sperm Motility
19–28	c	p. 523	Sperm Motility
19–29	b	p. 525	Genetic Testing of the Male
19–30	c	p. 525	Genetic Testing of the Male

CHAPTER 20

Treatment of the Infertile Couple

20-1. Which of the following is the most widely used pharmacologically active substance in the world?

    a. Caffeine

    b. Nicotine

    c. Marijuana

    d. Ethyl alcohol

20-2. All **EXCEPT** which of the following are true regarding smoking and fertility?

    a. Male smokers may have reduced sperm motility.

    b. Smoking increases the risk of miscarriage in assisted conception cycles.

    c. Smoking in pregnant women is associated with an increased risk of trisomy 21.

    d. The effects of smoking on fecundity can be overcome by fertility treatments such as in vitro fertilization (IVF).

20-3. This smoking cessation agent is considered what pregnancy category by the U.S. Food and Drug Administration?

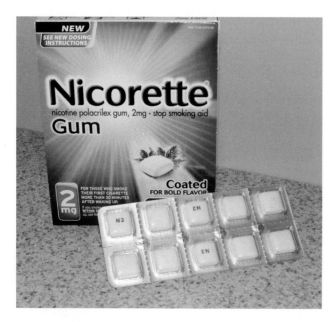

    a. A

    b. B

    c. C

    d. D

20-4. A 28-year-old obese female who is seeking pregnancy is recently diagnosed with polycystic ovarian syndrome (PCOS). Which of the following should be recommended as first-line management for her anovulation?

    a. Gonadotropins

    b. Clomiphene citrate

    c. Weight loss and exercise

    d. Insulin-sensitizing agents

20-5. In women with hyperprolactinemia caused by a pituitary microprolactinoma, which of the following is true?

    a. Surgical therapy is preferred over medical therapy.

    b. During pregnancy, cabergoline is preferred over bromocriptine.

    c. Clomiphene citrate may be ineffective for ovulation induction.

    d. Dopamine-agonist therapy should be increased once pregnancy is achieved.

20-6. Compared with clomiphene citrate therapy, gonadotropin therapy has which of the following characteristics?

    a. Higher ovulation rate

    b. Lower multiple pregnancy rate

    c. Lower ovarian hyperstimulation rate

    d. Greater negative effect on the endometrium

20-7. Which of the following is **LEAST** likely to be true regarding clomiphene citrate therapy?

    a. The typical starting dose is 100 mg.

    b. It is classified as a category X drug by the Food and Drug Administration (FDA).

    c. It can be initiated on the second day of the menstrual cycle.

    d. Most pregnancies will occur during the first three treatment cycles.

20-8. Which of the following gonadotropins is a recombinant product?

    a. Menopur

    b. Bravelle

    c. Repronex

    d. Follistim

20-9. As shown below, this treatment protocol is consistent with which of the following?

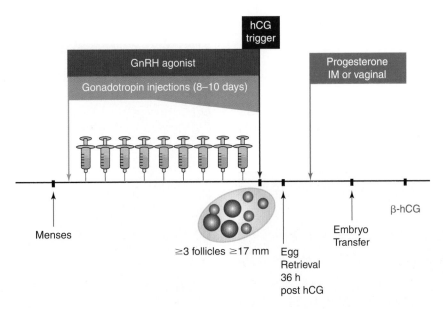

GnRH = gonadotropin-releasing hormone; hCG = human chorionic gonadotropin; IM = intramuscularly. Reproduced, with permission, from Doody KJ: Treatment of the infertile couple. In Schorge JO, Schaffer JI, Halvorson LM, et al (eds): Williams Gynecology, 1st ed. New York, McGraw-Hill, Figure 20-2C.

    a. GnRH antagonist protocol

    b. GnRH agonist flare protocol

    c. Downregulation GnRH agonist protocol

    d. None of the above

20-10. Which of the following is most likely true regarding letrozole?

    a. It is FDA approved for ovulation induction.

    b. It is typically used in doses of 10 mg daily.

    c. Compared with clomiphene citrate, it is associated with a thicker endometrium.

    d. It acts through inhibition of the estrogen receptor at the level of the hypothalamus.

20-11. Which of the following hormones is thought to play a major role in ovarian hyperstimulation syndrome?

    a. Progesterone

    b. Luteinizing hormone (LH)

    c. Human chorionic gonadotropin (hCG)

    d. Follicle-stimulating hormone (FSH)

20-12. A 38-year-old with infertility secondary to tubal blockage just underwent in vitro fertilization (IVF). Her peak estradiol was 4500 pg/mL. Seventeen oocytes were retrieved, and two embryos were transferred. She conceived with a singleton gestation. She developed ovarian hyperstimulation syndrome. Which of the following was a predisposing factor in developing ovarian hyperstimulation?

    a. Her age

    b. Estradiol level

    c. Etiology of her infertility

    d. Number of embryos transferred

20-13. If concern for ovarian hyperstimulation is present during ovulation induction, which of the following can be used to induce the endogenous luteinizing hormone (LH) surge?

    a. Urinary human chorionic gonadotropin (hCG)

    b. Recombinant human chorionic gonadotropin (hCG) (Ovidrel)

    c. Gonadotropin-releasing hormone (GnRH) agonist (Leuprolide)

    d. Gonadotropin-releasing hormone (GnRH) antagonist (Ganirelix)

20–14. Which of the following is **LEAST** likely required in the treatment of ovarian hyperstimulation syndrome?

   a. Oophorectomy

   b. Paracentesis

   c. Fluid resuscitation

   d. Thromboembolism prophylaxis

20–15. The image below is from a patient who just underwent in vitro fertilization (IVF). What is the concern based on this sonographic image?

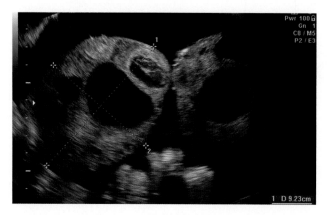

Reproduced, with permission, from Doody KJ: Treatment of the infertile couple. In Schorge JO, Schaffer JI, Halvorson LM, et al (eds): Williams Gynecology, 1st ed. New York, McGraw-Hill, Figure 20-5A.

   a. Bowel injury

   b. Vascular injury

   c. Ectopic gestation

   d. Ovarian hyperstimulation syndrome

20–16. Which of the following serum hormone levels are most likely to increase after ovarian drilling?

   a. Luteinizing hormone (LH)

   b. Follicle-stimulating hormone (FSH)

   c. Testosterone

   d. Androstenedione

20–17. Which of the following is the best treatment for a woman with a significant decline in ovarian reserve?

   a. Donor egg

   b. Clomid ovulation induction

   c. Gonadotropin ovulation induction

   d. In vitro fertilization (IVF) and intracytoplasmic sperm injection

20–18. Which of the following tubal obstruction locations is LEAST amenable to surgical repair?

   a. Isthmic

   b. Fimbrial

   c. Ampullary

   d. Interstitial

20–19. Which of the following treatment options would yield the highest pregnancy opportunity in a patient with the following problem?

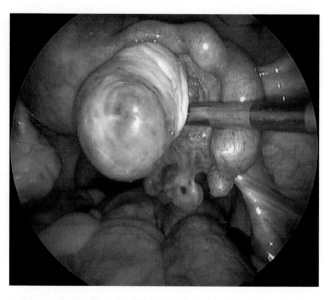

Photograph contributed by Dr. Karen Bradshaw. Reproduced, with permission, from Heinzman AB, Hoffman BL: Pelvic mass. In Hoffman BL, Schorge JO, Schaffer JI, et al (eds): Williams Gynecology, 2nd ed. New York, McGraw-Hill, 2012, Figure 9-25.

   a. In vitro fertilization (IVF)

   b. Clomid ovulation induction

   c. Gonadotropin ovulation induction

   d. Intracytoplasmic sperm injection (ICSI)

20–20. Compared with in vitro fertilization (IVF), bilateral tubal reanastomosis after tubal sterilization has higher rates of which of the following?

   a. Fetal malformation rate

   b. Multifetal gestation rate

   c. Cumulative pregnancy rate

   d. Intrauterine implantation rate in cases correcting fimbriectomy

20–21. Which of the following assisted reproductive technologies (ART) techniques is shown in the image below?

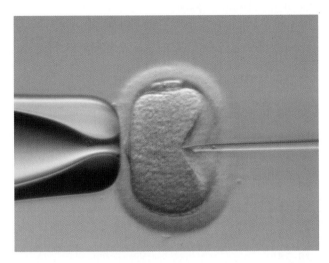

Reproduced, with permission, from Doody KJ: Treatment of the infertile couple. In Schorge JO, Schaffer JI, Halvorson LM, et al (eds): Williams Gynecology, 1st ed. New York, McGraw-Hill, Figure 20-10A.

    a. Intracytoplasmic sperm injection (ICSI)

    b. Embryo biopsy

    c. Assisted hatching

    d. Oocyte in vitro maturation

20–22. By definition, patients with severe oligospermia have sperm counts less than which of the following per milliliter of semen?

    a. <5 million/mL

    b. <15 million/mL

    c. <25 million/mL

    d. <35 million/mL

20–23. In cases of male hypogonadotropic hypogonadism, which of the following semen analysis abnormalities is most likely to be seen?

    a. Aspermia

    b. Oligospermia

    c. Asthenospermia

    d. Teratozoospermia

20–24. During in vitro fertilization (IVF), prevention of a premature luteinizing hormone (LH) surge is important. Which of the following medications achieves this goal?

    a. Recombinant LH

    b. Recombinant follicle-stimulating hormone (FSH)

    c. Leuprolide acetate

    d. Human menopausal gonadotropins

20–25. Which of the following infertility scenarios would warrant intracytoplasmic sperm injection (ICSI)?

    a. Infertility secondary to anovulation

    b. Infertility secondary to diminished ovarian reserve

    c. Infertility secondary to bilateral distal fallopian tube occlusion

    d. Infertility secondary to the male partner's severe oligospermia

20–26. Egg donor recipients typically discontinue progesterone supplementation at which time?

    a. Positive pregnancy test found

    b. 6 weeks' gestation

    c. 10 weeks' gestation

    d. 14 weeks' gestation

20–27. Which of the following avoids fertilization outside the body?

    a. In vitro fertilization (IVF)

    b. Intracytoplasmic sperm injection (ICSI)

    c. Gamete intrafallopian tube transfer (GIFT)

    d. Zygote intrafallopian tube transfer (ZIFT)

20–28. Lowest rates of successful cryopreservation are seen with which of the following?

    a. Sperm

    b. Oocytes

    c. Eight-cell embryo

    d. Blastocyst stage embryo

20–29. Which of the following assisted reproductive technologies (ART) techniques is shown in the image below?

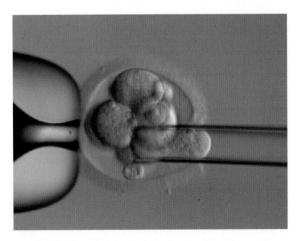

Reproduced, with permission, from Doody KJ: Treatment of the infertile couple. In Schorge JO, Schaffer JI, Halvorson LM, et al (eds): Williams Gynecology, 1st ed. New York, McGraw-Hill, Figure 20-15A.

    a. Embryo biopsy

    b. Assisted hatching

    c. Oocyte in vitro maturation

    d. Intracytoplasmic sperm injection (ICSI)

Chapter 20   ANSWER KEY

Question number	Letter answer	Page cited	Header cited
20-1	a	p. 529	Environmental Factors
20-2	d	p. 530	Smoking
20-3	d	p. 28	Table 1-23, Chapter 1
20-4	c	p. 530	Weight Optimization
20-5	c	p. 532	Hyperprolactinemia
20-6	a	p. 532	Correction of Ovarian Dysfunction
20-7	a	p. 533	Clomiphene Citrate
20-8	d	p. 534	Table 20-4
20-9	b	p. 534	Gonadotropins
20-10	c	p. 535	Aromatase Inhibitors
20-11	c	p. 535	Pathophysiology
20-12	b	p. 535	Pathophysiology
20-13	c	p. 537	Prevention
20-14	a	p. 535	Diagnosis and Treatment
20-15	d	p. 535	Diagnosis and Treatment

Question number	Letter answer	Page cited	Header cited
20-16	b	p. 539	Ovarian Drilling
20-17	a	p. 540	Correction of Diminished Ovarian Reserve
20-18	d	p. 540	Proximal Tubal Obstruction
20-19	a	p. 541	Distal Tubal Obstruction
20-20	c	p. 540	Proximal Tubal Obstruction
20-21	a	p. 544	Figure 20-9
20-22	a	p. 545	Oligospermia
20-23	b	p. 545	Oligospermia
20-24	c	p. 546	In Vitro Fertilization (IVF)
20-25	d	p. 546	Intracytoplasmic Sperm Injection (ICSI)
20-26	c	p. 546	Egg Donation
20-27	c	p. 548	Gamete Intrafallopian Transfer (GIFT)
20-28	b	p. 548	Oocyte Cryopreservation
20-29	a	p. 548	Preimplantation Genetic Diagnosis (PGD)

CHAPTER 21

Menopausal Transition

21-1. The menopausal transition is a progressive endocrinologic continuum that takes reproductive-aged women from regular, cyclic, predictable menses characteristic of ovulatory cycles to ovarian senescence and menopause. Most women can now expect to live what percentage of their lifetime in menopause?

a. 15

b. 20

c. 25

d. 33

21-2. Premature ovarian failure is associated with a persistently elevated follicle-stimulating hormone (FSH) level and refers to the cessation of menses before which of the following ages?

a. 35 years

b. 40 years

c. 45 years

d. 51 years

21-3. Characteristically, menopause begins with cycle irregularity that extends to 1 year after permanent cessation of menses. The more correct, scientific terminology for this time is *menopausal transition*, and it typically takes place over a span of how many years?

a. 1 to 2 years

b. 2 to 3 years

c. 4 to 7 years

d. 5 to 10 years

21-4. A number of environmental, genetic, and surgical influences may alter ovarian aging. Which of the following has been found to **INCREASE** the age of menopause?

a. Smoking

b. Chemotherapy

c. Ovarian surgery

d. Pelvic radiation

21-5. During the reproductive life of a woman, gonadotropin-releasing hormone is released in a pulsatile fashion from which of the following?

a. Corpus luteum

b. Ovarian follicle

c. Pituitary gonadotropes

d. Arcuate nucleus of the medial basal hypothalamus

21-6. With ovarian failure during menopausal transition, the negative-feedback loop is opened by cessation of ovarian steroid hormone release. This causes which of the following?

a. A rise in luteinizing hormone (LH) levels

b. A rise in follicle-stimulating hormone (FSH) levels

c. A maximal increase in the frequency and amplitude of gonadotropin-releasing hormone secretion

d. All of the above

21-7. This photomicrograph illustrates which of the following?

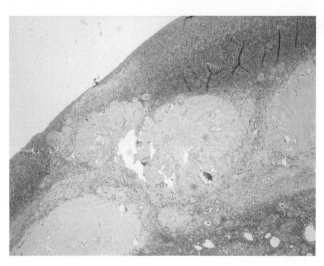

Reproduced, with permission, from Bradshaw KD: Menopausal transition. In Schorge JO, Schaffer JI, Halvorson LM, et al (eds): Williams Gynecology, 1st ed. New York, McGraw-Hill, 2008, Figure 21-3C.

a. Multiple corpora lutea

b. Multiple corpora albicans

c. Multiple primordial follicles

d. None of the above

21–8. An average woman is expected to experience how many ovulatory events during her reproductive lifetime?

    a. 100

    b. 400

    c. 700,000

    d. 6 to 7 million

21–9. Which of the following transvaginal sonographic images best illustrates a premenopausal ovary?

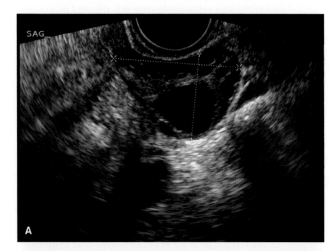

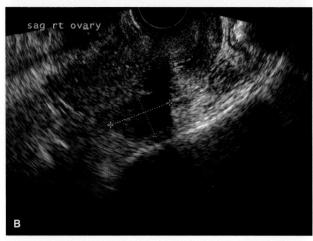

    a. A

    b. B

    c. A and B

    d. None of the above

21–10. In postmenopausal women, unopposed estrogen may be derived from which of the following sources?

    a. Exogenous estrogen

    b. Extragonadal endogenous estrogen production

    c. Decreased sex hormone-binding globulin levels

    d. All of the above

21–11. In the postmenopausal woman with uterine bleeding, evaluation of the endometrium may be accomplished by endometrial biopsy, hysteroscopy, or transvaginal sonography. Which of the following sonographic endometrial thickness measurements is commonly used as a threshold to indicate a low risk for endometrial hyperplasia or cancer?

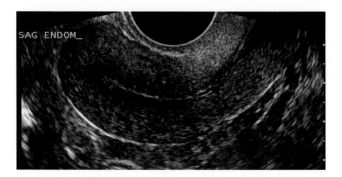

    a. 1 mm

    b. 5 mm

    c. 7 mm

    d. 10 mm

21–12. Less than 10 percent of postmenopausal women with abnormal uterine bleeding cannot be adequately evaluated by office biopsy, usually due to difficulty entering the uterine cavity. Which of the following pretreatment strategies may be warranted?

    a. Motrin, 400-mg dose taken orally the evening before the procedure

    b. Hydrocortisone, 25-mg vaginal suppository inserted the evening before the procedure

    c. Prostaglandin E_1 analog, misoprostol, 400-mg dose taken orally the night before the procedure

    d. Conjugated equine estrogen cream, 1-g dose inserted vaginally the evening before the procedure

21–13. What is the most common medical complaint of women during menopausal transition?

    a. Depression

    b. Painful intercourse

    c. Urinary incontinence

    d. Vasomotor symptoms characterized as hot flashes

21–14. A tabulation of published epidemiologic studies determined that up to what percent of menstruating women develop vasomotor symptoms during menopausal transition?

    a. 60

    b. 70

    c. 80

    d. 90

21-15. Thermoregulatory changes that accompany a hot flash have been well documented. An individual hot flash generally lasts which of the following?

    a. <1 minute

    b. 1 to 5 minutes

    c. 6 minutes

    d. 6 to 10 minutes

21-16. Hot flashes may be accompanied by which of the following?

    a. Panic

    b. Anxiety

    c. Palpitations

    d. All of the above

21-17. Physiologic increases during a hot flash include all **EXCEPT** which of the following?

    a. Core body temperature

    b. Mean skin temperature

    c. Respiratory exchange ratio

    d. Plasma levels of estradiol

21-18. Osteopenia and osteoporosis are disorders characterized by a progressive reduction in bone mass and predispose patients to fractures in the spine, hips, and other sites. What is the estimated mortality rate (percent) from hip fracture alone?

    a. 10

    b. 30

    c. 50

    d. 70

21-19. Bone mineral density (BMD) values for sex, age, and ethnicity have been determined. For diagnostic purposes, results of BMD testing are reported as *T-scores*. What T-score value is associated with osteopenia?

    a. T-score between + 2.5 and –1.0

    b. T-score between + 1.0 and –1.0

    c. T-score between + 1.0 and –2.5

    d. T-score between − 1.0 and –2.5

21-20. Which of the following are secondary causes of osteoporosis that should be screened for in any patient with osteoporosis?

    a. Hypothyroidism

    b. Hypoparathyroidism

    c. Chronic renal disease

    d. None of the above

21-21. Before menopausal transition, women have a much lower risk for cardiovascular events compared with men the same age. Reasons for protection from cardiovascular disease in premenopausal women are complex. However, a significant contribution can be assigned to an effect of estrogen that results in which of the following?

    a. Increased low-density lipoprotein levels

    b. Increased high-density lipoprotein levels

    c. Decreased high-density lipoprotein levels

    d. Increased total cholesterol and low-density lipoprotein levels

21-22. Weight gain during menopausal transition is associated with fat deposition in the abdomen, which increases the likelihood of developing which of the following metabolic changes?

    a. Diabetes mellitus

    b. Insulin resistance

    c. Cardiovascular disease

    d. All of the above

21-23. Decreasing estrogen levels seen in late menopausal transition result in which of the following dental changes?

    a. Increased salivation

    b. Buccal epithelium atrophy

    c. Increased oral alveolar bone osteoblasts

    d. All of the above

21-24. Estrogen receptors have been identified in the vulva, vagina, urethra, pelvic floor musculature, and endopelvic fascia. Which of the following is a result of the decreased estrogen trophic influence?

    a. Vaginal pH greater than 4.5

    b. Higher rates of abnormal Pap smear cytology

    c. Increased vaginal concentrations of lactobacilli

    d. Higher rates of Bartholin gland duct abscess formation

21-25. All **EXCEPT** which of the following changes is found during menopausal transition?

    a. Cognitive decline

    b. Skin thinning and wrinkling

    c. Decreased introital flexibility

    d. Predominance of cytologic parabasal cells

Chapter 21 ANSWER KEY

Question number	Letter answer	Page cited	Header cited
21–1	d	p. 554	Introduction
21–2	b	p. 554	Definitions
21–3	c	p. 554	Definitions
21–4	a	p. 555	Influential Factors
21–5	d	p. 555	Physiologic Changes
21–6	d	p. 555	Physiologic Changes
21–7	b	p. 557	Figure 21-3
21–8	b	p. 556	Ovarian Changes
21–9	a	p. 557	Figure 21-2
21–10	d	p. 558	Menstrual Disturbances
21–11	b	p. 558	Evaluation of Abnormal Bleeding
21–12	c	p. 558	Endometrial Biopsy
21–13	d	p. 560	Central Thermoregulation Changes; Incidence

Question number	Letter answer	Page cited	Header cited
21–14	a	p. 560	Central Thermoregulation Changes; Incidence
21–15	b	p. 560	Vasomotor Symptoms
21–16	d	p. 560	Vasomotor Symptoms
21–17	d	p. 561	Neurotransmitters
21–18	b	p. 565	Osteoporosis Sequelae
21–19	d	p. 565	Table 21-4
21–20	c	p. 566	Diagnosis of Osteoporosis
21–21	b	p. 570	Cardiovascular Disease Risk
21–22	d	p. 571	Weight Gain and Fat Distribution
21–23	b	p. 571	Dental Changes
21–24	a	p. 573	Lower Reproductive Tract Changes
21–25	a	p. 575	Physical Examination; Cognitive

CHAPTER 22

The Mature Woman

22–1. Menopause may be identified by which of the following?

    a. The point in time 1 year after cessation of menses

    b. The time when menstruation permanently stops due to loss of ovarian function

    c. The state associated with physical symptoms and with metabolic and structural changes related to declining estrogen levels

    d. All of the above

22–2. Regarding the large observational Nurses' Health Study from 1985, all **EXCEPT** which of the following are correct?

    a. It identified a significant reduction in heart disease among postmenopausal hormone users.

    b. It suggested at least a doubling of cerebrovascular disease among postmenopausal hormone users.

    c. Its findings likely were confounded by timing of the initiation of the postmenopausal hormone therapy.

    d. It likely was biased by including participants who were not representative of the U.S. postmenopausal population.

22–3. Which of the following is correct regarding the Heart and Estrogen/Progestin Replacement Study (HERS) and HERS II?

    a. They included healthy women without preexisting heart disease.

    b. They showed that estrogen was a useful medication for secondary prevention of cardiac disease progression.

    c. They showed (at 1 year) an increase in myocardial infarctions in women who received conjugated equine estrogen and continuous medroxyprogesterone acetate.

    d. They showed (at 4 years) a sustained increased risk of myocardial infarction in women receiving combined hormone therapy.

22–4. Results from the Women's Health Initiative (WHI) suggest which of following regarding coronary heart disease risk?

    a. It is decreased among older users (70–79 years).

    b. It is increased among younger users (50–59 years).

    c. It is universally increased among postmenopausal users of combined estrogen and progestin hormone replacement.

    d. It is likely decreased among women who initiate combined hormone therapy within 10 years of the menopause.

22–5. Results from the WHI suggest which of following regarding stroke risk?

    a. It is decreased among older users (70–79 years).

    b. It is decreased among younger users (50–59 years).

    c. It is universally increased among postmenopausal users of combined estrogen and progestin hormone replacement.

    d. It is likely decreased among women who initiate combined hormone therapy within 10 years of the menopause.

22–6. A summary of postmenopausal systemic hormone replacement risks and benefits indicates an increased risk of all **EXCEPT** which of the following?

    a. Stroke

    b. Breast cancer

    c. Colorectal cancer

    d. Venous thromboembolism

22–7. Estrogen replacement therapy is contraindicated in women with all **EXCEPT** which of the following?

    a. Vasomotor symptoms

    b. Active liver disease

    c. Known or suspected breast carcinoma

    d. Abnormal genital bleeding of unknown etiology

22–8. Which of the following is true of estrogen as treatment for hot flashes and sleep disturbances?

    a. It reduces hot flash frequency by 18 events per week (75 percent reduction compared with placebo).

    b. It is available in oral, parenteral, topical, and transdermal formulations.

    c. It should generally be prescribed at the lowest effective dose.

    d. All of the above

22–9. Which of the following is true of progestin-only hormone replacement therapy?

    a. It may attenuate estrogen's beneficial effects on lipids and blood flow.

    b. It provides protection against estrogen-induced endometrial hyperplasia and cancer.

    c. Its use may be limited by its adverse effects of weight gain and irregular vaginal bleeding.

    d. All of the above

22–10. Currently recommended alternatives to hormones for treatment of vasomotor symptoms include all **EXCEPT** which of the following?

    a. Bellergal

    b. Clonidine

    c. Gabapentin

    d. Selective serotonin-reuptake inhibitors

22–11. Which of the following is true of dong quai?

    a. It is rich in α-linolenic acid and touted to reduce inflammation, heart disease, and cancer.

    b. It contains addictive barbiturates and is not recommended for long-term use.

    c. It has been shown to significantly reduce vasomotor symptoms compared with placebo in double-blinded controlled trials.

    d. It is potentially photosensitizing and contains numerous coumarin-like derivatives that may cause excessive bleeding.

22–12. Decreasing central sympathetic tone by means such as paced respiration has which of the following effects?

    a. Increases intensity of hot flashes

    b. Increases symptoms of depression and anxiety

    c. May decrease frequency of common vasomotor symptoms

    d. Results in no significant reduction in hot-flash frequency compared with biofeedback and muscle relaxation techniques

22–13. Your patient is a 57-year-old G3P3 nonsmoking white woman who reached menopause at age 52. She has no family history of osteoporosis, no history of prolonged corticosteroid use, and no hyperparathyroidism or malabsorption syndrome. An evaluation for severe back pain reveals the anterior wedge fracture seen in this image. Bone mineral density screening was performed and gives a T-score of -1.7. Which of the following is the most effective and appropriate intervention?

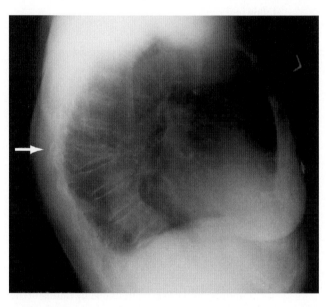

Reproduced, with permission, from Lindsay R, Cosman F: Osteoporosis. In Fauci AS, Braunwald E, Kasper DL, et al (eds): Harrison's Principles of Internal Medicine, 17th ed. New York, McGraw-Hill, 2008, Figure 348-2.

    a. Limit physical activity

    b. Initiate physical therapy and analgesia

    c. Initiate oral calcium, 1000 mg daily

    d. Initiate an oral bisphosphonate therapy for bone fracture prevention and treatment

22–14. Which of the following is the first Food and Drug Administration (FDA)-approved medication for osteoporosis treatment that works by stimulating bone formation rather than slowing bone resorption?

    a. Calcitonin

    b. Bisphosphonates

    c. Human parathyroid hormone

    d. Selective estrogen-receptor modulators

22–15. Which of the following is true of raloxifene?

    a. It is a potent bisphosphonate.

    b. It increases breast cancer risks.

    c. It increases thromboembolism risks.

    d. It significantly decreases *non*vertebral fracture risks.

22–16. Which of these oral bisphosphonates offers a dosing schedule (once monthly) that is more convenient for patients but still tolerated as well as daily dosing, thereby improving compliance?

    a. Alendronate

    b. Zoledronate

    c. Risedronate

    d. Teriparatide

22–17. Doctors of the patient from whom this image is taken hope to increase bone density, turnover, and size by increasing osteoblast numbers. Which of the following is true of the medication to be prescribed?

22–18. Vitamin D deficiency leads to which of the following?

    a. Decreased bone turnover

    b. Improved calcium absorption

    c. Decreased rate of bone loss

    d. Secondary hyperparathyroidism

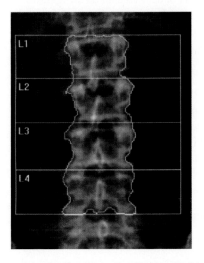

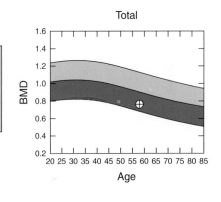

DXA Results Summary:

Region	Area (cm²)	BMC (g)	BMD (g/cm²)	T-Score	Z-Score
L1	11.73	8.03	0.684	–2.2	–1.0
L2	12.60	9.70	0.770	–2.3	–1.0
L3	14.59	11.70	0.802	–2.6	–1.1
L4	14.44	11.01	0.763	–3.2	–1.7
Total	**53.36**	**40.44**	**0.758**	**–2.6**	**–1.2**

Total BMD CV 1.0%, ACF = 1.028, BCF = 0.998, TH = 5.974
WHO Classification: Osteoporosis
Fracture Risk: High

Reproduced, with permission, from Bradshaw KD: Menopausal transition. In Schorge JO, Schaffer JI, Halvorson LM, et al (eds): Williams Gynecology, 1st ed. New York, McGraw-Hill, 2008, Figure 21-10D.

    a. It is given once weekly orally.

    b. It may be delivered by nasal spray.

    c. It is not recommended for patients at increased risk of skeletal malignancy.

    d. It may cause upper gastrointestinal inflammation, ulceration, and bleeding.

22–19. The image presents a schematic of the daily whole-body turnover of calcium. All **EXCEPT** which of the following interventions are expected to be beneficial to bone health and calcium absorption?

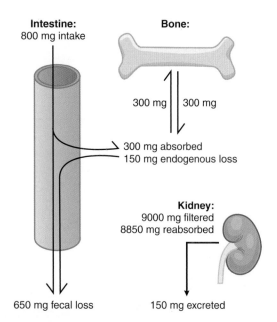

Intestine:
800 mg intake

Bone:

300 mg   300 mg

300 mg absorbed
150 mg endogenous loss

Kidney:
9000 mg filtered
8850 mg reabsorbed

650 mg fecal loss   150 mg excreted

Reproduced, with permission, from Friedman PA: Agents affecting mineral ion homeostasis and bone turnover. In Brunton LL, Chabner BA, Knollmann BC (eds): Goodman and Gilman's The Pharmacological Basis of Therapeutics, 12th ed. New York, McGraw-Hill, 2011, Figure 44-2.

a. Increasing caffeine intake

b. Increasing calcium intake to >1200 mg daily

c. Improving absorption by increasing daily vitamin D to >400–600 IU/d

d. Decreasing renal excretion by decreasing sodium excretion (i.e., low-sodium diet)

22–20. Vaginal products for estrogen replacement in postmenopausal women have which of the following effects?

a. Decrease vaginal mucosal sensorimotor responses

b. Increase vaginal mucosal fluid secretions and elasticity

c. Have lower patient-acceptance rates compared with systemic therapies

d. Have comparable systemic estradiol concentrations compared with systemic therapies

22–21. Which of the following statements are correct when agents are compared with daily or twice-weekly application of vaginal conjugated estrogen cream (Premarin)?

a. 17β-Estradiol tablet suppositories offer equivalent relief of atrophic vaginitis symptoms.

b. Continuous low-dose estradiol-releasing intravaginal rings are more acceptable to patients.

c. Continuous low-dose estradiol-releasing intravaginal rings are prescribed as a single unit and worn for 90 days.

d. All of the above

22–22. Prolonged treatment of decreased libido using androgens in postmenopausal women could contribute to all **EXCEPT** which of the following?

a. Acne and hirsutism

b. Clitoral hypertrophy

c. Worsening lipid profile

d. Decreased bone mineral density

22–23. All **EXCEPT** which of the following are among the top four causes of mortality in older women?

a. Cancer

b. Heart disease

c. Diabetes mellitus

d. Cerebrovascular disease

22–24. The incidence and prevalence of dementia increase as patients grow older. This would argue for routine dementia screening practices and identification/treatment of any reversible causes of dementia. Which of the following is a potentially reversible cause of dementia?

a. Hypothyroidism

b. Thiamine deficiency

c. Vitamin B_{12} deficiency

d. All of the above

22–25. Which of the following may be a reason to suggest estrogen therapy for a postmenopausal patient with mild urinary incontinence?

a. Periurethral vascularity is diminished by hypoestrogenism.

b. Estrogen receptors are found throughout the lower urinary tract.

c. Hypoestrogenism is associated with deleterious changes in collagen.

d. All of the above

Chapter 22   ANSWER KEY

Question number	Letter answer	Page cited	Header cited
22–1	d	p. 581	Introduction
22–2	b	p. 582	Estrogen as a Prevention Tool
22–3	c	p. 583	Heart and Estrogen/Progestin Replacement Study
22–4	d	p. 583	Women's Health Initiative
22–5	c	p. 583	Women's Health Initiative
22–6	c	p. 584	Summary of Risks and Benefits
22–7	a	p. 585	Summary of Current Use Indications
22–8	d	p. 585	Treatment of Vasomotor Symptoms
22–9	d	p. 586	Progestins
22–10	a	p. 588	Central Nervous System Agents for Vasomotor Symptoms
22–11	d	p. 589	Phytoestrogens
22–12	c	p. 590	Environmental and Lifestyle Changes

Question number	Letter answer	Page cited	Header cited
22–13	d	p. 590	Treatment Indications
22–14	c	p. 591	Pharmacologic Considerations
22–15	c	p. 591	Selective Estrogen Receptor Modulators
22–16	c	p. 592	Table 22-5
22–17	c	p. 595	Parathyroid Hormone
22–18	d	p. 595	Vitamin D
22–19	a	p. 595	Nonpharmacologic Therapy
22–20	b	p. 596	Dyspareunia
22–21	d	p. 596	Dyspareunia
22–22	d	p. 597	Testosterone
22–23	c	p. 598	Table 22-7
22–24	d	p. 599	Prevention of Alzheimer Senile Dementia
22–25	d	p. 600	Prevention of Urogynecologic Disease

FEMALE PELVIC MEDICINE AND RECONSTRUCTIVE SURGERY

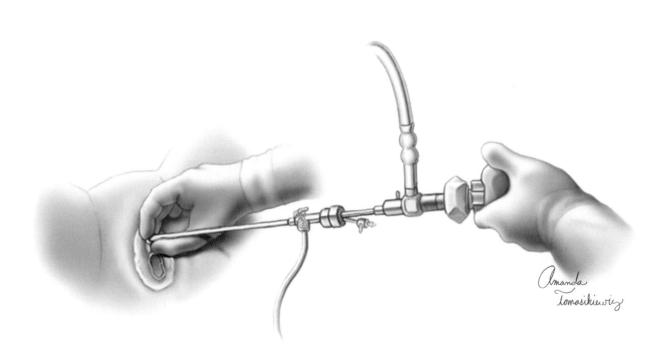

Urinary Incontinence

23-1. Involuntary loss of urine with coughing or sneezing typically reflects which of the following forms of incontinence?

a. Urge incontinence

b. Stress incontinence

c. Overflow incontinence

d. Functional incontinence

23-2. Involuntary loss of urine preceded by a strong sensation to void reflects which of the following forms of incontinence?

a. Urge incontinence

b. Stress incontinence

c. Overflow incontinence

d. Functional incontinence

23-3. If the symptoms of overactive bladder or urge incontinence are objectively demonstrated by urodynamic testing, which of the following terms is used?

a. Detrusor overactivity

b. Functional incontinence

c. Genuine urge incontinence

d. Verified urge incontinence

23-4. If stress incontinence is documented by urodynamic testing, which of the following terms is used?

a. Detrusor overactivity

b. Functional incontinence

c. Verified urge incontinence

d. Urodynamic stress incontinence

23-5. Of the forms of incontinence, which is the most common in the general ambulatory female population?

a. Urge

b. Stress

c. Overflow

d. Functional

23-6. A risk factor for urinary incontinence includes which of the following?

a. Nonsmoking

b. Nulliparity

c. Advanced age

d. Sickle cell anemia

23-7. Hypoestrogenism is linked to a greater risk of incontinence through which of the following mechanisms?

a. Increased urethral collagen volume

b. Atrophy of the urethral mucosal seal

c. Increased compliance of urethral sphincter musculature

d. All of the above

23-8. Childbirth likely contributes to urinary incontinence through which of the following mechanisms?

a. Nerve damage from stretch injury

b. Prolonged pudendal nerve latency

c. Direct injury to connective tissue attachments

d. All of the above

23–9. The layer indicated by the beige-highlighted label in the image below is responsible for what function(s)?

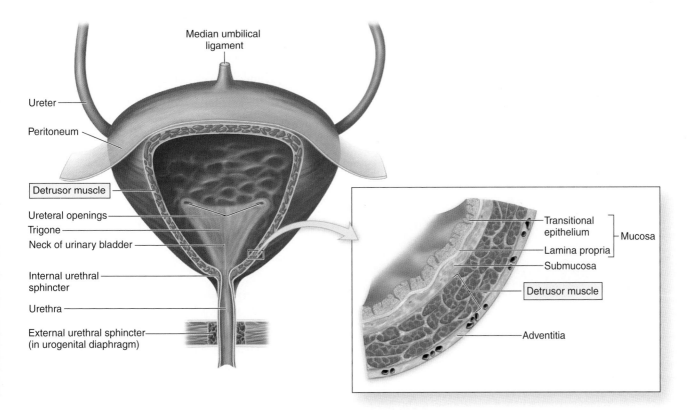

Reproduced, with permission, from McKinley M, O'Loughlin VD: Urinary system. In Human Anatomy. New York, McGraw-Hill, 2006, Figure 27-9.

    a. Aids greater permeability at the urine–plasma barrier

    b. Prohibits bacterial adherence and prevents urothelial damage

    c. Allows for rapid multidimensional expansion during bladder filling

    d. All of the above

23–10. Which statement correctly describes innervations of the bladder?

    a. The autonomic division of the peripheral nervous system innervates striated muscle.

    b. The sympathetic system acts via acetylcholine binding to α- or β-adrenergic receptors.

    c. The somatic component of the peripheral nervous system innervates smooth muscle.

    d. Autonomic fibers supplying the pelvic viscera course in the inferior and superior hypogastric plexi.

23-11. How do the structures whose label is highlighted in orange in this image contribute to the bladder's capacity for urine storage or emptying?

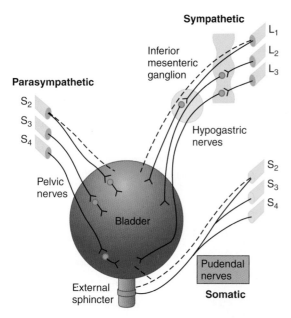

Reproduced, with permission, from Barrett KE, Barman SM, Boitano S, et al (eds): Renal function and micturition. In Ganong's Review of Medical Physiology, 23rd ed. New York, McGraw-Hill, 2010, Figure 38-20.

    a. Voluntary contraction or relaxation of the urogenital sphincter complex

    b. Involuntary relaxation of the detrusor muscle for bladder filling

    c. Involuntary contraction of the detrusor muscle for bladder emptying

    d. None of the above

23-12. Which of the following statements regarding the parasympathetic division of the autonomic nervous system and its innervation of the bladder is correct?

    a. Acetylcholine acts via α- or β-adrenergic receptors.

    b. The urethra's outlet must contract in concert with detrusor contraction to aid voiding.

    c. Muscarinic antagonist medications will augment detrusor contraction and worsen urinary incontinence.

    d. Of the five subtypes of muscarinic receptors, M_2 and M_3 are the ones predominantly responsible for detrusor smooth muscle contraction.

23-13. The urethra's ability to maintain a tight seal and prevent urinary incontinence requires which of the following?

    a. Urethral mucosal coaptation

    b. Healthy underlying vascular plexus

    c. Contraction of muscles surrounding the urethra

    d. All of the above

23-14. When the patient's history suggests an overlap in both stress and urge incontinence symptoms, which of the following terms is used?

    a. Overflow incontinence

    b. Mixed urinary incontinence

    c. Complex urinary incontinence

    d. Augmented urinary incontinence

23-15. Diabetes mellitus likely contributes to urinary incontinence through which mechanism?

    a. Decreased urine output

    b. Worsening peripheral edema

    c. Bladder mucosal inflammation

    d. Osmotic diuresis and polyuria

23-16. A urethral diverticulum is suggested by which of the following?

    a. Postvoid dribbling

    b. Suburethral bulging of the anterior vaginal wall

    c. Transurethral expression of fluid when compressing the anterior vaginal wall

    d. All of the above

23-17. Which of the following **CANNOT** be assessed or measured using simple cystometrics?

    a. Total bladder capacity

    b. Stress urinary incontinence

    c. Intrinsic sphincteric deficiency

    d. First sensation of bladder filling

23-18. The test depicted in the image, which graphically demonstrates a patient's maximum rate, duration, and pattern of flow during voiding, is known as which of the following?

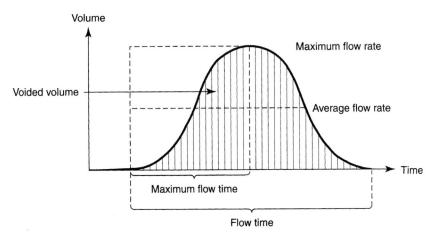

Reproduced, with permission, from Tanagho EA, Deng DY: Urodynamic studies. In Tanagho EA, McAninch JW (eds): Smith's General Urology, 17th ed. New York, McGraw-Hill, 2008, Figure 28-1.

a. Uroflowmetry

b. Cystometrography

c. Cystourethrography

d. Urethral pressure profile

23-19. Pressure flowmetry is useful for determining which of the following?

a. Maximum flow rate

b. Incomplete bladder emptying from obstructive causes

c. Incomplete bladder emptying from poor detrusor contractility

d. All of the above

23-20. All **EXCEPT** which of the following statements are true regarding pelvic floor muscle therapy (PFMT) for treatment of urinary incontinence?

a. Patients are asked to forcefully contract their abdominal muscles just before a cough or sneeze.

b. Over a series of weeks, patients steadily increase the duration of muscle contraction.

c. Rapid contraction and relaxation (i.e., "quick flicks") of the pelvic floor muscles may be helpful for treatment of urge urinary incontinence.

d. A predictor of likely poor response to PFMT is baseline prolapse beyond the hymenal ring.

23-21. Local estrogen therapy may help in the treatment of mild urinary incontinence via which mechanism?

a. Increased collagen deposition

b. Increased α-adrenergic receptor sensitivity

c. Increased vascularity of the periurethral capillary plexus

d. All of the above

23–22. Which of the following statements regarding the procedure depicted in the image is true?

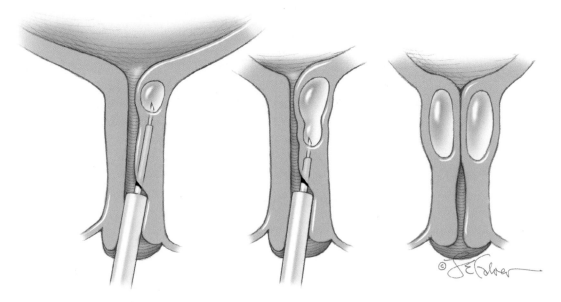

Reproduced, with permission, from Schaffer JI, Hoffman BL: Surgeries for female pelvic reconstruction. In Schorge JO, Schaffer JI, Halvorson LM, et al (eds): Williams Gynecology, 1st ed. New York, McGraw-Hill, 2008, Figure 42-6.1.

  a. This may only be performed for women with intrinsic sphincteric deficiency.

  b. It is best performed only in an operating room under adequate regional or general anesthesia.

  c. The injection location around and along the length of the urethra varies from patient to patient.

  d. The injectable material is designed to dissolve over time as it is frequently immunogenic.

23–23. The antiincontinence procedures described by Burch and Marshall-Marchetti-Krantz are examples of which of the following?

  a. Midurethral sling procedures

  b. Periurethral bulking techniques

  c. Retropubic urethropexy procedures

  d. Transvaginal needle suspension procedures

23–24. All **EXCEPT** which of the following statements are true regarding the two procedures demonstrated in the images below?

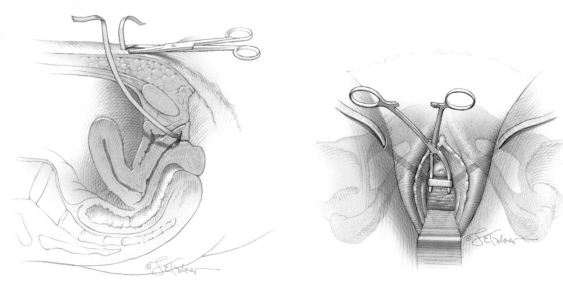

Reproduced, with permission, from Schaffer JI, Hoffman BL: Surgeries for female pelvic reconstruction. In Schorge JO, Schaffer JI, Halvorson LM, et al (eds): Williams Gynecology, 1st ed. New York, McGraw-Hill, 2008, Figures 42-3.5 and 42-4.4.

a. Long-term urinary incontinence cure rates are 75 to 85 percent.

b. This can usually be performed in a day-surgery/outpatient setting.

c. Bladder injury is more common in the transobturator route compared with the retropubic route.

d. Possible complications include worsening urinary urgency, mesh erosion, urinary retention, and vascular injury.

23–25. What are the most common side effects that patient complain about when using oral oxybutynin or tolterodine?

a. Nausea and vomiting

b. Headaches and tinnitus

c. Dry mouth and constipation

d. Skin irritation and pruritus

23–26. Before botulinum toxin A is used for idiopathic detrusor overactivity, the patient should be informed of which of the following true statements?

a. The effects will likely last for 3 to 4 years.

b. Temporary self-catheterization may be required if urinary retention occurs.

c. Postprocedural urinary retention usually leads to painful distension, urinary tract infections, or pyelonephritis.

d. All of the above

Chapter 23   ANSWER KEY

Question number	Letter answer	Page cited	Header cited	Question number	Letter answer	Page cited	Header cited
23–1	b	p. 606	Definitions	23–14	b	p. 616	Symptom Clustering
23–2	a	p. 606	Definitions	23–15	d	p. 618	Past Medical History
23–3	a	p. 606	Definitions	23–16	d	p. 616	Diagnosis
23–4	d	p. 606	Definitions	23–17	c	p. 621	Simple Cystometrics
23–5	b	p. 607	Epidemiology	23–18	a	p. 621	Uroflowmetry
23–6	c	p. 607	Risks for Urinary Incontinence	23–19	d	p. 623	Pressure Flowmetry
23–7	b	p. 607	Risks for Urinary Incontinence	23–20	a	p. 624	Pelvic Floor Muscle Training
23–8	d	p. 608	Childbirth and Pregnancy	23–21	d	p. 625	Estrogen Replacement
23–9	c	p. 609	Bladder Filling	23–22	c	p. 625	Urethral Bulking Agents
23–10	d	p. 609	Innervation Overview	23–23	c	p. 626	Retropubic Urethropexy
23–11	a	p. 609	Bladder Filling	23–24	c	p. 627	Midurethral Slings
23–12	d	p. 611	Innervation Related to Voiding	23–25	c	p. 628	Anticholinergic Medications
23–13	d	p. 616	Factors Affecting Urethral Integrity	23–26	b	p. 630	Botulinum Toxin A

CHAPTER 24

Pelvic Organ Prolapse

24-1. Which of the following are risk factors for the development of pelvic organ prolapse?

    a. Spina bifida

    b. Hypoestrogenism

    c. Prior hysterectomy

    d. All of the above

24-2. Compared with selective use, elective episiotomy during the second stage of labor has been associated with all **EXCEPT** which of the following?

    a. Periurethral tears

    b. Anal sphincter laceration

    c. Increased postpartum pain

    d. Postpartum anal incontinence

24-3. Which statement is true regarding measurements taken for the Pelvic Organ Prolapse Quantification (POP-Q) examination?

    a. All are taken at rest, except for total vaginal length, which is obtained during Valsalva.

    b. Point D is omitted in the absence of a cervix.

    c. GH is measured from the midline of the posterior hymenal ring to the mid-anal opening.

    d. Point Aa corresponds to the most distal portion of any part of the upper/proximal anterior vaginal wall.

24-4. As shown in this image of vaginal prolapse, when the leading edge of bulge is approximately even with the plane of the hymen or within 1 cm distal to the hymen, a patient is said to have which stage of prolapse?

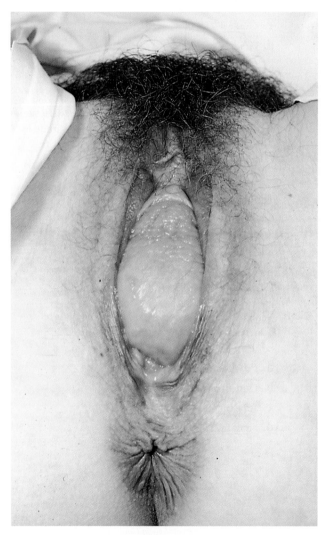

Reproduced, with permission, from Buckley RG, Knoop KJ: Gynecologic and obstetric conditions. In Knoop KJ, Stack LB, Storrow AB, et al (eds): The Atlas of Emergency Medicine, 3rd ed. New York, McGraw-Hill, 2010, Figure 10-17.

    a. Stage I

    b. Stage II

    c. Stage III

    d. Stage IV

24-5. Pelvic organ support is maintained in part by the levator ani muscle, which is composed of all **EXCEPT** which of the following?

a. Puborectalis

b. Iliococcygeus

c. Pubococcygeus

d. Obturator internus

24-6. Using the Baden-Walker Halfway System, decent of the prolapse to the level of the hymen is considered which of the following?

a. Grade 1

b. Grade 2

c. Grade 3

d. Grade 4

24-7. Which description of levels of vaginal support is accurate?

a. Level I support describes the upper/proximal vaginal support via lateral attachments to the arcus tendineus fascia pelvis.

b. Level II support describes midvaginal support via the cardinal and uterosacral ligaments.

c. Level III support describes attachment of the distal vagina to surrounding structures, namely, the perineal body and the superficial and deep perineal muscles.

d. Level IV describes the global support of an intact "endopelvic fascia."

24-8. Which of the following is the symptom that is reliably associated with prolapse and usually worsens as prolapse progresses?

a. Pelvic pain

b. Constipation

c. Anal incontinence

d. Sensation of pelvic pressure

24-9. Patients with this type of prolapse most commonly complain of which of the following?

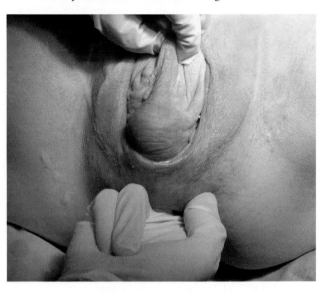

Photograph contributed by Dr. Marlene Corton.

a. Dyspareunia

b. Constipation

c. Anal incontinence

d. The need for digital decompression of the bulge for defecation

24-10. An anterior vaginal wall prolapse is noted that has sagging lateral vaginal sulci, but rugae are still present. This suggests which type of anatomic defect?

a. Central

b. Midline

c. Transverse

d. Paravaginal

24-11. An enterocele may definitively be diagnosed during examination by which of the following methods?

a. Assessing the vaginal apex with a bivalve speculum

b. Observing small bowel peristalsis behind the vaginal wall

c. Displacing the posterior vaginal wall with a split speculum

d. All of the above

24-12. Which of the following is true of the ring pessary?

a. It is an example of a space-filling pessary.

b. It works by creating suction between the vaginal walls and the pessary.

c. It is most effective for patients with stage III or IV prolapse.

d. It is appropriately fitted when positioned behind the pubic symphysis anteriorly and the cervix posteriorly.

24–13. Which of the following is true of this pessary type?

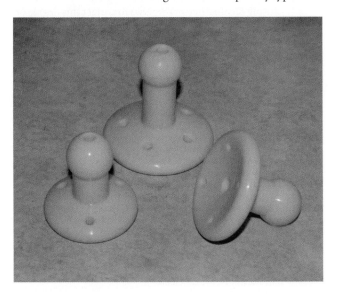

   a. It is a space-filling pessary.

   b. It creates a diameter larger than the genital hiatus.

   c. It is often used for moderate to severe prolapse or procidentia.

   d. All of the above

24–14. All **EXCEPT** which of the following statements regarding pessary management are correct?

   a. Ideally, the pessary is removed once every 4 to 6 months, washed with soap and water, and replaced the next morning.

   b. Ulcerations or abrasions on the vaginal wall may be from an ill-fitting pessary or from the initial prolapse itself.

   c. Pelvic pain with a pessary indicates its size is too large.

   d. Urinary leakage may occur due to new support of the vaginal wall.

24–15. Options for management of foul odors associated with pessary use include all **EXCEPT** which of the following?

   a. Warm water douches

   b. Broad-spectrum antibiotics

   c. Increased frequency of removal and washing

   d. Use of Trimo-San gel (Milex Products, Chicago, IL)

24–16. Which characteristics describe the typical operative candidate for the obliterative procedure demonstrated in the image?

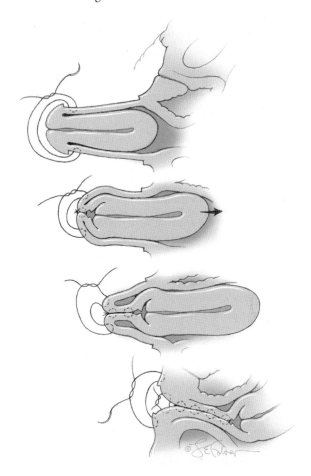

Reproduced, with permission, by Schaffer JI, Hoffman BL: Surgeries for female pelvic reconstruction. In Schorge JO, Schaffer JI, Halvorson LM, et al (eds): Williams Gynecology, 1st ed. New York, McGraw-Hill, 2008, Figure 42-23.1.

   a. Desiring future fertility

   b. Desiring future coital activity

   c. Medically compromised or elderly patient

   d. Abnormal uterine bleeding requiring concomitant hysterectomy

24–17. Compared with reconstructive procedures for prolapse correction, colpocleisis generally has which of the following characteristics?

   a. Is technically more difficult

   b. Requires greater operative time

   c. Has a less successful long-term anatomic outcome

   d. None of the above

24–18. A vaginal reconstructive procedure for prolapse correction may be preferable to an abdominal route for which of the following reasons?

  a. A prior vaginal approach has failed.

  b. A short total vaginal length is present.

  c. A higher risk of recurrent prolapse is expected.

  d. A quicker return to daily activities is desired.

24–19. Performing an abdominal sacrocolpopexy or uterosacral ligament suspension addresses the _____ detachment defect of anterior wall prolapse and should offer an improved repair over traditional anterior colporrhaphy alone.

  a. Central

  b. Midline

  c. Transverse

  d. Paravaginal

24–20. In the procedure depicted in this image, the fibromuscular layer of the anterior vaginal wall is reattached to which of the following?

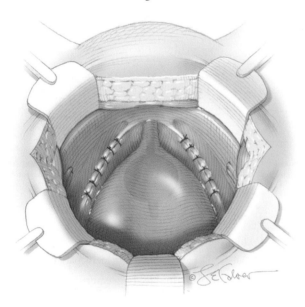

Reproduced, with permission, from Schaffer JI, Hoffman BL: Surgeries for female pelvic reconstruction. In Schorge JO, Schaffer JI, Halvorson LM, et al (eds): Williams Gynecology, 1st ed. New York, McGraw-Hill, 2008, Figure 42-14.3.

  a. Cardinal ligaments

  b. Uterosacral ligaments

  c. Arcus tendineus fascia pelvis

  d. Iliopectineal (Cooper) ligament

24–21. For this patient, which of the following is essential during reconstructive surgeries to correct this degree of prolapse?

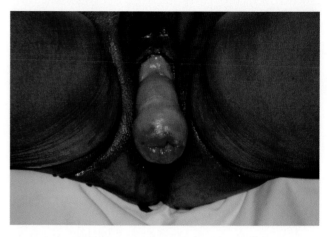

Photograph contributed by Dr. Marlene Corton.

  a. Perineorrhaphy

  b. Apical resuspension

  c. Burch colposuspension

  d. Paravaginal defect repair

24–22. Effective procedures for addressing prolapse at the vaginal apex include all **EXCEPT** which of the following?

  a. Simple hysterectomy

  b. Abdominal sacrocolpopexy

  c. Sacrospinous ligament fixation

  d. Uterosacral ligament vault suspension

24–23. Which of the following statements regarding sacrospinous ligament fixation are true?

  a. Requires an intraperitoneal approach

  b. May be performed unilaterally or bilaterally

  c. Results in buttock pain or vascular injury in 10 to 15 percent of cases

  d. Supports the apex well but results in frequent recurrent prolapse of the posterior vaginal wall

24–24. Regarding repair of posterior vaginal wall prolapse, all **EXCEPT** which of the following are correct?

  a. To achieve its high 76 to 96 percent anatomic cure rate, posterior colporrhaphy requires addition of biologic or synthetic mesh materials.

  b. Concurrent levator muscle plication narrows the genital hiatus but may increase dyspareunia.

  c. Site-specific repairs discretely close fibromuscular defects that may be midline, lateral, distal, or superior.

  d. Site-specific repairs have anatomic success rates comparable to those of traditional colporrhaphy.

24-25. In the surgery pictured here, with plication of tissues of the distal posterior vaginal wall, which of the following is true?

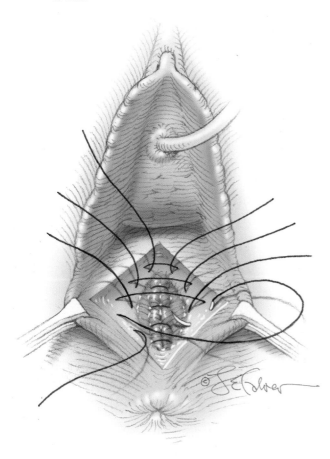

a. Level III support is being reestablished.

b. The risk of posterior wall prolapse recurrence is decreased.

c. Overly aggressive plication may narrow the introitus and lead to entry dyspareunia.

d. All of the above

24-26. Compared with type II or III mesh materials, type I mesh has which of the following characteristics?

a. Has smaller pore size of less than 1 μm

b. Has a higher rate of associated infection

c. Allows better tissue ingrowth, angiogenesis, and flexibility

d. Is harvested from another part of the body (e.g., rectus abdominis fascia)

24-27. Which statement correctly describes xenografts?

a. Synthetic, multifilament mesh material

b. Biologic graft from a human other than the patient

c. Biologic graft such as porcine dermis or bovine pericardium

d. Synthetic mesh with pore sizes less than 10 μm in at least one dimension

Chapter 24　ANSWER KEY

Question number	Letter answer	Page cited	Header cited
24–1	d	p. 633	Risk Factors
24–2	a	p. 634	Other Obstetric-related Risks
24–3	b	p. 636	Pelvic Organ Prolapse Quantification (POP-Q)
24–4	b	p. 638	Table 24-2
24–5	d	p. 637	Role of Levator Ani Muscle
24–6	b	p. 638	Table 24-3
24–7	c	p. 640	Levels of Vaginal Support
24–8	d	p. 641	Symptoms Associated with Pelvic Organ Prolapse
24–9	d	p. 643	Gastrointestinal Symptoms
24–10	d	p. 645	Vaginal Examination
24–11	b	p. 645	Vaginal Examination
24–12	d	p. 648	Types of Pessaries
24–13	d	p. 648	Types of Pessaries
24–14	a	p. 648	Pessary Use in Pelvic Organ Prolapse

Question number	Letter answer	Page cited	Header cited
24–15	b	p. 649	Complications with Pessary Use
24–16	c	p. 651	Obliterative Procedures
24–17	d	p. 651	Obliterative Procedures
24–18	d	p. 651	Reconstructive Procedures
24–19	c	p. 652	Anterior Compartment
24–20	c	p. 652	Anterior Compartment
24–21	b	p. 652	Vaginal Apex
24–22	a	p. 652	Vaginal Apex
24–23	b	p. 653	Sacrospinous Ligament Fixation
24–24	a	p. 653	Posterior Compartment
24–25	d	p. 654	Perineum
24–26	c	p. 655	Mesh Material
24–27	c	p. 655	Mesh Material

CHAPTER 25

CHAPTER 25

Anal Incontinence and Functional Anorectal Disorders

25–1. The definition of anal incontinence includes all **EXCEPT** which of the following?

   a. Anal mucoid seepage

   b. Incontinence to flatus

   c. Incontinence to liquid

   d. Incontinence to solid stool

25–2. Which of these statements regarding the epidemiology of anal incontinence in adults is true?

   a. Anal incontinence prevalence decreases with age.

   b. Anal incontinence is more common in men than in women.

   c. There are wide variations in the estimated prevalence of anal incontinence.

   d. Anal incontinence including flatal incontinence is uncommon, affecting fewer than 1 percent of community-dwelling adults.

25–3. Which of the following are required for normal defecation to occur?

   a. Normal anorectal sensation

   b. Competent anal sphincter complex

   c. Adequate rectal capacity and compliance

   d. All of the above

25–4. The anal sphincter complex includes all **EXCEPT** which of the following?

   a. Puborectalis muscle

   b. Pubococcygeus muscle

   c. External anal sphincter

   d. Internal anal sphincter

25–5. This image illustrates a *physiologic* contraction of pelvic floor muscles in response to increasing intraabdominal pressure. *Paradoxical* contraction of these muscles during defecation may cause which of the following?

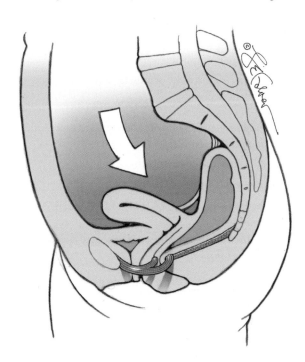

Reproduced, with permission, from Corton MM: Anatomy. In Hoffman BL, Schorge JO, Schaffer JI, et al (eds): Williams Gynecology, 2nd ed. New York, McGraw-Hill, 2012, Figure 38-10B.

   a. Anal incontinence

   b. Anal mucoid seepage

   c. Impaired evacuation

   d. A greater (less obtuse) anorectal angle

25-6. Which of the following is true of the rectoanal inhibitory reflex?

    a. Allows "sampling" of the rectum's contents

    b. Is mediated by the middle rectal branch of the pudendal nerve

    c. Disappears in patients with cauda equina lesions or spinal cord transection

    d. Involves transient relaxation of the external anal sphincter and contraction of the internal anal sphincter

25-7. Anorectal manometry allows assessment of all **EXCEPT** which of the following?

    a. Anal reflexes

    b. Rectal sensation

    c. Rectal compliance

    d. Electrical activity of muscles at rest and during contraction

25-8. Decreased perception of balloon insufflation during anorectal manometry

    a. May indicate neuropathy

    b. Occurs with decreased rectal compliance

    c. Will likely occur with ulcerative or radiation proctitis

    d. Indicates a rectal reservoir unable to appropriately store stool

25-9. This endoanal sonogram demonstrates which of the following?

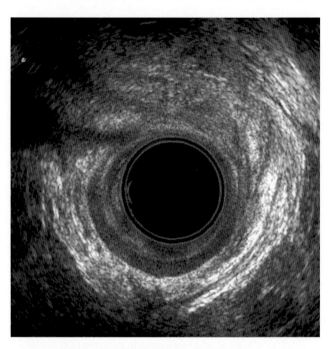

Reproduced, with permission, from Bullard Dunn KM, Rothenberger DA: Colon, rectum, and anus. In Brunicardi FC, Andersen DK, Billiar TR, et al (eds): Schwartz's Principles of Surgery, 9th ed. New York, McGraw-Hill, 2010, Figure 29-8.

    a. Increased anorectal angle

    b. Increased pudendal nerve motor latency

    c. Disruption of the puborectalis muscle

    d. Disruption of the external and internal anal sphincters

25-10. Compared with endoanal sonography, which of the following is true of magnetic resonance imaging?

    a. Is less expensive

    b. Allows better detection of external anal sphincter atrophy

    c. Is more sensitive for detecting abnormalities of the internal anal sphincter

    d. None of the above

25-11. Defecography may be helpful for the evaluation of which of the following?

    a. Enteroceles

    b. Intussusception

    c. Internal rectal prolapse

    d. All of the above

25–12. The angle measured in this image, which illustrates straining for defecation, is best captured using which test?

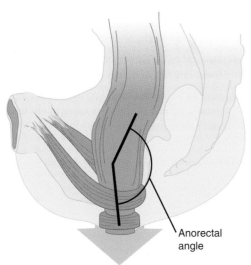

Anorectal angle

Descent of the pelvic floor

Reproduced, with permission, from Barrett KE, Barman SM, Boitano S, et al (eds): Gastrointestinal motility. In Ganong's Review of Medical Physiology, 23rd ed. New York, McGraw-Hill, 2010, Figure 28-9B.

   a. Defecography

   b. Electromyography

   c. Anorectal manometry

   d. Pudendal nerve motor latency testing

25–13. Loperamide hydrochloride may be helpful for treatment of fecal incontinence by which of the following mechanisms?

   a. Reducing stool volume

   b. Increasing anal resting tone

   c. Slowing fecal intestinal transit time

   d. All of the above

25–14. Which of the following is true of agents such as methylcellulose and psyllium?

   a. May cause abdominal distension and bloating

   b. Improve bowel control via their anticholinergic properties

   c. Increase the time available for the intestines to remove fluid from stool

   d. All of the above

25–15. Which of the following anal incontinence treatment surgeries requires an implantable generator device to stimulate muscle?

   a. Secca procedure

   b. Artificial anal sphincter

   c. Gracilis muscle transposition

   d. Overlapping anal sphincteroplasty

25–16. Which of the following anal incontinence treatment surgeries uses temperature-controlled radiofrequency energy directed to the anal sphincter muscles?

   a. Secca procedure

   b. Sacral nerve stimulation

   c. Gracilis muscle transposition

   d. Overlapping anal sphincteroplasty

25–17. All **EXCEPT** which of the following are examples of functional anorectal disorders?

   a. Proctalgia fugax

   b. Dyssynergic defecation

   c. External anal sphincter defect

   d. Inadequate defecatory propulsion

25–18. Functional fecal incontinence may be due to which of the following?

   a. Poor rectal compliance

   b. Abnormal intestinal motility

   c. Weakened pelvic floor muscles

   d. All of the above

25–19. A 37-year-old G3P3 woman presents to her gynecologist at the time of her annual examination with complaints of severe anal pain every few months that is incapacitating but lasts only approximately 2 minutes. After exclusion of organic pathology, this condition is best managed how?

   a. Reassurance

   b. Secca procedure

   c. Opioid analgesics

   d. Sacral nerve stimulation

25–20. Which of the following is true of dyssynergic defecation?

   a. Is associated with mucoid seepage and anal incontinence

   b. May be confirmed by anorectal manometry or electromyography

   c. Accounts for less than 5 percent of cases of chronic constipation

   d. May be treated with diphenoxylate hydrochloride or loperamide hydrochloride

25–21. What is the most common rectovaginal fistula location?

   a. High (the upper third of the vaginal wall)

   b. Mid (the middle third of the vaginal wall)

   c. Low (the distal third of the vaginal wall)

   d. These three occur with approximately equivalent frequency.

25–22. In addition to developing as an obstetric complication, rectovaginal fistula may be associated with which of the following?

    a. Coital trauma

    b. Cervical cancer

    c. Tuberculosis infection

    d. All of the above

25–23. All **EXCEPT** which of the following may aid in diagnosis of a rectovaginal fistula?

    a. Vaginoscopy

    b. Barium enema

    c. Noncontrast computed tomography

    d. Tampon in the vagina with methylene blue instilled in the rectum

25–24. The rectovaginal fistula repair depicted here is which of the following?

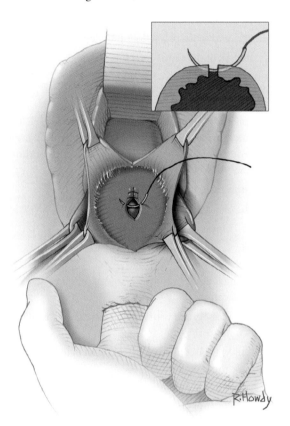

Reproduced, with permission, from Schaffer JI, Hoffman BL: Surgeries for female pelvic reconstruction. In Schorge JO, Schaffer JI, Halvorson LM, et al (eds): Williams Gynecology, 1st ed. New York, McGraw-Hill, 2008, Figure 42-26.4.

    a. Transanal episioproctotomy

    b. Endorectal flap advancement

    c. Transvaginal episioproctotomy

    d. Fistulotomy with tension-free layered closure

25–25. All **EXCEPT** which of the following are true statements regarding surgical repair of rectovaginal fistulas?

    a. Success of repair after obstetrical injury is usually very good: 78 to 100 percent.

    b. Generally, successful repair rates are highest with the first surgical attempt.

    c. Surgical repair should be delayed until surrounding tissues are free of edema and infection.

    d. Fistulas in the midvagina commonly are repaired by a transabdominal approach using bowel resection and primary reanastomosis.

Chapter 25   ANSWER KEY

Question number	Letter answer	Page cited	Header cited	Question number	Letter answer	Page cited	Header cited
25–1	a	p. 659	Anal Incontinence	25–14	a	p. 669	Medical Management
25–2	c	p. 659	Epidemiology	25–15	c	p. 671	Gracilis Muscle Transposition
25–3	d	p. 660	Pathophysiology of Defecation and Anal Continence	25–16	a	p. 671	Secca Procedure
				25–17	c	p. 672	Functional Anorectal Disorders
25–4	b	p. 660	Anal Sphincter Complex	25–18	d	p. 672	Functional Fecal Incontinence
25–5	c	p. 660	Anal Sphincter Complex				
25–6	a	p. 661	Anorectal Sensation	25–19	a	p. 672	Functional Anorectal Pain
25–7	d	p. 665	Anorectal Manometry				
25–8	a	p. 665	Anorectal Manometry	25–20	b	p. 672	Functional Defecation Disorders
25–9	d	p. 666	Figure 25-7 Endoanal Ultrasonography				
				25–21	c	p. 673	Definition and Classification
25–10	b	p. 668	Magnetic Resonance Imaging				
25–11	d	p. 668	Evacuation Proctography	25–22	d	p. 674	Table 25-8 Rectovaginal Fistula Risk Factors
25–12	a	p. 667	Table 25-5 Functional Testing for Patients with Fecal Incontinence	25–23	c	p. 674	Diagnostic Testing
				25–24	d	p. 674	Treatment
25–13	d	p. 669	Medical Management	25–25	d	p. 674	Treatment

CHAPTER 25

Genitourinary Fistula and Urethral Diverticulum

26-1. What is the most common type of genitourinary fistula?

   a. Vesicovaginal

   b. Vesicouterine

   c. Ureterovaginal

   d. Urethrovaginal

26-2. Which of the following is the correct sequence of events in wound healing?

   a. Angiogenesis → fibrosis → remodeling

   b. Angiogenesis → remodeling → fibrosis

   c. Fibrosis → remodeling → angiogenesis

   d. Remodeling → angiogenesis → fibrosis

26-3. All **EXCEPT** which of the following anatomic communications have been described?

   a. Vesicocervical

   b. Ureterouterine

   c. Urethrouterine

   d. Ureterocervical

26-4. All **EXCEPT** which of the following are examples of *complicated* vesicovaginal fistulas?

   a. Concurrent pelvic malignancy

   b. Prior pelvic radiation therapy

   c. Posthysterectomy fistula distant from the vaginal cuff

   d. High posthysterectomy fistula with normal vaginal length

26-5. According to the more comprehensive fistula classification system introduced by Goh in 2004, how would one classify a 2-cm diameter fistula with moderate-to-severe surrounding fibrosis located 5 cm from the external urethral meatus?

   a. Type 1 a i

   b. Type 1 b ii

   c. Type 3 a ii

   d. Type 2 c iii

26-6. In developing countries, most genitourinary fistulas (approximately 90 percent) are attributable to which of the following?

   a. Malignancy

   b. Pelvic surgery

   c. Obstetric trauma

   d. Sexual trauma or foreign body

26-7. In developed countries, most genitourinary fistulas (approximately 90 percent) are attributable to which of the following?

   a. Malignancy

   b. Pelvic surgery

   c. Obstetric trauma

   d. Sexual trauma or foreign body

26-8. Which of the following diagnostic tools or techniques would help identify a ureterovaginal fistula?

   a. Cystourethroscopy

   b. Intravenous pyelogram

   c. Voiding cystourethrogram

   d. "Three-swab" or tampon test with diluted solution of methylene blue instilled (retrograde) into the bladder

26-9. This image is of a normal female voiding cystourethrogram. This modality, when viewed laterally, may help in the diagnosis of all **EXCEPT** which of the following?

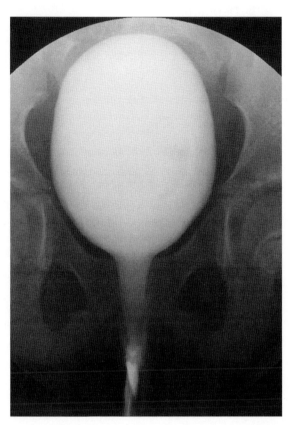

Reproduced, with permission, from Gash JR, Noe J: Radiology of the urinary tract. In Chen MYM, Pop TL, Ott DJ (eds): Basic Radiology, 2nd ed. New York, McGraw-Hill, 2011, Figure 9-14.

a. Urethral diverticulum

b. Vesicovaginal fistula

c. Ureterouterine fistula

d. Urethrovaginal fistula

26-10. Spontaneous healing of a genitourinary fistula via continuous bladder drainage using an indwelling urinary catheter is more likely to happen in which of the following settings?

a. The fistula is large, greater than 2 cm.

b. The fistula is small, 2 to 3 mm.

c. The fistula is related to pelvic radiation.

d. The catheter is left in place for a minimum of 8 weeks.

26-11. Compared with an abdominal (transperitoneal) approach for genitourinary fistula repair, the route of surgery depicted in this figure is associated with which of the following?

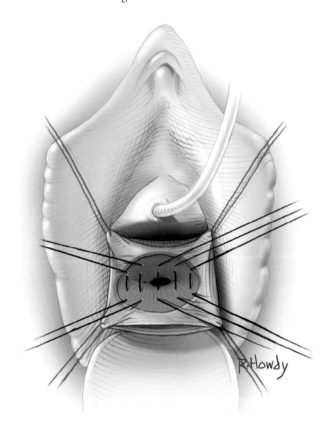

Reproduced, with permission, from Schaffer JI, Hoffman BL: Surgeries for female pelvic reconstruction. In Schorge JO, Schaffer JI, Halvorson LM, et al (eds): Williams Gynecology, 1st ed. New York, McGraw-Hill, 2008, Figure 42-10.3.

a. Greater blood loss

b. Greater operative time

c. Less overall morbidity

d. Increased duration of hospitalization

26-12. Indications for an abdominal approach to genitourinary fistula repair include which of the following?

a. Recurrent fistula

b. Complex or large fistula

c. Concomitant ureteric fistula or fistula in close proximity to ureteral orifices

d. All of the above

26–13. If intervening tissues for surgical closure of a fistula are poorly vascularized and weak, which of the following would be an appropriate intervention?

  a. Use synthetic graft material to reinforce the repair

  b. Consider an abdominal approach with an omental interpositional flap

  c. Abort the procedure in favor of conservative management with a long-term indwelling urinary catheter

  d. All of the above

26–14. In developed countries, urethrovaginal fistulas are most commonly attributed to which of the following?

  a. Obstetric trauma

  b. Pelvic infection

  c. Prior hysterectomy

  d. Prior anterior colporrhaphy or urethral diverticulectomy

26–15. Which of the following statements regarding urethral diverticula is correct?

  a. They commonly are associated with urethral cancer.

  b. They may be associated with infectious urethritis.

  c. They are identified almost exclusively in reproductive-aged women.

  d. They develop with equal frequency in men and women.

26–16. Which of the following statements is true regarding calculi that develop within urethral diverticula?

  a. They result from stagnation of urine and precipitation of salts.

  b. They are usually composed of calcium oxalate or calcium phosphate.

  c. They are associated with approximately 10 percent of urethral diverticula.

  d. All of the above

26–17. Urethral cancers related to urethral diverticula are usually which histologic type?

  a. Sarcomas

  b. Adenocarcinomas

  c. Squamous cell carcinomas

  d. Transitional cell carcinomas

26–18. A predominance of paraurethral glands are found along the which portion of the urethra?

  a. Distal third

  b. Middle third

  c. Proximal third

  d. At the bladder neck

26–19. The communication point between the diverticular ostium and the urethra most commonly occurs at which location?

  a. Midurethra

  b. Distal urethra

  c. Proximal urethra

  d. Mid- and distal urethra with approximately equal frequency

26–20. Among women presenting with symptomatic urethral diverticula, which of the following statements is correct?

  a. Urinary retention is the most common complaint.

  b. The mass is soft and pliable and is almost always nontender.

  c. Associated urinary incontinence or postvoid dribbling is rare, occurring in less than 10 percent of patients.

  d. Dyspareunia may be either with entry or deeper penetration, depending on whether the diverticulum is distal or proximal.

26–21. Cystourethroscopy for the detection of urethral diverticula is best performed with which of the following endoscopes?

  a. 0-degree rigid telescope

  b. 30-degree rigid telescope

  c. 70-degree rigid telescope

  d. 120-degree rigid telescope

26–22. Use of cystourethroscopy for the diagnosis of urethral diverticula is beneficial for all **EXCEPT** which of the following?

  a. May be performed as an office-based procedure

  b. Generally allows for identification of diverticular ostium location

  c. Allows for exclusion of other pathology such as lower urinary tract calculi

  d. Allows for characterization of diverticular size and circumferential extent

26-23. A 51-year-old G3P3 woman presents with voiding difficulties and recurrent bladder infections. A voiding cystourethrogram is performed, and a large, irregular urethral diverticulum is identified (*arrow*). Which of the statements is true regarding this diagnostic modality?

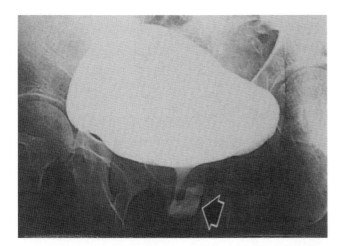

Reproduced, with permission, from Gerst SR, Hricak H: Radiology of the urinary tract. In Tanagho EA, McAninch JW (eds): Smith's General Urology, 17th ed. New York, McGraw-Hill, 2008, Figure 6-13B.

a. Is no longer available in most hospital centers

b. Is painful for patients and complicated to perform

c. Requires exposure of the patient to ionizing radiation

d. Is more sensitive for detection of diverticula compared with positive-pressure urethrography

26-24. Which of the following is true regarding magnetic resonance imaging of periurethral pathology?

a. Requires ionizing radiation and contrast exposure

b. Is generally less expensive than other imaging modalities

c. Has limited utility in identifying location, extent, and internal characteristics of masses

d. Has comparable or superior sensitivity for detecting urethral diverticula compared with other imaging modalities

26-25. The procedure depicted here places patients at risk for which of the following?

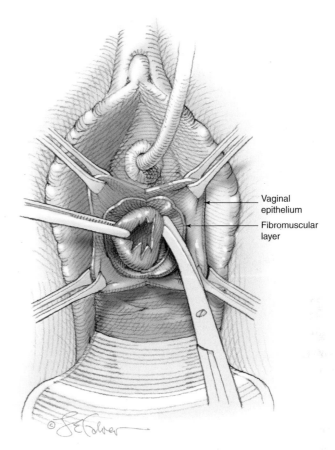

Vaginal epithelium

Fibromuscular layer

Reproduced, with permission, from Schaffer JI, Hoffman BL: Surgeries for female pelvic reconstruction. In Schorge JO, Schaffer JI, Halvorson LM, et al (eds): Williams Gynecology, 1st ed. New York, McGraw-Hill, 2008, Figure 42-9.3.

a. Urinary leakage

b. Urethral stenosis

c. Urethrovaginal fistula

d. All of the above

Reference:

Goh JT: A new classification for female genital tract fistula. Aust N Z J Obstet Gynaecol 44:502, 2004

Chapter 26   ANSWER KEY

Question number	Letter answer	Page cited	Header cited	Question number	Letter answer	Page cited	Header cited
26–1	a	p. 677	Genitourinary Fistula	26–14	d	p. 683	Urethrovaginal and Other Genitourinary Fistulas
26–2	a	p. 677	Pathophysiology	26–15	b	p. 683	Urethral Diverticulum
26–3	c	p. 678	Table 26-1	26–16	d	p. 685	Calculi
26–4	d	p. 677	Classification	26–17	b	p. 685	Cancer
26–5	b	p. 679	Table 26-3	26–18	b	p. 685	Classification
26–6	c	p. 678	Obstetric Trauma	26–19	a	p. 685	Classification
26–7	b	p. 679	Pelvic Surgery	26–20	d	p. 686	Signs and Symptoms
26–8	b	p. 680	Diagnosis	26–21	a	p. 686	Cystourethroscopy
26–9	c	p. 681	Diagnosis	26–22	d	p. 686	Cystourethroscopy
26–10	b	p. 681	Conservative Treatment	26–23	c	p. 687	Voiding Cystourethrogram
26–11	c	p. 682	Route of Repair, Vaginal	26–24	d	p. 688	Magnetic Resonance Imaging
26–12	d	p. 682	Route of Repair, Abdominal	26–25	d	p. 688	Surgical
26–13	b	p. 682	Interpositional Flaps				

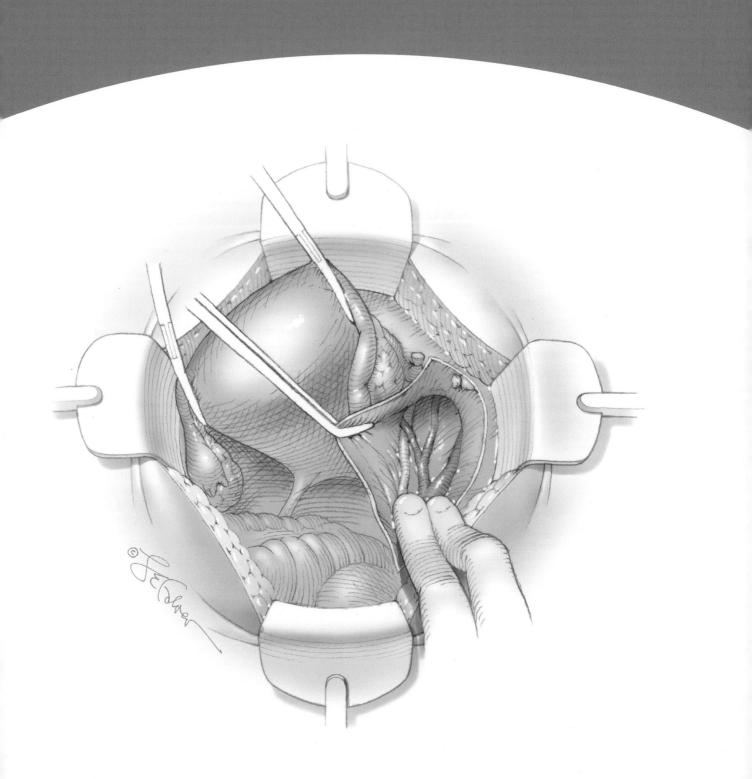

CHAPTER 27

Principles of Chemotherapy

27-1. Compared with normal cells within the same tissue, tumor cells have which characteristic that leaves them more vulnerable to chemotherapy?

  a. Greater cell membrane permeability

  b. Faster completion of the cell cycle

  c. Slower completion of the cell cycle

  d. A greater percentage of cells progressing through the cell cycle

27-2. Cells in which phase of the cell cycle are **LEAST** sensitive to chemotherapeutic agents?

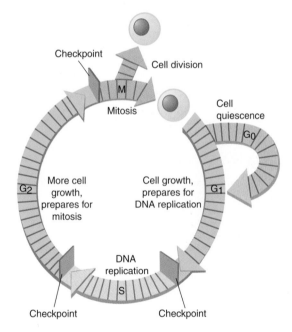

Reproduced, with permission, from Nguyen PD: Principles of Radiation Therapy. In Hoffman BL, Schorge JO, Schaffer JI, et al (eds): Williams Gynecology, 2nd ed. New York, McGraw-Hill, 2012, Figure 28-8.

  a. S

  b. G_0

  c. G_1

  d. G_2

27-3. Which of the following tumor qualities decreases a tumor's susceptibility to chemotherapy?

  a. Metastatic lesion

  b. Slow doubling time

  c. High growth fraction

  d. No gross residual disease after debulking surgery

27-4. Which term is used to describe drugs that can kill at several cell cycle phases?

  a. Omnicyclic

  b. Generational

  c. Broad spectrum

  d. Cell cycle nonspecific

27-5. Which term is used to describe chemotherapy used as primary treatment of advanced malignancy when no feasible alternative treatment exists?

  a. Salvage

  b. Adjuvant

  c. Induction

  d. Neoadjuvant

27-6. Which term is used to describe chemotherapy used preoperatively to decrease the extent of subsequent resection?

  a. Salvage

  b. Adjuvant

  c. Induction

  d. Neoadjuvant

27-7. Combination chemotherapy is commonly used to provide maximum cell kill. When drugs are selected, agents should have which of the following characteristics?

  a. Overlapping toxicities

  b. Similar mechanisms of action

  c. Effectiveness as a sole agent

  d. Lower dosages required when used solely

27-8. Patients with advanced endometrial cancer may receive both adjuvant chemotherapy and radiation. Which of the following is true when patients are treated with both modalities?

  a. Toxicity is increased.

  b. A decrease in chemotherapy dose due to toxicity is seldom required.

  c. Tumor within a previously irradiated field is more sensitive to chemotherapy.

  d. All of the above

27–9. Most chemotherapy drugs are typically dosed using what patient parameter?

a. Height

b. Weight

c. Body mass index

d. Body surface area

27–10. Intraperitoneal chemotherapy efficacy may be limited by all **EXCEPT** which of the following?

a. Ascites

b. Slower drug clearance than intravenous administration

c. Intraabdominal adhesions

d. Fibrotic tumor encapsulation

27–11. Special care should be taken if administering a chemotherapeutic agent capable of causing skin ulceration and tissue necrosis. Which term describes this group?

a. Irritant

b. Vesicant

c. Exfoliant

d. Inflammant

27–12. Which of the following chemotherapeutic agents is considered a vesicant?

a. Etoposide

b. Methotrexate

c. Dactinomycin

d. Cyclophosphamide

27–13. In defining chemotherapy response, a decrease of at least 30 percent in the sum of diameters of all target lesions is termed which of the following?

a. Progression

b. Stable disease

c. Partial response

d. Complete response

27–14. Methotrexate binds tightly to which enzyme to exert its antimetabolite effects?

a. Topoisomerase

b. RNA polymerase

c. Dihydrofolate reductase

d. Receptor tyrosine kinase

27–15. In the United States, methotrexate is commonly used as a sole primary agent to treat which of the following?

a. Partial mole

b. Complete mole

c. Gestational trophoblastic neoplasia

d. All of the above

27–16. Concurrent leucovorin administration in women treated with methotrexate achieves which of the following goals?

a. Decreases drug clearance

b. Minimizes myelosuppression

c. Expands cell-cycle specificity

d. Enhances tumor radiosensitivity

27–17. Cyclophosphamide and ifosfamide have which of the following classic side effects, which is paired with the pretreatment agent used to attenuate this problem?

a. Anemia; leucovorin

b. Neuropathy; amifostine

c. Hemorrhagic cystitis; mesna

d. Ovarian suppression; gonadotropin-releasing hormone agonist

27–18. Your patient is a 25-year-old G1P0A1 who underwent dilatation and curettage for treatment of the condition shown here. During postoperative surveillance, low-risk gestational trophoblastic neoplasia is diagnosed. Which of the following is a suitable single agent for primary treatment?

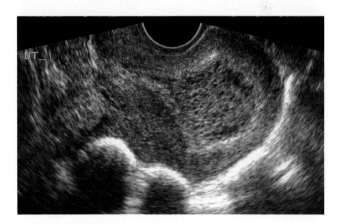

a. Cisplatin

b. Doxorubicin

c. Gemcitabine

d. Dactinomycin

27–19. These preoperative images show a tumor-enlarged uterus and para-aortic node involvement. Which combination of agents is commonly used as adjuvant treatment of advanced endometrial cancer?

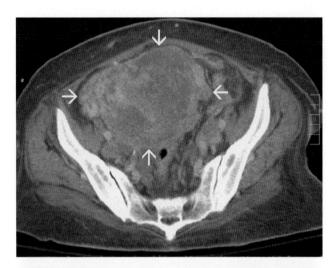

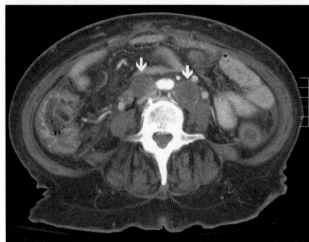

Images contributed by Dr. Diane Twickler. Reproduced, with permission, from Miller DS, Schorge JO: Endometrial cancer. In Schorge JO, Schaffer JI, Halvorson LM, et al (eds): Williams Gynecology, 1st ed. New York, McGraw-Hill, 2008, Figure 33-5.

    a. Cisplatin, ifosfamide

    b. Taxol, Adriamycin, cisplatin (TAP)

    c. Bleomycin, etoposide, cisplatin (BEP)

    d. Etoposide, methotrexate, Adriamycin D, cyclophosphamide, Oncovin (EMA-CO)

27–20. Which combination of agents is commonly used as adjuvant treatment of advanced epithelial ovarian cancer? Extensive omental involvement is seen here.

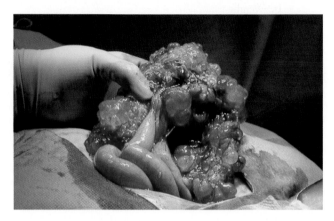

Reproduced, with permission, from Schorge JO: Epithelial ovarian cancer. In Schorge JO, Schaffer JI, Halvorson LM, et al (eds): Williams Gynecology, 1st ed. New York, McGraw-Hill, 2008, Figure 35-16.

    a. Carboplatin, paclitaxel

    b. Taxol, Adriamycin, cisplatin (TAP)

    c. Bleomycin, etoposide, cisplatin (BEP)

    d. Etoposide, methotrexate, Adriamycin D, cyclophosphamide, Oncovin (EMA-CO)

27–21. Which of the following is used commonly as a radiosensitizing agent in the primary treatment of cervical cancer such as the clinical stage 1B2 cancer shown here?

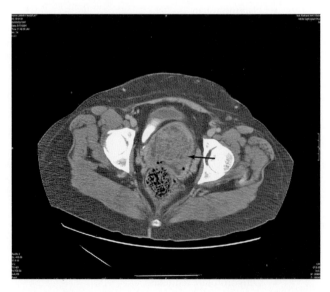

Photograph contributed by Dr. John Schorge. Reproduced, with permission, from Lea JS: Cervical cancer. In Schorge JO, Schaffer JI, Halvorson LM, et al (eds): Williams Gynecology, 1st ed. New York, McGraw-Hill, 2008, Figure 30-14.

    a. Cisplatin

    b. Doxorubicin

    c. Gemcitabine

    d. Dactinomycin

27–22. Risks and side effects of tamoxifen include all **EXCEPT** which of the following?

   a. Osteoporosis

   b. Thromboembolism

   c. Endometrial cancer

   d. Vasomotor symptoms

27–23. Which of the following biologic agents does not have VEGF as a direct or indirect target of action?

   a. Sunitinib

   b. Bevacizumab

   c. Poly(ADP) ribose polymerase (PARP) inhibitor

   d. Mammalian target of rapamycin (mTOR) inhibitor

27–24. Which of the following agents commonly used in gynecologic oncology is associated with a high risk for nausea and vomiting?

   a. Bleomycin

   b. Cisplatin

   c. Etoposide

   d. Paclitaxel

27–25. Which of the following is an agent used to stimulate granulocyte production in those with chemotherapy-induced neutropenia?

   a. Leucovorin

   b. Filgrastim

   c. Darbepoetin alfa

   d. None of the above

Chapter 27 ANSWER KEY

Question number	Letter answer	Page cited	Header cited	Question number	Letter answer	Page cited	Header cited
27–1	d	p. 692	The Cell Cycle	**27–14**	c	p. 698	Methotrexate
27–2	b	p. 692	The Cell Cycle	**27–15**	c	p. 698	Methotrexate
27–3	b	p. 692	Cancer Cell Growth; Doubling Time	**27–16**	b	p. 698	Prescribing Information and Toxicity
27–4	d	p. 694	Cell Kinetics	**27–17**	c	p. 699	Alkylating Agents
27–5	c	p. 694	Clinical Setting	**27–18**	d	p. 700	Dactinomycin
27–6	d	p. 694	Clinical Setting	**27–19**	b	p. 701	Doxorubicin
27–7	c	p. 694	Combination Therapy	**27–20**	a	p. 704	Carboplatin
27–8	a	p. 694	Multimodality Treatment	**27–21**	a	p. 705	Cisplatin
27–9	d	p. 695	Drug Dosing	**27–22**	a	p. 705	Tamoxifen
27–10	b	p. 696	Route of Administration	**27–23**	c	p. 706	Biological and Targeted Therapy
27–11	b	p. 696	Table 27-2	**27–24**	b	p. 708	Table 27-10
27–12	c	p. 696	Table 27-2	**27–25**	b	p. 709	Filgrastim
27–13	c	p. 697	Evaluating Response to Chemotherapy				

CHAPTER 28

Principles of Radiation Therapy

28-1. In gynecology, radiation therapy is most commonly used for which of the following?

   a. Cervical cancer

   b. Endometrial cancer

   c. Epithelial ovarian cancer

   d. Gestational trophoblastic neoplasia

28-2. Which is a clinically used radionuclide?

   a. Cobalt-60

   b. Iodine-125

   c. Cesium-137

   d. All of the above

28-3. Linear accelerators can produce which of the following?

   a. Photon and electron beams

   b. Photon beams and gamma rays

   c. Neutron beams and gamma rays

   d. Electron beams and gamma rays

28-4. When electromagnetic radiation impacts target tissues, this energy is transferred to the target tissues by several mechanisms. Which of the following mechanisms is shown here?

28-5. For treatment of inguinal lymph node metastasis, which of the following modalities is preferred due to its energy-transfer properties?

   a. Photon beam therapy

   b. Electron beam therapy

   c. Intracavity brachytherapy

   d. Interstitial brachytherapy

28-6. When quantifying the absorbed dose of electromagnetic radiation, which of the following units of measure is currently preferred?

   a. Rad

   b. Gray

   c. Curie

   d. Becquerel

28-7. Within irradiated tissues, which of the following is the effective biologic target?

   a. DNA

   b. Ribosomes

   c. Mitochondria

   d. Endoplasmic reticulum

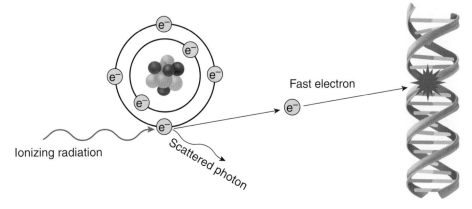

Reproduced, with permission, from Nguyen PD: Principles of Radiation Therapy. In Hoffman BL, Schorge JO, Schaffer JI, et al (eds): Williams Gynecology, 2nd ed. New York, McGraw-Hill, 2012, Figure 28-4B.

   a. Poiseuille law

   b. Compton effect

   c. Werner equation

   d. Bernoulli principle

28-8. With radiation therapy, most tissue damage is caused by electromagnetic radiation impacting water to create which DNA-damaging molecule?

a. Nitric oxide

b. Carboxyl group

c. Hydroxyl radical

d. Hydrogen peroxide

28-9. The four Rs of radiation biology include which of the following?

a. Reassortment

b. Recavitation

c. Recolumnization

d. Restandardization

28-10. Radiation therapy simulation allows which of the following?

a. Maximize radiation dose to tumor

b. Minimize damage to late-responding normal tissue

c. Minimize damage to early-responding normal tissue

d. All of the above

28-11. By definition, during which of the following are radionuclides inserted directly into the cancer?

a. Interstitial brachytherapy

b. Intracavitary brachytherapy

c. Intralymphatic brachytherapy

d. Intraperitoneal brachytherapy

28-12. During brachytherapy with tandem and ovoid use, the tandem fits into which of the following?

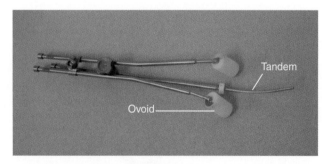

Reproduced, with permission, from Nguyen PD: Principles of radiation therapy. In Schorge JO, Schaffer JI, Halvorson LM, et al (eds): Williams Gynecology, 1st ed. New York, McGraw-Hill, 2008, Figure 28-10.

a. Vagina

b. Uterus

c. Rectum

d. Posterior cul-de sac

28-13. The factor that most commonly leads to poor tumor control achieved by radiotherapy includes which of the following?

a. Hypertension

b. Hyperglycemia

c. Tissue hypoxia

d. Hyperlipidemia

28-14. In combination, carbogen and which other agent are used to improve tissue oxygenation and responsiveness to radiotherapy?

a. Nicotinamide

b. Nitric oxide

c. Nitroprusside

d. Nitroglycerin

28-15. For patients undergoing radiotherapy, improved tumor control has been associated with which of the following?

a. Hypertension control

b. Heparin anticoagulation

c. Antibiotic administration

d. Blood transfusion for anemia

28-16. Radiation therapy combined with cisplatin chemotherapy is the standard treatment for newly diagnosed, locally advanced cases of which cancer type?

a. Cervical

b. Clear cell endometrial cancer

c. Nongestational choriocarcinoma

d. None of the above

28-17. Regarding their response to radiotherapy, early-responding tissues include which of the following?

a. Lung

b. Brain

c. Kidney

d. Bone marrow

28-18. Long-term consequences of radiotherapy include which of the following?

a. Ovarian failure

b. Secondary malignancy

c. Vesicovaginal fistula

d. All of the above

28-19. An early skin response to radiotherapy includes which of the following?

    a. Necrosis

    b. Erythema

    c. Ichthyosis

    d. Depigmentation

28-20. Immediate vaginal changes following radiotherapy may include which of the following?

    a. Mucositis

    b. Synechiae

    c. Shortening

    d. None of the above

28-21. In premenopausal women, which of the following has been shown to reduce radiation exposure to the ovaries during treatment of gynecologic cancer?

    a. Omental flap overlay

    b. Ovarian transposition

    c. Ovarian transplantation

    d. None of the above

28-22. Following pelvic radiation, early bladder response includes which of the following?

    a. Fistula

    b. Cystitis

    c. Stone formation

    d. All of the above

28-23. Which of the following is commonly used to effectively relieve acute bladder symptoms from radiotherapy?

    a. Oxybutynin

    b. Prednisone

    c. Nitroglycerin

    d. Phenylpropanolamine

28-24. This patient suffered a postradiation small bowel obstruction. Preventative approaches to minimize radiotherapy-associated bowel injury include administration of which of the following?

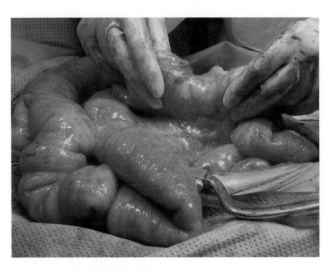

Photograph contributed by Dr. David Miller.

    a. Sulfasalazine

    b. Erythropoietin

    c. Hyperbaric oxygen

    d. Third-generation cephalosporin

28-25. Later effects of radiotherapy on the rectosigmoid include all **EXCEPT** which of the following?

    a. Fistula

    b. Stricture

    c. Hemorrhage

    d. Diverticulum

28-26. For a cancer to be considered the secondary result of radiotherapy, which of the following criteria must be met?

    a. Cancer should develop outside the irradiated area.

    b. Cancer differs from the original tumor pathology type.

    c. Cancer develops within the first year following treatment.

    d. None of the above

Chapter 28   ANSWER KEY

Question number	Letter answer	Page cited	Header cited	Question number	Letter answer	Page cited	Header cited
28–1	a	p. 712	Introduction	28–15	d	p. 723	Blood Transfusion
28–2	d	p. 714	Table 28-2	28–16	a	p. 723	Combination of Ionizing Radiation and Chemotherapy
28–3	a	p. 714	Linear Accelerator (Linac)				
28–4	b	p. 715	Figure 28-4	28–17	d	p. 725	Normal Tissue Response to Radiation Therapy
28–5	b	p. 716	Depth-dose Curve				
28–6	b	p. 716	Radiation Unit	28–18	d	p. 725	Normal Tissue Response to Radiation Therapy
28–7	a	p. 716	Direct versus Indirect Actions of Ionizing Radiation				
				28–19	b	p. 725	Skin
28–8	c	p. 716	Direct versus Indirect Actions of Ionizing Radiation	28–20	a	p. 725	Vagina
				28–21	b	p. 726	Ovary and Pregnancy Outcomes
28–9	a	p. 718	Five Rs of Radiation Biology				
28–10	d	p. 720	External Beam Radiation Therapy	28–22	b	p. 726	Bladder
				28–23	a	p. 726	Bladder
28–11	a	p. 721	Intracavitary, Interstitial, and Intraperitoneal Brachytherapy	28–24	a	p. 726	Small Bowel
				28–25	d	p. 726	Rectosigmoid
28–12	b	p. 721	Equipment	28–26	b	p. 727	Radiation-Induced Carcinogenesis
28–13	c	p. 723	Tumor Hypoxia				
28–14	a	p. 723	Hyperbaric Oxygen				

CHAPTER 29

Preinvasive Lesions of the Lower Genital Tract

29-1. The location of the cervical squamocolumnar junction (SCJ) varies with age and hormonal status. The SCJ tends to move outward onto the ectocervix, as in the example below, with which of the following conditions?

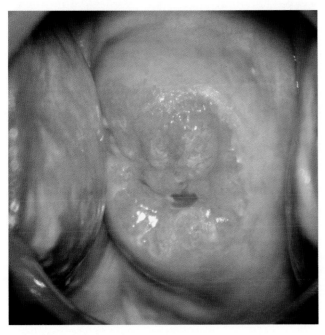

Reproduced, with permission, from Cunningham FG, Leveno KL, Bloom SL et al (eds): Williams Obstetrics, 23rd ed. New York, McGraw-Hill, 2010, Figure 5-1.

   a. Menopause

   b. Pregnancy

   c. Prolonged lactation

   d. Use of progestin-only contraceptives

29-2. All **EXCEPT** which of the following are true statements regarding the cervical transformation zone (TZ)?

   a. Squamous metaplasia occurring within the TZ is abnormal.

   b. Most cervical neoplasia arises within the TZ.

   c. The TZ lies between the original squamous epithelium and columnar epithelium of the cervix.

   d. The location and size of the TZ changes through the process of squamous metaplasia.

29-3. *L1* and *L2*, which are the two late genes of the human papillomavirus (HPV), encode proteins responsible for which of the following?

   a. Capsid construction

   b. Regulatory functions

   c. DNA synthesis and replication

   d. Conformational changes aiding entry into the host cell

29-4. More than 100 human papillomavirus (HPV) types have been identified to date. Clinically, HPV types are classified as high risk (HR) or low risk based upon their oncogenic potential. Which two HR HPV types together account for approximately 70 percent of cervical cancers worldwide?

   a. 6 and 11

   b. 11 and 45

   c. 16 and 18

   d. 18 and 31

29-5. Which of the following is the **LEAST** common outcome of cervical human papillomavirus (HPV) infection?

   a. Condylomata

   b. Latent infection

   c. Subclinical infection

   d. Neoplasia (dysplasia or cancer)

29-6. A 40-year-old woman has been in a mutually monogamous relationship for 25 years. She is upset that her recent Pap test result is low-grade squamous intraepithelial neoplasia (LSIL), consistent with human papillomavirus (HPV) changes. HPV infection is reliably diagnosed by which of the following clinical tests?

   a. Cytology

   b. Histology

   c. Colposcopy

   d. HPV DNA testing

29-7. Which of the following is true of the two prophylactic human papillomavirus (HPV) vaccines currently available?

    a. They require one initial dose followed by a booster dose 2 years later.

    b. Both use HPV type-specific virus-like particles to induce immunity.

    c. They are theoretically protective against the HPV types that account for 90% of cervical cancers.

    d. They are Food and Drug Administration (FDA) approved for the prevention of cervical, vulvar, and vaginal neoplasia.

29-8. What approximate percentage of women in the United States who undergo cervical cancer screening will have an abnormal cervical cytology result?

    a. 1

    b. 7

    c. 11

    d. 17

29-9. The natural history of cervical intraepithelial neoplasia (CIN) lesions is better known than in the past. Respectively, what percentages of CIN 1 lesions are expected to spontaneously regress and progress to invasive malignancy without treatment?

    a. 60, 1

    b. 50, 5

    c. 40, 10

    d. 20, 15

29-10. A 22-year-old woman with a low-grade squamous intraepithelial neoplasia (LSIL) Pap result is subsequently diagnosed with cervical intraepithelial neoplasia (CIN) 2 by colposcopy (as shown) and directed biopsy. Colposcopy is satisfactory, and the endocervical curettage is negative for dysplasia or cancer. She is given the option of undergoing treatment or observation. She should be counseled that CIN 2 may spontaneously regress without treatment. Approximately what percentage of CIN 2 shows spontaneous regression?

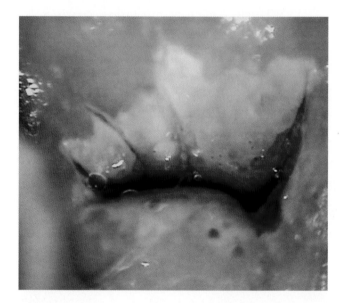

    a. 20

    b. 40

    c. 60

    d. 80

29-11. A 42-year-old multipara has negative screening Pap test and positive human papillomavirus (HPV) DNA test results. These were repeated 1 year later with the same results. She is a long-time cigarette smoker and has had six lifetime sexual partners. She has not had a new sexual partner for 7 years. What is her strongest risk factor for cervical cancer?

    a. Parity

    b. Tobacco use

    c. Persistent HPV infection

    d. Multiple lifetime sexual partners

29-12. Cervical cytology screening is one of modern medicine's success stories. Although the sensitivity of an individual Pap test is imperfect, organized screening programs have generally decreased the incidence of cervical cancer by what percentage?

  a. 20 to 30

  b. 40 to 50

  c. 60 to 70

  d. 80 to 90

29-13. Clinical studies have conclusively shown which of the following to be increased by liquid-based Pap tests compared with conventional (glass slide) Pap testing?

  a. Cost

  b. Sensitivity

  c. Specificity

  d. Cervical cancers prevented

29-14. Which of the following patients should be offered initiation of cervical cancer screening according to 2009 American College of Obstetricians and Gynecologists (ACOG) guidelines?

  a. 19-year-old female who has never been sexually active

  b. 17-year-old female with multiple sexual partners since age 14 years

  c. 18-year-old female who has one lifetime partner and who has recently been diagnosed with human immunodeficiency virus (HIV) infection

  d. 20-year-old primigravida who present for her first prenatal examination and who has been sexually active with her first partner for 1 year

29-15. Based on 2009 American College of Obstetricians and Gynecologists (ACOG) guidelines, at what interval should a 52-year-old woman undergo cervical cancer cytologic screening if she has an average risk for this cancer and if her three previous, consecutive Pap test results are negative?

  a. Annually

  b. Every 2 years

  c. Every 3 years

  d. Every 5 years

29-16. For which of the following women would discontinuation of cervical cancer screening be acceptable? All of their Pap tests to date have been negative and performed at intervals adherent to current screening guidelines.

  a. 42-year-old woman with past hysterectomy for leiomyomas

  b. 72-year-old woman in good health with one long-standing sexual partner

  c. 55-year-old woman with metastatic breast cancer refusing further therapeutic cancer interventions

  d. All of the above are reasonable candidates for discontinuation of cervical cancer screening.

29-17. Your patient is a healthy 38-year-old woman with a history of total hysterectomy 1 year ago for uterine leiomyomas and menorrhagia. She has no prior history of abnormal Pap test results or lower genital tract neoplasia. She smokes cigarettes and has a new sexual partner. Her physical examination is without abnormalities. Which of the following strategies for prevention of lower genital tract neoplasia is indicated?

  a. Vaginal cytology every 3 years

  b. Vaginal cytology and human papillomavirus (HPV) DNA testing every 3 years

  c. Vaccination against high-risk HPV infection (types 16 and 18)

  d. Discontinue screening for neoplasia with Pap tests or HPV DNA testing

29-18. Which of the following is an appropriate clinical use of human papillomavirus (HPV) DNA testing according to current evidence-based guidelines?

  a. Determine eligibility for HPV vaccination in females aged 9 to 26 years

  b. Cervical cancer screening of women aged 30 years and older in conjunction with cervical cytology

  c. Reflex testing of atypical glandular cell Pap results to determine triage for further evaluation

  d. Cervical testing for posttreatment surveillance 4 to 6 weeks after ablation or excision with negative margins

29-19. A 42-year-old patient with normal, cyclic menses is referred for colposcopy for an "AGC (atypical glandular cells), not otherwise specified" Pap result. Your evaluation of her should include which of the following?

  a. Colposcopy

  b. Human papillomavirus (HPV) DNA test

  c. Endometrial biopsy

  d. All of the above

29–20. Deferral of colposcopy should be considered for which of the following conditions?

   a. Mucopurulent cervicitis

   b. Anticoagulation for a mechanical heart valve

   c. Unscheduled, intermenstrual bleeding on the day of examination

   d. Last menstrual period began 20 days ago; negative urine pregnancy test; condoms for contraception

29–21. A 32-year-old presents for evaluation of an abnormal Pap test result. This is a colpophotograph of her cervix before and after application of 5-percent acetic acid. It does **NOT** demonstrate which of the following?

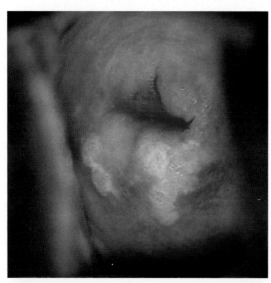

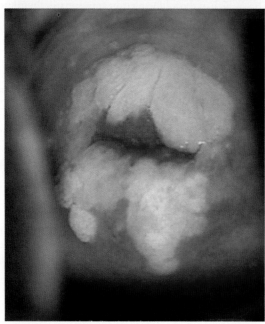

   a. Acetowhite change

   b. Columnar epithelium

   c. Squamous epithelium

   d. Unsatisfactory colposcopy

29–22. Your patient is a 45-year-old with a Pap test result of high-grade squamous intraepithelial lesion (HSIL). Subsequent colposcopy is unsatisfactory due to incomplete visualization of the squamocolumnar junction. Cervical biopsy confirms a CIN 3 lesion; there is also histologic CIN 2 present in the endocervical curettage specimen. Which of the following is the most appropriate procedure for further diagnosis and/or treatment?

   a. Cryosurgery

   b. Hysterectomy

   c. Loop excision

   d. Laser ablation

29–23. A 27-year-old nulligravida is referred to you for evaluation of a Pap test result indicating low-grade squamous intraepithelial neoplasia (LSIL). Colposcopy is negative for lesions, but vaginal lesions (shown here) are observed in numerous locations along the vaginal walls after application of 5-percent acetic acid. A biopsy of a representative lesion shows features characteristic of human papillomavirus (HPV) infection and low-grade vaginal intraepithelial neoplasia (VaIN 1). The patient is asymptomatic. Which of the following is the best option for management of these vaginal lesions?

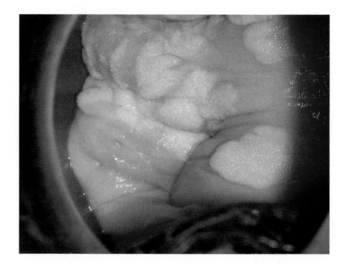

   a. Observation

   b. Laser ablation

   c. HPV vaccination

   d. Intravaginal fluorouracil (5-FU) cream

29–24. A 48-year-old multiparous woman presents with a vulvar lesion and itching and burning. She estimates that it has been present and growing in size and number for the past 2 years. She has no medical problems but is a heavy cigarette smoker. She was treated for cervical intraepithelial neoplasia (CIN) 3 in the past. Her lesion (shown here) is most likely histologically to show which of the following?

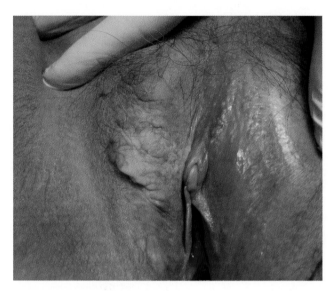

Photograph contributed by Dr. David Miller.

a. Paget disease

b. Condyloma acuminata

c. Squamous cell hyperplasia

d. Vulvar intraepithelial neoplasia (VIN) 3

29–25. Which of the following are risk factors for anal intraepithelial neoplasia, seen here with high-resolution anoscopy?

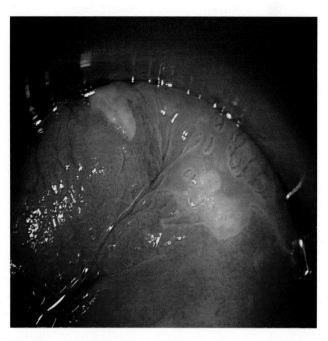

Photography contributed by Naomi Jay, RN, NP, PhD. Reproduced, with permission, from Werner CL, Griffith WF: Preinvasive lesions of the lower genital tract. In Schorge JO, Schaffer JI, Halvorson LM, et al (eds): Williams Gynecology, 1st ed. New York, McGraw-Hill, 2008, Figure 29-17.

a. Human immunodeficiency virus (HIV) infection

b. Tobacco smoking

c. Anal receptive intercourse

d. All of the above

Reference:

American College of Obstetricians and Gynecologists: Cervical cytology screening. Practice Bulletin No. 109, December 2009.

Chapter 29 ANSWER KEY

Question number	Letter answer	Page cited	Header cited	Question number	Letter answer	Page cited	Header cited
29–1	b	p. 732	Squamocolumnar Junction	**29–15**	c	p. 742	Screening Interval
29–2	a	p. 733	Squamous Metaplasia	**29–16**	d	p. 743	Discontinuation of Screening
29–3	a	p. 734	HPV Life Cycle	**29–17**	d	p. 743	Hysterectomy
29–4	c	p. 734	HPV Types	**29–18**	b	p. 743	Cytology and HPV Cotesting
29–5	d	p. 735	Outcomes of HPV Infection	**29–19**	d	p. 746	Glandular Cell Abnormalities
29–6	d	p. 736	Diagnosis of HPV Infection				
29–7	b	p. 737	Prophylactic HPV Vaccines	**29–20**	a	p. 747	Preparation; Biopsy
29–8	b	p. 738	Incidence	**29–21**	d	p. 750	Satisfactory Colposcopy
29–9	a	p. 738	Table 29-1	**29–22**	c	p. 753	Excisional Treatment Modalities
29–10	b	p. 738	Natural History	**29–23**	a	p. 755	Low-Grade Vaginal Intraepithelial Neoplasia
29–11	c	p. 738	Risk Factors				
29–12	c	p. 740	Efficacy of Cervical Cancer Screening				
29–13	a	p. 741	Comparison of Conventional and Liquid-Based Cytology	**29–24**	d	p. 758	Vulvoscopy
29–14	c	p. 742	Initiation of Screening	**29–25**	d	p. 761	Risk Factors

CHAPTER 30

Cervical Cancer

30-1. Which human papillomavirus (HPV) subtype is most commonly associated with adenocarcinoma of the cervix?

    a. HPV 6

    b. HPV 16

    c. HPV 18

    d. HPV 31

30-2. Which of the following is associated with a higher risk of squamous cell carcinoma of the cervix but not adenocarcinoma of the cervix?

    a. Smoking

    b. Age at first intercourse

    c. Number of lifetime sexual partners

    d. Combination oral contraceptive pills

30-3. The protein product of the human papillomavirus (HPV) E6 oncogene binds to which of the following tumor-suppressor proteins? After binding, the tumor-suppressor protein is degraded and leads to immortalization of the cell.

    a. Rb

    b. p16

    c. p53

    d. Cyclin D1

30-4. Which histologic subtype is represented in the micrograph?

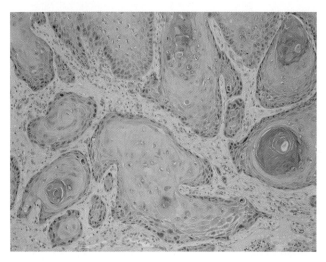

Photograph contributed by Dr. Kelley Carrick.

    a. Melanoma

    b. Adenocarcinoma

    c. Squamous cell carcinoma

    d. Neuroendocrine carcinoma

30-5. Which of the following should not be used for hemostasis in cases of life-threatening hemorrhage from cervical cancer?

    a. Lugol solution

    b. Emergent radiation

    c. Uterine artery embolization

    d. Monsel (ferric subsulfate) solution

30-6. In patients with stage I cervical cancer, what percentage of their Pap smears are read as cancer?

    a. 10

    b. 20

    c. 50

    d. 80

30-7. A woman comes in for an annual gynecologic examination. During speculum examination, you see the following. What is the most appropriate next step?

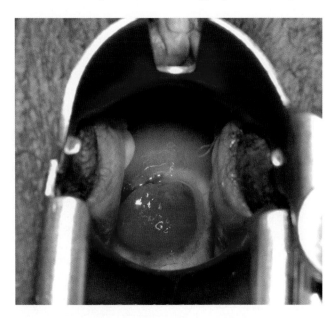

a. Perform a pap smear

b. Perform a cervical biopsy

c. Refer to a gynecologic oncologist

d. Obtain a computed tomography (CT) scan

30-8. A woman undergoes a radical hysterectomy with bilateral pelvic and para-aortic lymph node dissection for a 4-cm squamous cell carcinoma. On final pathologic evaluation of the surgical specimen, the parametria are positive for cancer involvement. Based on these findings, which International Federation of Gynecology and Obstetrics (FIGO) clinical stage is she assigned?

a. IB1

b. IB2

c. IIA1

d. IIB2

30-9. Which of the following tests cannot be used for staging cervical cancer per International Federation of Gynecology and Obstetrics (FIGO) criteria?

a. Cystoscopy

b. Chest radiograph

c. Computed tomography

d. Intravenous pyelogram

30-10. A woman has a 6-cm adenocarcinoma of the cervix, positive para-aortic nodes found on positron emission tomography (PET) scan, and hydronephrosis. Based on these findings, which FIGO stage is she assigned?

a. IB2

b. IIB

c. IIIB

d. IVB

30-11. What is the most significant prognostic factor for early stage cervical cancer?

a. Grade

b. Histology

c. Depth of invasion

d. Lymph node metastasis

30-12. What is the most appropriate surgical procedure for a woman who has completed childbearing with a stage IA1 squamous cell carcinoma of the cervix?

a. Cold knife conization

b. Extrafascial hysterectomy

c. Type III radical hysterectomy

d. Modified (type II) radical hysterectomy

30-13. What is the most appropriate treatment for a 30-year-old G1P1 with stage IA1 adenocarcinoma of the cervix who desires future fertility?

a. Trachelectomy

b. Cold knife conization

c. Extrafascial hysterectomy and later, gestational surrogacy

d. Modified (type II) radical hysterectomy and later, gestational surrogacy

30–14. For a 37-year-old woman who has completed child-bearing, you perform cold knife conization for CIN 3 found in ectocervical biopsies and in endocervical curettage (ECC) samples. The specimen is shown in the photograph, with a stitch at 12:00. The final pathologic analysis reveals a grade 2 invasive squamous cell carcinoma, with a depth of invasion of 2 mm and a width of 8 mm, and CIN 3 at the margins. What is the most appropriate next step?

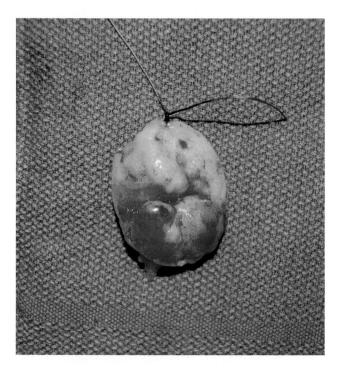

Photograph contributed by Dr. Sasha Andrews.

    a. Extrafascial hysterectomy

    b. Type III radical hysterectomy

    c. Repeat cold knife conization and ECC

    d. Radiation with concomitant chemotherapy

30–15. Where is the uterine artery ligated during a type III radical hysterectomy?

    a. At the uterine isthmus

    b. At the level of the ureter

    c. At the origin of the uterine artery

    d. At the level of the uterosacral ligament

30–16. Which of the following arrows depicts where the uterosacral ligament is ligated during a type II radical hysterectomy?

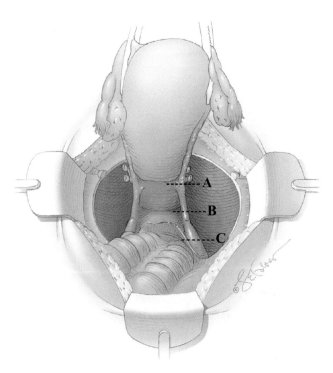

Reproduced, with permission, from Schorge JO: Surgeries for gynecologic malignancies. In Schorge JO, Schaffer JI, Halvorson LM, et al (eds): Williams Gynecology, 1st ed. New York, McGraw-Hill, 2008, Figure 43-2.3.

    a. A

    b. B

    c. C

    d. None of the above

30–17. Patients with which of the following would not require adjuvant chemoradiation after radical hysterectomy and lymph node dissection?

    a. Positive parametria

    b. Positive lymph nodes

    c. 3-cm tumor with deep-third stromal invasion and lymphovascular space invasion

    d. 4-cm tumor with inner-third stromal invasion and no lymphovascular space invasion

30-18. Which of the following patients should be treated with chemoradiation rather than radical hysterectomy for a stage IB1 squamous cell carcinoma of the cervix (shown here)?

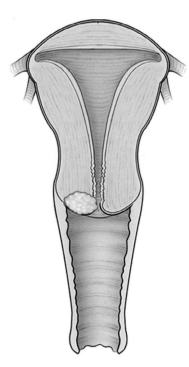

Reproduced, with permission, from Richardson DL: Cervical cancer. In Hoffman BL, Schorge JO, Schaffer JI, et al (eds): Williams Gynecology, 2nd ed. New York, McGraw-Hill, 2012, Figure 30-10.

    a. 35-year-old woman with a body mass index (BMI) of 37

    b. 55-year-old woman with diabetes mellitus, chronic hypertension, and a BMI of 30

    c. 40-year-old woman with moderate to severe pulmonary hypertension and a BMI of 22

    d. 65-year-old woman with systemic lupus erythematosus, chronic renal insufficiency, and a BMI of 24

30-19. What percentage of women who have adenocarcinoma of the cervix also have ovarian metastasis?

    a. 2

    b. 12

    c. 22

    d. 32

30-20. In brachytherapy, how is point A defined?

    a. 2 cm lateral and 2 cm superior to the external os

    b. 5 cm lateral and 2 cm superior to the external os

    c. 2 cm lateral and 5 cm superior to the external os

    d. 5 cm lateral and 2 cm superior to the internal os

30-21. Which of the following is the most commonly used radiation sensitizer for the treatment of cervical cancer?

    a. Cisplatin

    b. Paclitaxel

    c. Carboplatin

    d. Fluorouracil (5-FU)

30-22. If a patient with stage IB1 squamous cell carcinoma recurs at the vagina after a radical hysterectomy with pelvic lymph node dissection, what is the most appropriate treatment?

    a. Radiation alone

    b. Systemic chemotherapy

    c. Total pelvic exenteration

    d. Radiation with concomitant chemotherapy

30-23. Which of the following is the most appropriate chemotherapy regimen for newly diagnosed stage IVB adenocarcinoma of the cervix?

    a. Cisplatin and topotecan

    b. Cisplatin and Navelbine

    c. Cisplatin and paclitaxel

    d. Cisplatin and gemcitabine

30-24. Which of the following is the most appropriate treatment of menopausal symptoms in a 47-year-old treated with chemoradiation for a stage IIB squamous cell carcinoma of the cervix?

    a. Clonadine

    b. Conjugated estrogen

    c. Vaginal estrogen cream

    d. Conjugated estrogen with progesterone

30-25. In a woman with recurrent cervical cancer after radiation, which of the following signs or symptoms is not part of a triad that suggests she has sidewall disease and is not a candidate for pelvic exenteration?

    a. Lymphedema

    b. Hydronephrosis

    c. Pelvic lymphadenopathy

    d. Back pain which radiates down the leg

Chapter 30   ANSWER KEY

Question number	Letter answer	Page cited	Header cited	Question number	Letter answer	Page cited	Header cited
30–1	c	p. 770	Human Papillomavirus Infection	**30–15**	c	p. 786	Table 30-9
				30–16	b	p. 786	Table 30-9
30–2	a	p. 770	Risks	**30–17**	d	p. 785	Recurrence Risk
30–3	c	p. 771	Tumorigenesis	**30–18**	c	p. 784	Treatment of Stage IB to IIA Tumors
30–4	c	p. 773	Histologic types				
30–5	a	p. 775	Symptoms	**30–19**	a	p. 784	Treatment of Stage IB to IIA Tumors
30–6	c	p. 776	Pap Smear				
30–7	b	p. 776	Pap Smear	**30–20**	a	p. 787	Radiation Therapy
30–8	a	p. 777	Clinical Staging	**30–21**	a	p. 787	Chemoradiation
30–9	c	p. 777	Clinical Staging	**30–22**	d	p. 788	Radiotherapy for Secondary Disease
30–10	c	p. 777	Radiologic Imaging				
30–11	d	p. 780	Prognostic Factors	**30–23**	c	p. 787	Stage IVB; Chemotherapy for Secondary Disease
30–12	b	p. 781	Treatment				
30–13	b	p. 781	Treatment				
30–14	b	p. 781	Treatment	**30–24**	d	p. 788	Hormone Replacement
				30–25	c	p. 788	Pelvic Exenteration

CHAPTER 31

Vulvar Cancer

31-1. Squamous cell carcinoma is the most common histologic subtype of vulvar cancer. What is the second most common histologic type?

    a. Sarcoma

    b. Melanoma

    c. Basal cell

    d. Adenocarcinoma

31-2. Approximately how many women are diagnosed with vulvar cancer annually in the United States?

    a. 1,000

    b. 4,000

    c. 8,000

    d. 15,000

31-3. The internal pudendal artery is a branch of which artery?

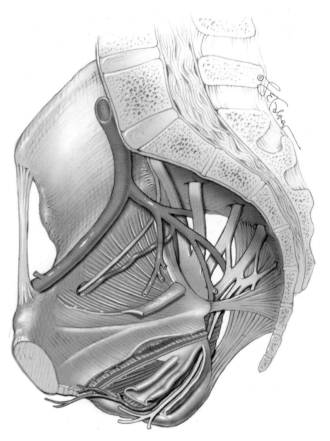

Reproduced, with permission, from Corton MM: Anatomy. In Hoffman BL, Schorge JO, Schaffer JI, et al (eds): Williams Gynecology, 2nd ed. New York, McGraw-Hill, 2012, Figure 38-6.

    a. Femoral artery

    b. External iliac artery

    c. Internal iliac artery

    d. Superficial pudendal artery

31-4. Which of the following is not part of the femoral triangle?

    a. Gracilis muscle

    b. Sartorius muscle

    c. Inguinal ligament

    d. Adductor longus muscle

31–5. What is the structure at the arrow tip?

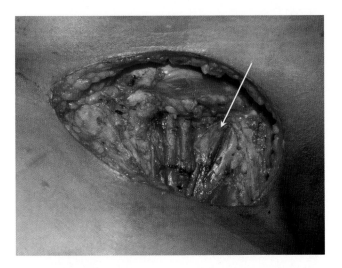

    a. Gracilis muscle

    b. Sartorius muscle

    c. Adductor brevis muscle

    d. Adductor longus muscle

31–6. Which of the following is not a risk factor for vulvar cancer?

    a. Lichen planus

    b. Tobacco abuse

    c. Lichen sclerosus

    d. Human papillomavirus

31–7. What is the most accurate description of Cloquet node?

    a. It is a deep inguinofemoral node.

    b. It is the most superior node in the femoral triangle.

    c. If negative, no pelvic lymph node dissection is indicated.

    d. All of the above

31–8. What percentage of vulvar cancers is positive for human papillomavirus (HPV)?

    a. 0

    b. 5

    c. 30

    d. 60

31–9. A 39-year-old woman is referred to you for a painful 3-cm vulvar mass. You biopsy the mass, and it reveals invasive squamous cell carcinoma. Which of the following tests should you perform prior to definitive surgery?

    a. Pap smear

    b. Vulvoscopy

    c. Human immunodeficiency virus (HIV) test

    d. All of the above

31–10. A 62-year-old woman presents for her annual well woman examination and complains of vulvar pruritis. During examination, you note an area of thickened white plaque. What is the most appropriate next step?

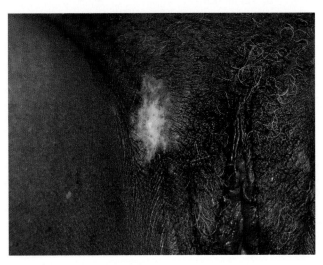

Photograph contributed by Dr. Elaine Duryea.

    a. Biopsy the lesion in your office

    b. Prescribe estrogen cream and follow up in 3 months

    c. Perform a wide local excision in the operating room

    d. Prescribe clobetasol cream and follow up in 3 months

31–11. What is the maximum depth of invasion to still be considered minimally invasive vulvar cancer?

    a. 1 mm

    b. 3 mm

    c. 5 mm

    d. 7 mm

31–12. You perform a radical vulvectomy and bilateral inguinofemoral lymph node dissection for a 3-cm invasive squamous cell carcinoma of the vulva involving the lower third of the vagina. Final pathologic analysis of the specimen reveals margins and lymph nodes that are negative for cancer. Based on these findings, which International Federation of Gynecology and Obstetrics (FIGO) stage is she assigned?

    a. I

    b. II

    c. III

    d. IVA

31–13. Which of the following is not associated with an increased risk of lymph node metastasis?

    a. High grade

    b. Increasing age

    c. Clitoral lesion

    d. Lymphovascular space invasion

31–14. What is the most important prognostic factor in vulvar cancer?

  a. Grade

  b. Tumor size

  c. Depth of invasion

  d. Lymph node metastasis

31–15. What is the risk of recurrence (percent) if the tumor-free margin around a resected vulvar cancer is less than 8 mm?

  a. 5

  b. 25

  c. 33

  d. 50

31–16. What is the most common complication of an inguinofemoral lymph node dissection?

  a. Lymphocele

  b. Lymphedema

  c. Groin infection

  d. Wound dehiscence

31–17. What technique can decrease the risk of lymphedema?

  a. Spare the saphenous vein

  b. Use compression stockings

  c. Transpose the sartorius muscle

  d. Avoid drain placement at the time of inguinofemoral dissection

31–18. You perform a radical vulvectomy with bilateral inguinofemoral lymphadenectomy on a woman with a 4-cm squamous cell carcinoma tumor of the vulva. Margins are negative for cancer, but there are three positive lymph nodes. What is the most appropriate treatment?

  a. Radiation alone

  b. Chemoradiation

  c. Close observation

  d. Pelvic lymph node dissection

31–19. What is the most appropriate treatment for a 55-year-old patient with a 4-cm squamous cell carcinoma of the vulva involving the urethral meatus and a medical history significant for systemic lupus erythematosus?

  a. Chemoradiation

  b. Pelvic exenteration

  c. Chemoradiation followed by radical vulvectomy

  d. Radical vulvectomy with bilateral inguinofemoral lymph node dissection

31–20. What is the correct term for the lesion depicted by the arrow?

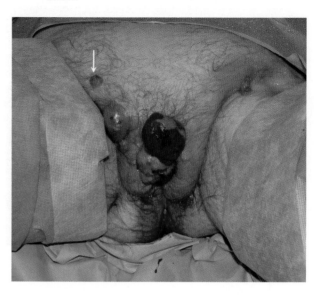

  a. Primary tumor

  b. Satellite lesion

  c. In-transit metastasis

  d. None of the above

31–21. Which of the following is **FALSE** regarding the tumor shown here involving the outer surface of the right labia minora?

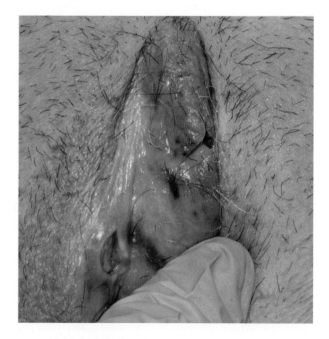

  a. It is typically a disease of the elderly.

  b. It commonly arises from the labia minora and clitoris.

  c. Differential diagnoses include seborrheic keratosis and dysplastic nevi.

  d. It is more common in African American women than Caucasian women.

31–22. What is the most appropriate treatment for a 3-cm basal cell carcinoma of the right vulva, 2 cm from the midline?

    a. Wide local excision with a 1-cm margin

    b. Wide local excision with a 2-cm margin

    c. Radical vulvectomy with right inguinofemoral lymph node dissection

    d. Radical vulvectomy with bilateral inguinofemoral lymph node dissection

31–23. A 54-year-old woman presents with the persistent vulvar mass seen in the picture below and complaints of dyspareunia. She denies previous Bartholin gland abscess or mass in the past. What is the most appropriate management?

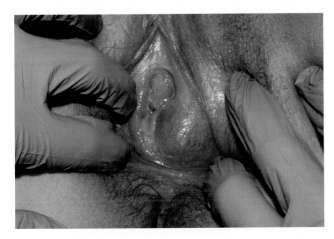

Photograph contributed by Dr. William N. Denson.

    a. Antibiotics

    b. Resection of the Bartholin gland

    c. Incision and drainage, Word catheter placement

    d. Incision and drainage, cyst wall biopsy, and Word catheter placement

31–24. Which vulvar lesion can be associated with a primary cancer at a distant site?

    a. Lichen planus

    b. Lichen sclerosus

    c. Vulvar Paget disease

    d. Vulvar basal cell carcinoma

31–25. What condition is illustrated in these photographs? Grossly, one would expect to see an erythematous, eczematoid, possibly weeping lesion of the vulva. Histologically, cells pathognomonic to this condition are found (*arrow*).

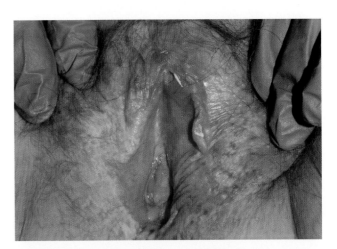

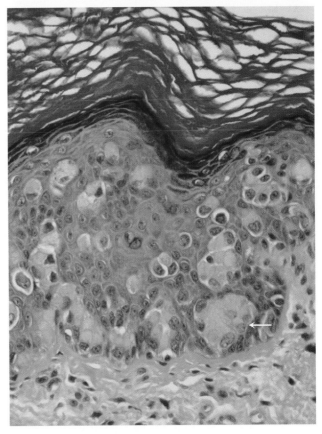

Photographs contributed by Drs. Claudia Werner and Kelley Carrick.

    a. Vulvar melanoma

    b. Lichen sclerosus

    c. Vulvar Paget disease

    d. Vulvar squamous cell carcinoma

SECTION 4

Chapter 31   ANSWER KEY

Question number	Letter answer	Page cited	Header cited	Question number	Letter answer	Page cited	Header cited
31–1	b	p. 794	Table 31-1	31–14	d	p. 797	Lymph Node Metastasis
31–2	b	p. 793	Incidence	31–15	d	p. 798	Surgical Margins
31–3	c	p. 795	Vulvar Blood Supply	31–16	b	p. 801	Table 31-5
31–4	a	p. 794	Vulvar Lymphatics	31–17	a	p. 800	Inguinofemoral Lymphadenectomy
31–5	d	p. 794	Vulvar Lymphatics				
31–6	a	p. 795	Epidemiology and Risk Factors	31–18	b	p. 801	Stage III Vulvar Cancer
				31–19	d	p. 799	Treatment
31–7	d	p. 794	Vulvar Lymphatics	31–20	c	p. 794	Vulvar Lymphatics
31–8	c	p. 795	Human Papillomavirus	31–21	d	p. 803	Melanoma
31–9	d	p. 795	Immunosuppression	31–22	a	p. 804	Basal Cell Carcinoma
31–10	a	p. 796	Symptoms	31–23	d	p. 805	Bartholin Gland Adenocarcinoma
31–11	a	p. 797	Table 31-2				
31–12	b	p. 797	Table 31-2	31–24	c	p. 805	Vulvar Paget Disease
31–13	c	p. 797	Lymph Node Metastasis	31–25	c	p. 805	Vulvar Paget Disease

CHAPTER 32

Vaginal Cancer

32-1. Primary vaginal cancer comprises what percentage of gynecologic malignancies?

a. 1 to 2

b. 5 to 7

c. 9 to 11

d. 13 to 15

32-2. Most vaginal cancers are which of the following?

a. Primary vaginal leiomyosarcoma

b. Primary vaginal adenocarcinoma

c. Squamous cell cancer metastatic from the cervix

d. Endometrioid adenocarcinoma metastatic from the endometrium

32-3. The caudal ends of the fused müllerian tubes (shown here) are originally lined by which of the following epithelia?

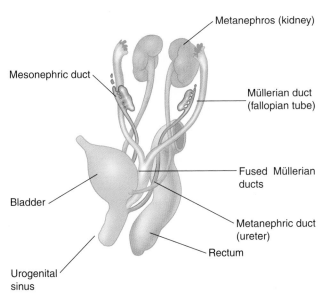

Reproduced, with permission, from Bradshaw KD: Anatomic disorders. In Schorge JO, Schaffer JI, Halvorson LM, et al (eds): Williams Gynecology, 1st ed., New York, McGraw-Hill, 2008, Figure 18-1E.

a. Columnar

b. Transitional cell

c. Stratified squamous

d. None of the above

32-4. Which of the following is a common form of primary vaginal cancer spread?

a. Lymphatic

b. Exfoliative

c. Hematogenous

d. None of the above

32-5. Shown here, which is the most common histologic type of primary vaginal cancer?

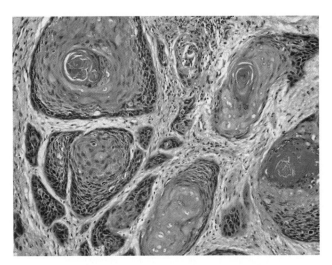

Photograph contributed by Dr. Kelley Carrick. Reproduced, with permission, from Nishida KJ: Vaginal cancer. In Schorge JO, Schaffer JI, Halvorson LM, et al (eds): Williams Gynecology, 1st ed. New York, McGraw-Hill, 2008, Figure 32-1B.

a. Melanoma

b. Adenocarcinoma

c. Squamous cell carcinoma

d. Clear cell adenocarcinoma

32-6. Of the following, which has been most closely linked with primary squamous cell cancer of the vagina?

a. *BRCA1* mutation

b. Human papillomavirus

c. Diethylstilbestrol exposure

d. Hereditary nonpolyposis colon cancer (HNPCC)

32–7. Which of the following is the most common presenting complaint in women with primary vaginal cancer?

a. Bleeding

b. Constipation

c. Vaginal mass

d. Urinary retention

32–8. Most vaginal cancers develop in which part of the vagina?

a. Upper third

b. Middle third

c. Lower third

d. None of the above

32–9. In a woman with vaginal cancer, which procedures are used to determine the International Federation of Gynecology and Obstetrics (FIGO) stage?

a. Vaginectomy alone

b. Physical examination

c. Computed tomography alone

d. Vaginectomy with pelvic lymphadenectomy

32–10. The tumor shown here corresponds to which International Federation of Gynecology and Obstetrics (FIGO) stage?

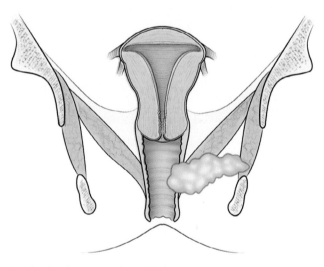

Reproduced, with permission, from Richardson DL: Vaginal cancer. In Hoffman BL, Schorge JO, Schaffer JI, et al (eds): Williams Gynecology, 2nd ed. New York, McGraw-Hill, 2012, Figure 32-3.

a. Stage I

b. Stage II

c. Stage III

d. Stage IV

32–11. In addition to an advanced International Federation of Gynecology and Obstetrics (FIGO) stage, which of the following is associated with a poorer prognosis for survival with primary vaginal cancer?

a. Nulliparity

b. Younger age

c. Adenocarcinoma cell type

d. All of the above

32–12. Which of the following is **NOT** considered appropriate sole therapy for this stage of squamous cell vaginal cancer?

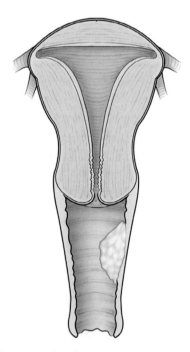

Reproduced, with permission, from Richardson DL: Vaginal cancer. In Hoffman BL, Schorge JO, Schaffer JI, et al (eds): Williams Gynecology, 2nd ed. New York, McGraw-Hill, 2012, Figure 32-3.

a. Cisplatin chemotherapy

b. External beam radiation

c. Radial vaginectomy plus pelvic lymphadenectomy

d. All of the above

32–13. Which chemotherapeutic agent is commonly paired with radiotherapy for the treatment of primary vaginal cancer?

a. Cisplatin

b. Doxorubicin

c. Vincristine

d. Methotrexate

32–14. Which of the following is commonly used to treat stage IVA squamous cell vaginal cancer?

a. Cisplatin chemotherapy alone

b. External beam radiation plus cisplatin chemotherapy

c. Radical vaginectomy plus lymphadenectomy, then cisplatin chemotherapy alone

d. Radical vaginectomy plus lymphadenectomy, then external beam radiation alone

32–15. Which of the following is among the most common sites of distant spread of primary squamous cell cancer?

a. Bone

b. Brain

c. Spleen

d. Omentum

32–16. During surveillance for recurrent disease, which of the following findings suggests pelvic sidewall disease?

a. Sciatica

b. Lymphedema

c. Hydronephrosis

d. All of the above

32–17. For women with a central tumor recurrence following radiotherapy, which of the following are treatment options?

a. Brachytherapy

b. Wide local excision

c. Pelvic exenteration

d. External beam radiation plus cisplatin

32–18. In addition to cervical abnormalities, such as the cervical hood shown here, which of the following are linked to diethylstilbestrol exposure?

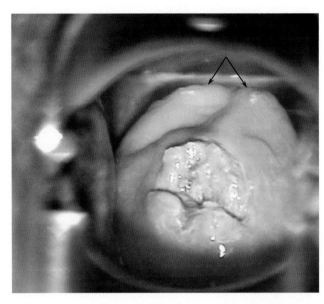

Reproduced, with permission, from Nishida KJ: Vaginal cancer. In Schorge JO, Schaffer JI, Halvorson LM, et al (eds): Williams Gynecology, 1st ed. New York, McGraw-Hill, 2008, Figure 32-7.

a. Vaginal adenosis

b. Müllerian uterine anomalies

c. Vaginal clear cell carcinoma

d. All of the above

32–19. Which of the following is true of vaginal adenocarcinoma?

a. Primary adenocarcinoma is believed to arise from vaginal adenosis.

b. Primary adenocarcinoma is less common than cancer metastatic to the vagina.

c. Endometrial cancer is the most common source of adenocarcinoma metastatic to the vagina.

d. All of the above

32–20. Which of the following is the most common malignancy of the vagina in infants and children?

a. Melanoma

b. Chondrosarcoma

c. Leiomyosarcoma

d. Embryonal rhabdomyosarcoma

32–21. Sarcoma botryoides most commonly presents with which of the following symptoms?

a. Uremia

b. Hemoptysis

c. Vaginal bleeding

d. Urinary retention

32–22. Which of the following is currently considered appropriate treatment for sarcoma botryoides?

　　a. Chemotherapy alone

　　b. Radiotherapy alone

　　c. Pelvic exenteration

　　d. Radiotherapy followed by radical excision

32–23. A Schiller-Duval body, found during histologic evaluation, and an elevated alpha-fetoprotein (AFP) level may be found with which type of vaginal cancer?

　　a. Yolk sac tumor

　　b. Leiomyosarcoma

　　c. Clear cell adenocarcinoma

　　d. Embryonal rhabdomyosarcoma

32–24. Although a benign nevus was identified by histologic evaluation, this upper right vaginal wall lesion was biopsied to exclude melanoma. Which of the following is true of vaginal melanoma?

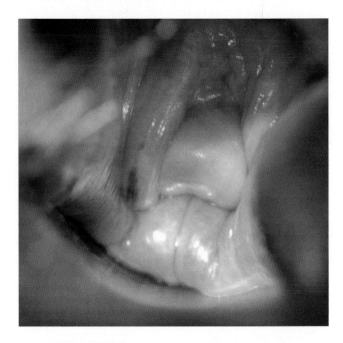

　　a. It is most commonly diagnosed in young women.

　　b. It is most frequently found in the distal vagina.

　　c. It is the most common site for reproductive tract melanoma.

　　d. All of the above

32–25. Which melanoma staging system is **NOT** applicable for vaginal melanoma?

　　a. Clark

　　b. Chung

　　c. Breslow

　　d. All of the above

Chapter 32   ANSWER KEY

Question number	Letter answer	Page cited	Header cited	Question number	Letter answer	Page cited	Header cited
32–1	a	p. 808	Introduction	**32–16**	d	p. 812	Recurrent Disease
32–2	c	p. 808	Introduction	**32–17**	c	p. 812	Recurrent Disease
32–3	a	p. 808	Vaginal Epithelium	**32–18**	d	p. 813	Vaginal Adenosis- and DES-Related Tumors
32–4	a	p. 808	Vascular and Lymphatic Supply	**32–19**	d	p. 813	Adenocarcinoma
32–5	c	p. 809	Incidence	**32–20**	d	p. 813	Embryonal Rhabdomyosarcoma (Sarcoma Botryoides)
32–6	b	p. 809	Squamous Cell Carcinoma				
32–7	a	p. 809	Diagnosis	**32–21**	c	p. 813	Embryonal Rhabdomyosarcoma (Sarcoma Botryoides)
32–8	a	p. 809	Diagnosis				
32–9	b	p. 810	Table 32-1	**32–22**	a	p. 813	Embryonal Rhabdomyosarcoma (Sarcoma Botryoides)
32–10	c	p. 810	Table 32-2				
32–11	c	p. 810	Prognosis	**32–23**	a	p. 814	Yolk Sac Tumor (Endodermal Sinus Tumor)
32–12	a	p. 811	Stage I				
32–13	a	p. 811	Stage II	**32–24**	b	p. 815	Melanoma
32–14	b	p. 811	Stage III and IVA	**32–25**	a	p. 815	Melanoma
32–15	a	p. 812	Stage IVB				

CHAPTER 33

Endometrial Cancer

33-1. What is a woman's lifetime risk of developing uterine cancer in the United States?

    a. 1 in 8

    b. 1 in 20

    c. 1 in 38

    d. 1 in 77

33-2. Which of the following does not increase a woman's risk of developing endometrial cancer?

    a. Obesity

    b. Smoking

    c. Tamoxifen

    d. Unopposed estrogen

33-3. What is the primary mechanism by which obesity increases the risk of endometrial cancer?

    a. Androstenedione is aromatized by adipose tissue to estrone.

    b. Androstenedione is aromatized by adipose tissue to estradiol.

    c. Higher levels of insulin-like growth factor lead to anovulation, which results in unopposed estrogen.

    d. None of the above

33-4. What is the most common genetic syndrome associated with endometrial cancer?

    a. Li-Fraumeni syndrome

    b. Hereditary nonpolyposis colorectal cancer (HNPCC)

    c. Hereditary breast ovarian cancer syndrome (BRCA1/BRCA2)

    d. Cowden syndrome (phosphatase and tensin homolog [PTEN] mutation)

33-5. A 60-year-old woman has abnormal uterine bleeding. A transvaginal ultrasound reveals a 15-mm endometrial stripe and an 8-cm solid right adnexal mass. An office endometrial biopsy shows grade 1 endometrioid adenocarcinoma of the uterus. What is the most likely diagnosis?

    a. Endometrial cancer metastatic to the ovary

    b. Synchronous ovarian and endometrial cancer

    c. Pedunculated leiomyoma and endometrial cancer

    d. Ovarian granulosa cell tumor and endometrial cancer

33-6. Which of the following is appropriate treatment of a 35-year-old woman with the diagnosis of complex hyperplasia without atypia?

    a. Medroxyprogesterone acetate

    b. Combination oral contraceptive pills

    c. Levonorgestrel-releasing intrauterine system (IUD)

    d. All of the above

33-7. What is the clinical success rate (percent) of the treatment of simple and complex hyperplasia without atypia with progestins?

    a. 50

    b. 75

    c. 90

    d. 100

33-8. A 30-year-old nulligravida has a body mass index (BMI) of 35 kg/m^2 and desires fertility. An endometrial biopsy performed for abnormal bleeding reveals complex atypical hyperplasia. What is the most appropriate next step?

    a. Magnetic resonance (MR) imaging

    b. Dilatation and curettage (D&C)

    c. Medroxyprogesterone acetate 10mg orally daily × 10 days monthly

    d. Total laparoscopic hysterectomy with bilateral salpingo-oophorectomy

33-9. What is the underlying risk of endometrial cancer (percent) in a woman diagnosed with complex atypical hyperplasia by endometrial biopsy?

a. 29

b. 43

c. 52

d. 61

33-10. Which of the following is the most appropriate surgical approach to a 51-year-old woman with a BMI of 35 kg/m² and a preoperative diagnosis of complex atypical hyperplasia?

a. Transvaginal hysterectomy, bilateral salpingo-oophorectomy

b. Total abdominal hysterectomy, bilateral salpingo-oophorectomy, pelvic washings

c. Total laparoscopic hysterectomy, bilateral salpingo-oophorectomy, pelvic washings, intraoperative frozen section

d. None of the above

33-11. Which of the following women should undergo annual endometrial biopsy?

a. 36-year-old woman with hereditary nonpolyposis colorectal cancer (HNPCC)

b. 45-year-old woman on tamoxifen for a personal history of breast cancer

c. 40-year-old woman with a BMI of 40 kg/m², and a family history of colon cancer in her father at age 60, and uterine cancer in her paternal aunt at age 55

d. All of the above

33-12. Which patient below should be referred to genetics for possible hereditary nonpolyposis colon cancer (HNPCC)?

a. 35-year-old with endometrial cancer, and family history of breast cancer in her sister, age 52, and colon cancer in her maternal grandmother at age 60

b. 39-year-old with endometrial cancer, and family history of endometrial cancer in her mother at age 50 and colon cancer in her maternal grandmother at age 55

c. 35-year-old with complex atypical hyperplasia, and family history of colon cancer in her maternal grandmother at age 48 and small bowel cancer in her maternal grandfather at age 70

d. 39-year-old with endometrial cancer, and family history of colon cancer in her maternal grandfather at age 65 and endometrial cancer in her paternal grandmother at age 58

33-13. The histology shown below demonstrates less than 5% solid growth with severe nuclear atypia. What grade endometrioid adenocarcinoma of the uterus does this patient have?

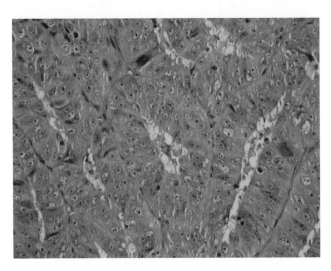

Photograph contributed by Dr. Kelley Carrick.

a. Grade 1

b. Grade 2

c. Grade 3

d. This is not endometrioid adenocarcinoma, but rather papillary serous carcinoma of the uterus

33-14. Which of the following subtypes is **NOT** a type II endometrial cancer?

a. Clear cell carcinoma

b. Papillary serous carcinoma

c. Endometrioid adenocarcinoma

d. None of the above

SECTION 4

33–15. Which of the following is true regarding the type of uterine cancer shown in the photomicrograph below?

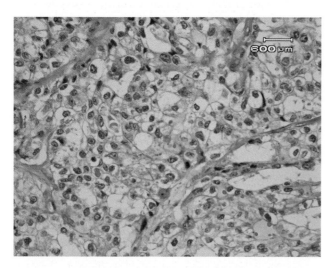

Reproduced, with permission, from Miller DS, Schorge JO: Endometrial cancer. In Schorge JO, Schaffer JI, Halvorson LM, et al (eds): Williams Gynecology, 1st ed. New York, McGraw-Hill, 2008, Figure 33-13.

a. It is the most common cell type of uterine cancer.

b. It is the least common cell type of uterine cancer.

c. Most patients with this cell type are cured with surgery alone.

d. This is an aggressive type II uterine cancer, managed by a combination of surgery and chemotherapy, with or without radiation therapy.

33–16. What is the most common way endometrioid adenocarcinoma of the uterus spreads?

a. Lymphatic

b. Hematogenous

c. Intraperitoneal

d. Direct extension

33–17. A 60-year-old woman undergoes a robotic assisted hysterectomy, bilateral salpingo-oophorectomy, and bilateral pelvic and paraaortic lymph node dissection. Her pathology reveals a grade 2 endometrioid adenocarcinoma with greater than 50% myometrial invasion, lymphovascular space invasion (LVSI), and positive washings. All the other pathology is benign. What stage is she assigned according 2009 International Federation of Gynecology and Obstetrics (FIGO) criteria?

a. Stage IB

b. Stage IC

c. Stage IIIA

d. Stage IIIC

33–18. A 52-year-old woman undergoes a robotic hysterectomy and bilateral salpingo-oophorectomy for grade 1 endometrioid adenocarcinoma of the uterus. The uterus is opened (shown below). On frozen section, there is no myometrial invasion and no lymphovascular space invasion (LVSI). Which of the following is **FALSE**?

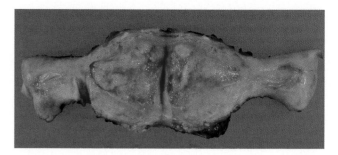

Reproduced, with permission, from Miller DS, Schorge JO: Endometrial cancer. In Schorge JO, Schaffer JI, Halvorson LM, et al (eds): Williams Gynecology, 1st ed. New York, McGraw-Hill, 2008, Figure 33-6C.

a. There is an approximately 20% chance that the frozen section is inaccurate.

b. Many experts recommend a complete pelvic and paraaortic lymphadenectomy in this patient, although this is controversial.

c. If the final pathology concurs with the frozen section, she will need postoperative radiation if a lymph node dissection is not done.

d. None of the above

33–19. For the endometrial cancer shown here, which International Federation of Gynecology and Obstetrics (FIGO) 2009 stage is represented?

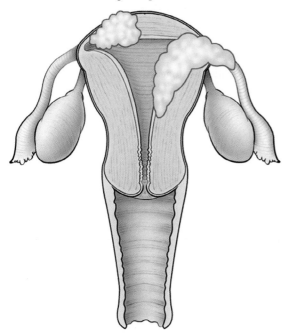

Reproduced, with permission, from Miller DS, Schorge JO: Endometrial cancer. In Hoffman BL, Schorge JO, Schaffer JI, et al (eds): Williams Gynecology, 2nd ed. New York, McGraw-Hill, 2012, Figure 33-12.

    a. IIIA

    b. IIIB

    c. IIIC1

    d. IIIC2

33–20. Which of the following is **NOT** an advantage of laparoscopy compared with laparotomy for the surgical management of uterine cancer?

    a. Shorter hospital stay

    b. Improved quality of life

    c. Lower rate of intraoperative injuries

    d. Fewer moderate to severe complications

33–21. Which of the following women needs continued Pap smears after a hysterectomy, bilateral salpingo-oophorectomy, and bilateral pelvic and para-aortic lymph node dissection for a stage IB grade 1 endometrioid adenocarcinoma of the uterus?

    a. A 50-year-old woman with no history of abnormal Pap smears

    b. A 50-year-old woman with a history of CIN 2 in the past 3 years, whose most recent Pap smear was normal

    c. A 50-year-old woman with a remote history of cervical intraepithelial neoplasia (CIN) 2 treated with a loop electrosurgical excision procedure (LEEP) and no abnormal Pap smears in the last 10 years

    d. All of the above

33–22. A 60-year-old woman is diagnosed with a grade 1 endometrioid adenocarcinoma of the uterus by office endometrial biopsy. She has a BMI of 45 kg/m², uncontrolled type 2 diabetes mellitus, and a myocardial infarction within the past 3 months. She has undergone placement of two drug-eluting stents in her coronary arteries and takes clopidogrel (Plavix). What is the most appropriate management?

    a. Tamoxifen

    b. Progesterone

    c. Vaginal hysterectomy

    d. Robotic hysterectomy, bilateral salpingo-oophorectomy, bilateral pelvic and paraaortic lymph node dissection, pelvic washings

33–23. A 65-year-old otherwise healthy woman has an episode of postmenopausal bleeding. You perform an endometrial biopsy, which reveals papillary serous carcinoma. At exploration, she has carcinomatosis and an omental cake (shown here). What is the most appropriate management of this patient?

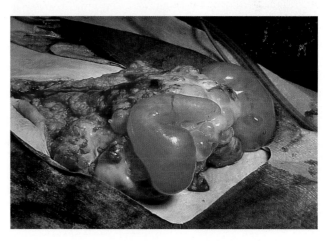

Photograph contributed by Dr. David Miller.

    a. Total abdominal hysterectomy, bilateral salpingo-oophorectomy, omentectomy, adjuvant chemotherapy

    b. Total abdominal hysterectomy, bilateral salpingo-oophorectomy, omental biopsy, adjuvant chemotherapy

    c. Total abdominal hysterectomy, bilateral salpingo-oophorectomy, omentectomy, maximal effort at tumor debulking, adjuvant chemotherapy

    d. Total abdominal hysterectomy, bilateral salpingo-oophorectomy, omentectomy, maximal effort at tumor debulking, adjuvant hormonal therapy

33–24. A 34-year-old nulligravida with polycystic ovarian syndrome (PCOS) who desires fertility has undergone a hysteroscopy, dilatation and curettage (D&C), and placement of a levonorgestrel-releasing intrauterine system (IUD) for grade 1 endometrioid adenocarcinoma of the uterus. Findings at the time of surgery are depicted below. How should she be followed?

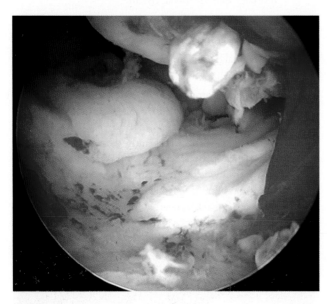

Photograph contributed by Dr. Mayra Thompson.

  a. Remove IUD in 3 months and perform an office biopsy

  b. Repeat endometrial biopsy in 3 months with IUD in place

  c. Remove IUD in 3 months and perform a hysteroscopy, D&C

  d. None of the above

33–25. What is the most important prognostic factor for a woman with endometrioid adenocarcinoma of the uterus?

  a. Age

  b. Grade

  c. Stage

  d. Positive peritoneal washings

Chapter 33 ANSWER KEY

Question number	Letter answer	Page cited	Header cited
33–1	c	p. 817	Epidemiology and Risk Factors
33–2	b	p. 817	Epidemiology and Risk Factors
33–3	a	p. 817	Epidemiology and Risk Factors
33–4	b	p. 817	Epidemiology and Risk Factors
33–5	d	p. 821	Clinical features
33–6	d	p. 822	Nonatypical Endometrial Hyperplasia
33–7	c	p. 822	Response of Nonatypical Endometrial Hyperplasia to Progestins
33–8	b	p. 822	Atypical Endometrial Hyperplasia
33–9	b	p. 822	Atypical Endometrial Hyperplasia
33–10	c	p. 822	Atypical Endometrial Hyperplasia

Question number	Letter answer	Page cited	Header cited
33–11	a	p. 823	Prevention; Screening
33–12	b	p. 823	Prevention; Screening
33–13	b	p. 825	Histologic Grade
33–14	c	p. 825	Histologic Type
33–15	d	p. 826	Clear Cell Carcinoma
33–16	d	p. 827	Patterns of Spread
33–17	a	p. 829	Surgical Staging
33–18	c	p. 829	Surgical Staging
33–19	a	p. 830	Figure 33-10
33–20	c	p. 830	Laparoscopic Staging
33–21	b	p. 831	Surveillance
33–22	b	p. 832	Hormonal Therapy
33–23	c	p. 832	Management of UPSC
33–24	b	p. 833	Fertility-Sparing Management
33–25	c	p. 833	Prognostic Factors

CHAPTER 34

Uterine Sarcoma

34-1. Which of the following sarcomas demonstrates both malignant epithelial and malignant stromal components?

    a. Adenosarcoma

    b. Carcinosarcoma

    c. Leiomyosarcoma

    d. Endometrial stromal sarcoma

34-2. Which of the following was previously termed malignant mixed müllerian tumor (MMMT)?

    a. Adenosarcoma

    b. Leiomyosarcoma

    c. Endometrial stroma sarcoma

    d. None of the above

34-3. Sarcomas account for approximately what percentage of uterine cancer?

    a. 1 to 2

    b. 3 to 8

    c. 11 to 15

    d. 17 to 23

34-4. Which of the following is the most common presenting symptom of women with uterine sarcoma?

    a. Infertility

    b. Shortness of breath

    c. Abnormal uterine bleeding

    d. Abnormal screening PAP smear result

34-5. Of the sarcoma types, the technique shown here could be most effective for diagnosing which of the following sarcomas?

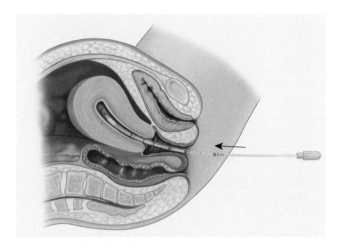

Reproduced, with permission, from Sharma M, Hoffman BL: Abnormal uterine bleeding. In Hoffman BL, Schorge JO, Schaffer JI, et al (eds): Williams Gynecology, 2nd ed. New York, McGraw-Hill, 2012, Figure 8-6A.

    a. Adenosarcoma

    b. Carcinosarcoma

    c. Leiomyosarcoma

    d. Endometrial stromal sarcoma

34-6. This is the preoperative computed tomography scan of a woman with suspected leiomyosarcoma. Which of the following is an advantage to this type of imaging preoperatively?

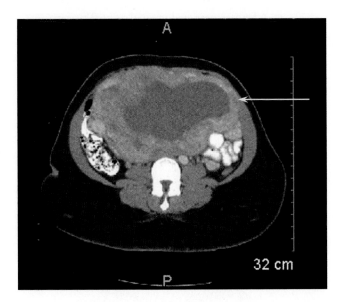

a. Operative treatment plans may be altered according to findings.

b. If varying tissue densities are found, then leiomyosarcoma is reliably diagnosed.

c. If individual tumors within the uterus measure greater than 10 cm, then leiomyosarcoma is reliably diagnosed.

d. All of the above

34-7. Following a total abdominal hysterectomy (TAH) for presumed benign disease, the final pathologic evaluation reveals leiomyosarcoma. After referral to a gynecologic oncologist, subsequent appropriate management may include which of the following?

a. Surveillance

b. Chemotherapy

c. Chemoradiation

d. All of the above

34-8. Most leiomyosarcomas are diagnosed at what International Federation of Gynecology and Obstetrics (FIGO) stage?

a. Stage I

b. Stage II

c. Stage III

d. Stage IV

34-9. As shown in this figure, leiomyosarcomas (A) compared with benign leiomyomas (B) show higher rates of all **EXCEPT** which of the following histologic criteria?

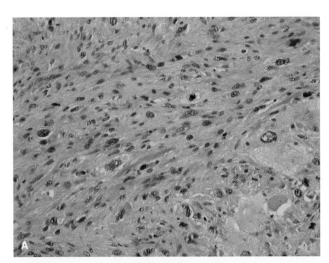

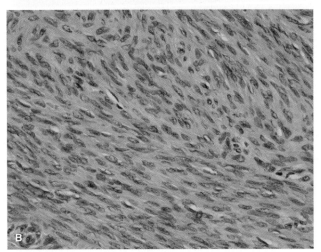

Photographs contributed by Dr. Kelley Carrick.

a. Cell necrosis

b. Cytologic atypia

c. Bland spindle-shaped cells

d. More than 15 mitoses per high-powered field

34–10. Which stromal tumor is benign and in many cases may be adequately treated by this procedure alone?

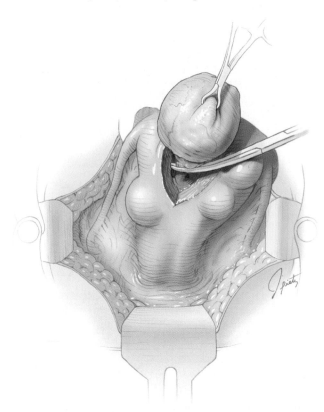

Reproduced, with permission, from Hoffman BL: Surgeries for benign gynecologic conditions. In Schorge JO, Schaffer JI, Halvorson LM, et al (eds): Williams Gynecology, 1st ed. New York, McGraw-Hill, 2008, Figure 41-18.3.

   a. Adenosarcoma

   b. Carcinosarcoma

   c. Leiomyosarcoma

   d. Endometrial stromal nodule

34–11. Microscopically, which of the following resembles the stromal cells of proliferative phase endometrium?

   a. Adenosarcoma

   b. Carcinosarcoma

   c. Leiomyosarcoma

   d. Endometrial stromal sarcoma

34–12. An adenosarcoma is typified by which of the following?

   a. Benign epithelial and malignant mesenchymal components

   b. Malignant epithelial and benign mesenchymal components

   c. Borderline epithelial and benign mesenchymal components

   d. Malignant epithelial and malignant mesenchymal components

34–13. Which of the following pairs is typified by an indolent growth pattern with long disease-free intervals?

   a. Leiomyosarcoma, adenosarcoma

   b. Leiomyosarcoma, carcinosarcoma

   c. Adenosarcoma, endometrial stromal sarcoma

   d. Leiomyosarcoma, endometrial stromal sarcoma

34–14. Which of the sarcomas is staged using the same criteria as for endometrial carcinoma?

   a. Adenosarcoma

   b. Leiomyosarcoma

   c. Endometrial stromal sarcoma

   d. None of the above

34–15. This figure of an adenosarcoma depicts which International Federation of Gynecology and Obstetrics (FIGO) stage?

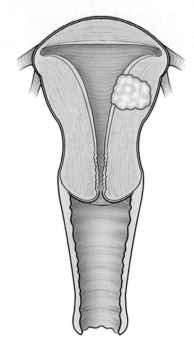

Reproduced, with permission, from Miller DS, Schorge JO: Uterine sarcoma. In Hoffman BL, Schorge JO, Schaffer JI, et al (eds): Williams Gynecology, 2nd ed. New York, McGraw-Hill, 2012, Figure 34-11.

   a. Stage IC

   b. Stage IIB

   c. Stage IIIA

   d. Stage IVA

34–16. This figure of a leiomyosarcoma depicts which International Federation of Gynecology and Obstetrics (FIGO) stage?

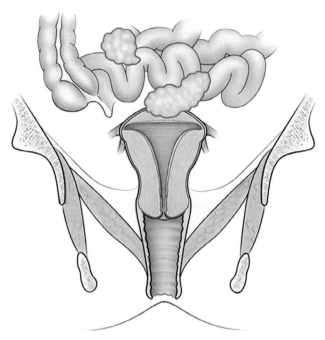

Reproduced, with permission, from Miller DS, Schorge JO: Uterine sarcoma. In Hoffman BL, Schorge JO, Schaffer JI, et al (eds): Williams Gynecology, 2nd ed. New York, McGraw-Hill, 2012, Figure 34-11.

   a. Stage IB
   b. Stage IIB
   c. Stage IIIB
   d. Stage IVB

34–17. This figure of a carcinosarcoma depicts which International Federation of Gynecology and Obstetrics (FIGO) stage?

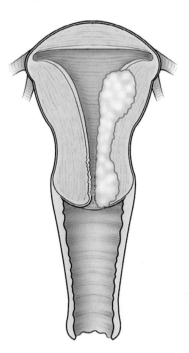

Reproduced, with permission, from Miller DS, Schorge JO: Endometrial cancer. In Hoffman BL, Schorge JO, Schaffer JI, et al (eds): Williams Gynecology, 2nd ed. New York, McGraw-Hill, 2012, Figure 33-12.

   a. Stage IB
   b. Stage II
   c. Stage IIIA
   d. Stage IVA

34–18. Which of the following sarcomas is least likely to have lymph node involvement?
   a. Adenosarcoma
   b. Carcinosarcoma
   c. Leiomyosarcoma
   d. Endometrial stromal sarcoma

34–19. Following total abdominal hysterectomy (TAH) for a presumed benign diagnosis, the final pathologic evaluation reveals a "smooth muscle tumor of uncertain malignant potential." Subsequent management typically includes which of the following?
   a. Surveillance
   b. Chemotherapy
   c. Radiation therapy
   d. Radiotherapy with adjuvant chemotherapy

34–20. Which of the following sarcomas is most likely to have lymph node involvement?

    a. Adenosarcoma

    b. Carcinosarcoma

    c. Leiomyosarcoma

    d. Endometrial stromal sarcoma

34–21. Following total abdominal hysterectomy (TAH) with bilateral salpingo-oophorectomy and complete surgical staging for early stage disease, estrogen replacement therapy may be considered for suitable symptomatic candidates with which of the following sarcoma types?

    a. Leiomyosarcoma

    b. Carcinosarcoma

    c. Endometrial stromal sarcoma

    d. All of the above

34–22. Improved survival benefit has been shown with which of the following postoperative adjuvant modalities for stage I or II sarcoma?

    a. Cisplatin chemotherapy

    b. Pelvic radiation treatment

    c. Whole abdominal radiotherapy

    d. None of the above

34–23. For advanced-stage leiomyosarcoma, which of the following chemotherapy combinations has the highest proven response rate?

    a. Bleomycin, etoposide

    b. Ifosfamide, paclitaxel

    c. Gemcitabine, docetaxel

    d. Etoposide, actinomycin D

34–24. For which of the following sarcoma types is oral progestin therapy effective in the treatment of recurrent disease?

    a. Adenosarcoma

    b. Leiomyosarcoma

    c. Endometrial stromal sarcoma

    d. High-grade undifferentiated sarcoma

34–25. For advanced-stage carcinosarcoma, which of the following chemotherapy combinations has the highest proven response rate?

    a. Bleomycin, etoposide

    b. Ifosfamide, paclitaxel

    c. Gemcitabine, docetaxel

    d. Etoposide, actinomycin D

34–26. Which of the following based on tumor histology has the worst prognosis?

    a. Leiomyosarcoma

    b. Endometrial stromal sarcoma

    c. Endometrial stromal nodules

    d. High-grade undifferentiated sarcoma

Chapter 34   ANSWER KEY

Question number	Letter answer	Page cited	Header cited
34–1	b	p. 839	Introduction
34–2	d	p. 839	Introduction
34–3	b	p. 839	Epidemiology and Risk Factors
34–4	c	p. 840	Signs and Symptoms
34–5	b	p. 840	Endometrial Sampling
34–6	a	p. 841	Imaging Studies
34–7	a	p. 841	Role of the Generalist
34–8	a	p. 842	Leiomyosarcoma
34–9	c	p. 842	Leiomyosarcoma
34–10	d	p. 843	Endometrial Stromal Nodule
34–11	d	p. 843	Endometrial Stromal Sarcoma
34–12	a	p. 845	Adenosarcoma
34–13	c	p. 846	Patterns of Spread
34–14	d	p. 847	Staging

Question number	Letter answer	Page cited	Header cited
34–15	a	p. 848	Figure 34-11
34–16	c	p. 848	Figure 34-11
34–17	b	p. 830	Figure 33-12
34–18	c	p. 848	Surgery
34–19	a	p. 848	Surgery
34–20	b	p. 848	Surgery
34–21	a	p. 849	Surveillance
34–22	d	p. 849	Adjuvant Radiation; Adjuvant Chemotherapy
34–23	c	p. 849	Leiomyosarcoma
34–24	c	p. 850	Endometrial Stromal Tumors
34–25	b	p. 850	Carcinosarcoma
34–26	a	p. 850	Survival and Prognostic Factors

CHAPTER 34

CHAPTER 35

Epithelial Ovarian Cancer

35-1. What percentage of epithelial ovarian cancers are hereditary?

   a. 1

   b. 10

   c. 15

   d. 20

35-2. Which of the following is not a risk factor for ovarian cancer?

   a. Nulliparity

   b. Late menopause

   c. Combination oral contraceptive pill use

   d. Hereditary nonpolyposis colon cancer (HNPCC)

35-3. Which of the following genetic mutations is associated with the highest risk of developing ovarian cancer?

   a. Phosphatase and tensin homolog (PTEN)

   b. Hereditary Breast Ovarian Cancer Syndrome 1 (BRCA1)

   c. Hereditary Breast Ovarian Cancer Syndrome 2 (BRCA2)

   d. MutL homolog 1, colon cancer, nonpolyposis type 2 (MLH1)

35-4. A 40-year-old woman with a BRCA1 mutation undergoes a laparoscopic bilateral salpingo-oophorectomy (BSO) for risk reduction. By what percentage is her breast cancer risk reduced by her BSO?

   a. 25

   b. 50

   c. 75

   d. 90

35-5. What is the main histologic difference between a low malignant potential tumor and epithelial ovarian cancer?

   a. Stromal invasion

   b. Mitotic activity

   c. Degree of nuclear atypia

   d. Nuclear-to-cytoplasmic ratio

35-6. A 55-year-old healthy woman undergoes exploration for a large pelvic mass (shown below). Frozen section analysis of her right ovary notes "mucinous low malignant potential, cannot exclude invasion." There is no other obvious disease. What surgical procedures should be performed, in addition to total abdominal hysterectomy and bilateral salpingo-oophorectomy?

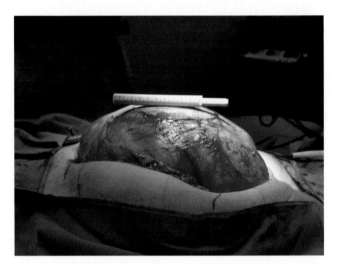

   a. Pelvic washings, omentectomy, multiple peritoneal biopsies

   b. Pelvic washings, omentectomy, multiple peritoneal biopsies, bilateral pelvic and para-aortic lymph node dissection

   c. Pelvic washings, omentectomy, multiple peritoneal biopsies, bilateral pelvic and para-aortic lymph node dissection, appendectomy

   d. None of the above

35–7. A 27-year-old nulligravida who desires future fertility underwent a laparoscopic left salpingo-oophorectomy for a 7-cm cyst. The cyst was removed intact, and washings were negative. Final pathology revealed a serous low malignant potential tumor. What is the most appropriate management?

   a. Close observation

   b. Right salpingo-oophorectomy (RSO), omentectomy, multiple peritoneal biopsies

   c. RSO, omentectomy, multiple peritoneal biopsies, bilateral pelvic and para-aortic lymph node dissection

   d. Hysterectomy, RSO, omentectomy, multiple peritoneal biopsies, bilateral pelvic and para-aortic lymph node dissection

35–8. Which of the following is the worst prognostic feature associated with low malignant potential (LMP) tumors?

   a. Advanced stage

   b. Invasive implants

   c. Mucinous histology

   d. Stromal microinvasion

35–9. Which of the following is **FALSE** regarding ovarian cancer symptoms?

   a. Most women with ovarian cancer experience symptoms 20 to 30 days per month.

   b. Women with ovarian cancer do not have symptoms until the disease is very advanced.

   c. The most frequent symptoms associated with ovarian cancer include urinary urgency, pelvic pain, and bloating.

   d. None of the above

35–10. What percentage of patients with stage I ovarian cancer have a normal cancer antigen 125 (CA125) level?

   a. 5

   b. 15

   c. 25

   d. 50

35–11. Which of the following conditions can create an elevated CA125 level?

   a. Leiomyomas

   b. Endometriosis

   c. Congestive heart failure

   d. All of the above

35–12. Which of the following radiologic tests is most helpful in a patient with suspected advanced ovarian cancer?

   a. Transvaginal ultrasound

   b. Positron emission tomography (PET) scan

   c. Magnetic resonance (MR) imaging of the pelvis

   d. Computed tomography (CT) scan of the abdomen and pelvis

35–13. Which one of the following women does not need referral to a gynecologic oncologist?

   a. A 35-year-old with a complex 7-cm adnexal mass and a CA125 level of 75

   b. A 60-year-old with a complex 7-cm adnexal mass and a CA125 level of 75

   c. A 35-year-old with a complex 7-cm adnexal mass, ascites, and a CA125 level of 75

   d. A 50-year-old with a complex 7-cm fixed adnexal mass and a CA125 level of 25

35–14. In the photomicrograph below, to what structures are the white arrows pointing? (Hint—this finding is pathognomonic for the most common histologic cell type of epithelial ovarian cancer.)

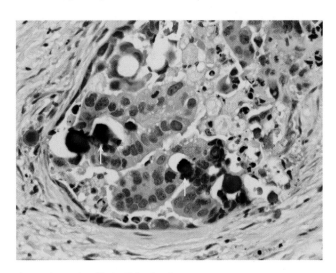

Photograph contributed by Dr. Kelley Carrick.

   a. Signet rings

   b. Hobnail cells

   c. Keratin pearls

   d. Psammoma bodies

35–15. Shown here, what is the most common cell type of epithelial ovarian cancer associated with endometriosis?

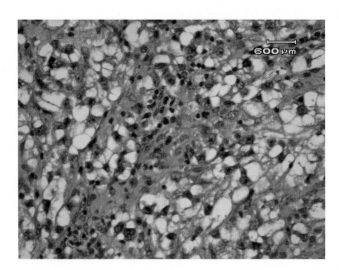

Reproduced, with permission, from Schorge JO: Epithelial ovarian cancer. In Schorge JO, Schaffer JI, Halvorson LM, et al (eds): Williams Gynecology, 1st ed. New York, McGraw-Hill, 2008, Figure 35-14.

   a. Mucinous

   b. Clear cell

   c. Endometrioid

   d. Papillary serous

35–16. A 27-year-old presents to the emergency department with a complaint of increasing abdominal distension, constipation, and weight loss. A computed tomographic (CT) scan reveals a 10-cm right adnexal mass and retroperitoneal lymphadenopathy. Her serum CA125 level is 45, β-human chorionic gonadotropin (β-hCG) concentration is less than 5, and alpha-fetoprotein (AFP) and lactate dehydrogenase (LDH) levels are normal. Her serum calcium level is 15. What is the most likely diagnosis?

   a. Lymphoma

   b. Small cell ovarian cancer

   c. Primary hyperparathyroidism

   d. Malignant germ cell tumor of the ovary with bone metastasis

35–17. Which of the following is **NOT** a characteristic of Krukenberg tumors?

   a. They are bilateral.

   b. They usually arise from primary gastric tumors.

   c. They are usually the only site of metastatic disease.

   d. They are comprised of mucinous and signet ring cells.

35–18. What is the most common method of ovarian cancer spread?

   a. Lymphatic

   b. Hematogenous

   c. Direct extension

   d. Tumor exfoliation

35–19. Which of the following correctly indicates the cephalad border of the para-aortic lymph node dissection for ovarian cancer clinically confined to the ovary?

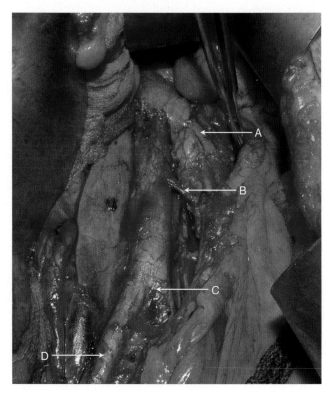

Photograph contributed by Dr. Jayanthi Lea.

   a. A

   b. B

   c. C

   d. D

35-20. A 40-year-old woman with a right-sided pleural effusion undergoes exploratory laparotomy for a pelvic mass and elevated CA125 level. Cytologic analysis of the pleural fluid reveals no malignant cells. Upon exploration, the finding below is seen. Which International Federation of Gynecology and Obstetrics (FIGO) stage is she?

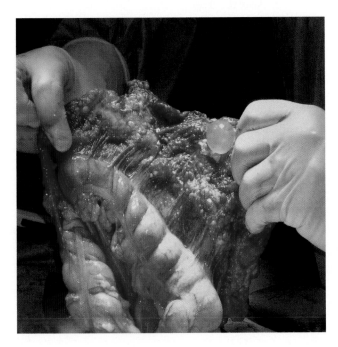

Photograph contributed by Dr. John Schorge.

    a. IIA

    b. IIC

    c. IIIA

    d. IIIC

35-21. What percentage of women with ovarian cancer clinically confined to the ovaries will be upstaged by surgery?

    a. 10

    b. 25

    c. 33

    d. 50

35-22. Which of the following patients does not need adjuvant chemotherapy following surgery for epithelial ovarian cancer?

    a. A 65-year-old following total abdominal hysterectomy, bilateral salpingo-oophorectomy, omentectomy, multiple peritoneal biopsies, and pelvic and para-aortic lymph node dissection for a stage IC clear cell ovarian cancer

    b. A 45-year-old following total abdominal hysterectomy, bilateral salpingo-oophorectomy, omentectomy, multiple peritoneal biopsies, and pelvic lymph node dissection for a stage IA grade 1 endometrioid adenocarcinoma of the ovary

    c. A 55-year-old following total abdominal hysterectomy, bilateral salpingo-oophorectomy, omentectomy, multiple peritoneal biopsies, and pelvic and para-aortic lymph node dissection for a stage IB grade 1 papillary serous carcinoma of the ovary

    d. A 70-year-old following total abdominal hysterectomy, bilateral salpingo-oophorectomy, omentectomy, multiple peritoneal biopsies, and pelvic and para-aortic lymph node dissection for a stage IC grade 1 papillary serous carcinoma of the ovary

35-23. What is the goal of cytoreductive surgery for advanced ovarian cancer?

    a. Remove all tumors larger than 1 cm

    b. Remove all tumors larger than 2 cm

    c. Remove all tumors larger than 0.5 cm

    d. Remove all gross disease

35-24. Which of the following chemotherapy regimens is associated with the longest overall survival for women with optimally debulked (less than 1 cm residual disease) stage III epithelial ovarian cancer?

    a. Single agent carboplatin

    b. Intravenous (IV) carboplatin and paclitaxel

    c. Intraperitoneal (IP) cisplatin and paclitaxel

    d. Intravenous (IV) carboplatin, paclitaxel, and bevacizumab

35–25. A woman with a history of stage IIIC ovarian cancer who underwent optimal cytoreductive surgery followed by six cycles of intraperitoneal (IP) cisplatin and paclitaxel recurs 4 months after completion of chemotherapy. She complains of bloating and decreased appetite. Which of the following is the most appropriate treatment?

a. Tamoxifen

b. Intravenous (IV) carboplatin

c. IV carboplatin and paclitaxel

d. Pegylated liposomal doxorubicin

35–26. Which of the following chemotherapy regimens is appropriate treatment of a patient with recurrent platinum-sensitive ovarian cancer?

a. Carboplatin with paclitaxel

b. Carboplatin with gemcitabine

c. Carboplatin with pegylated liposomal doxorubicin

d. All of the above

Chapter 35   ANSWER KEY

Question number	Letter answer	Page cited	Header cited	Question number	Letter answer	Page cited	Header cited
35–1	b	p. 853	Epidemiology and Risk Factors	35–14	d	p. 863	Serous Tumors
35–2	c	p. 853	Epidemiology and Risk Factors	35–15	b	p. 865	Clear Cell Adenocarcinoma
35–3	b	p. 854	Hereditary Breast and Ovarian Cancer	35–16	b	p. 866	Small Cell Carcinoma
				35–17	c	p. 867	Secondary Tumors
35–4	b	p. 857	Prophylactic Surgery	35–18	d	p. 867	Patterns of Spread
35–5	a	p. 857	Low malignant Potential Tumors	35–19	a	p. 868	Staging
35–6	c	p. 857	Low malignant Potential Tumors	35–20	d	p. 868	Staging
				35–21	c	p. 868	Staging
35–7	a	p. 858	Treatment	35–22	c	p. 868	Management of Early-Stage Ovarian Cancer
35–8	b	p. 858	Treatment	35–23	d	p. 870	Primary Cytoreductive Surgery
35–9	b	p. 860	Signs and Symptoms				
35–10	d	p. 861	Laboratory Testing	35–24	c	p. 871	Adjuvant Chemotherapy
35–11	d	p. 861	Laboratory Testing	35–25	d	p. 873	Management of Recurrent Ovarian Cancer
35–12	d	p. 861	Imaging				
35–13	a	p. 862	Role of the Generalist	35–26	d	p. 873	Salvage Chemotherapy

CHAPTER 36

Ovarian Germ Cell and Sex Cord-Stromal Tumors

36-1. What percentage of all ovarian cancers are germ cell and sex cord-stromal tumors?

   a. 1

   b. 10

   c. 20

   d. 30

36-2. Which of the following is the most commonly diagnosed International Federation of Gynecology and Obstetrics (FIGO) stage for women with germ cell tumors?

   a. I

   b. II

   c. III

   d. IV

36-3. What is the most common presenting symptom in a woman with a germ cell tumor?

   a. Bloating

   b. Abdominal pain

   c. Abdominal distention

   d. Menstrual abnormality

36-4. Which of the following is not a tumor marker for germ cell tumors?

   a. Inhibin

   b. Alpha-fetoprotein (AFP)

   c. Lactate dehydrogenase (LDH)

   d. Human chorionic gonadotropin (hCG)

36-5. Which of the following is the most commonly diagnosed ovarian malignancy during pregnancy?

   a. Dysgerminoma

   b. Choriocarcinoma

   c. Immature teratoma

   d. Granulosa cell tumor

36-6. A 19-year-old female college student is diagnosed with a pelvic mass and an elevated lactate dehydrogenase (LDH) level. She reports that she was amenorrheic until she started taking combination oral contraceptive pills (COCs). She undergoes surgical exploration, and frozen section analysis of the surgical specimen reveals ovarian dysgerminoma. Which of the following is **FALSE**?

   a. Her karyotype is most likely 46,XX.

   b. Regardless of stage, she has an excellent prognosis.

   c. Her other ovary may contain a gonadoblastoma and should be removed.

   d. She should undergo complete surgical staging, but her uterus may be preserved.

36-7. What percentage of gonadoblastomas undergo malignant transformation?

   a. 10

   b. 20

   c. 40

   d. 60

36-8. Which germ cell tumor is most likely to be bilateral?

   a. Dysgerminoma

   b. Mature teratoma

   c. Immature teratoma

   d. Embryonal carcinoma

36-9. The structure shown in the photomicrograph below is pathognomonic for which germ cell tumor?

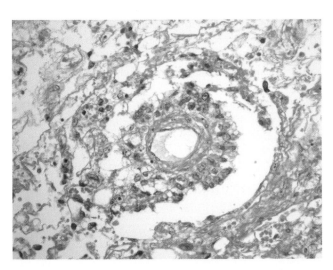

Photograph contributed by Dr. Kelley Carrick.

   a. Dysgerminoma

   b. Yolk sac tumor

   c. Immature teratoma

   d. Nongestational choriocarcinoma

36-10. Which of the following malignant germ cell tumors has the worst prognosis?

   a. Dysgerminoma

   b. Yolk sac tumor

   c. Immature teratoma

   d. Nongestational choriocarcinoma

36-11. What is the most common germ cell malignancy of the ovary?

   a. Dysgerminoma

   b. Yolk sac tumor

   c. Mature teratoma

   d. Immature teratoma

36-12. How are immature teratomas graded?

   a. Amount of solid component present

   b. Amount of immature elements present

   c. Amount of immature neural tissue present

   d. None of the above

36-13. An 18-year-old female has a history of a stage IC grade 3 immature teratoma. She received adjuvant chemotherapy with bleomycin, etoposide, and cis-platin (BEP). At her 6-month follow-up, she is noted to have an enlarging pelvic mass. Which of the following is the most appropriate management?

   a. Chemotherapy

   b. Radiation therapy

   c. Continued observation

   d. Exploratory laparotomy with removal of masses

36-14. What is the most common cancer found in a mature teratoma?

   a. Struma ovarii

   b. Basal cell carcinoma

   c. Neuroectodermal tumors

   d. Squamous cell carcinoma

36-15. Which of the following patients does **NOT** need adjuvant chemotherapy after unilateral salpingo-oophorectomy (USO) with surgical staging?

   a. Stage IA dysgerminoma

   b. Stage IA yolk sac tumor

   c. Stage IA grade 3 immature teratoma

   d. All of the above

36-16. Which of the following is **NOT** a protective factor against the development of a sex cord-stromal tumor?

   a. Smoking

   b. Obesity

   c. Multiparity

   d. Combination oral contraceptive (COC) pills

36-17. What is the most common presenting symptom of a sex cord-stromal tumor in a prepubescent girl?

   a. Hirsutism

   b. Abdominal pain

   c. Primary amenorrhea

   d. Isosexual precocious puberty

36–18. A 35-year-old nulligravida who desires future fertility is found during frozen section analysis of a right salpingo-oophorectomy (RSO) specimen to have a granulosa cell tumor. What is the appropriate surgical management of this patient?

a. RSO alone

b. RSO, omentectomy, multiple peritoneal biopsies, consider pelvic and para-aortic lymph node dissection

c. RSO, omentectomy, multiple peritoneal biopsies, consider pelvic and para-aortic lymph node dissection, dilatation and curettage (D&C)

d. Total abdominal hysterectomy (TAH), bilateral salpingo-oophorectomy (BSO), omentectomy, multiple peritoneal biopsies, consider pelvic and para-aortic lymph node dissection

36–19. Which of the following is true regarding the tumor represented in the photomicrograph?

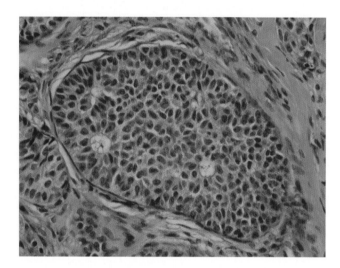

Reproduced, with permission, from Schorge JO: Ovarian germ cell and sex cord-stromal tumors. In Schorge JO, Schaffer JI, Halvorson LM, et al (eds): Williams Gynecology, 1st ed. New York, McGraw-Hill, 2008, Figure 36-6A.

a. Inhibin B is often elevated.

b. The tumor can often exceed 10 cm in size.

c. The characteristic feature is the Call-Exner body.

d. All of the above

36–20. Which of the following tumors are hormonally active and most often secrete estrogen?

a. Thecoma

b. Fibroma

c. Sertoli-Leydig tumor

d. None of the above

36–21. A woman undergoes an exploratory laparotomy, total abdominal hysterectomy (TAH), bilateral salpingo-oophorectomy (BSO) for a solid pelvic mass, ascites, and an elevated serum cancer antigen 125 (CA125) level. Her preoperative chest radiograph is shown below. Frozen section demonstrates a benign ovarian neoplasm. What is the most likely diagnosis?

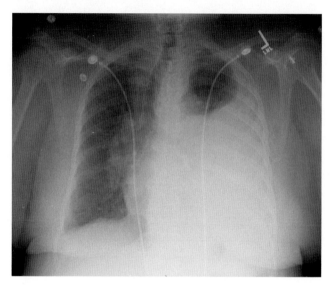

a. Meigs syndrome

b. Benign ovarian neoplasm and cirrhosis

c. Metastatic cancer with a benign adnexal mass

d. Ovarian cancer—the frozen section was inaccurate.

36–22. A 22-year-old woman has the vulvar finding demonstrated below, and an 8-cm pelvic mass is palpated during bimanual examination. What is the most likely diagnosis?

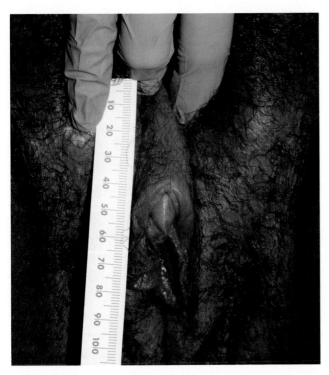

Reproduced, with permission, from Wilson EE: Polycystic ovarian syndrome and hyperandrogenism. In Hoffman BL, Schorge JO, Schaffer JI, et al (eds): Williams Gynecology, 2nd ed. New York, McGraw-Hill, 2012, Figure 17-11.

  a. Sertoli tumor

  b. Swyer syndrome

  c. Leydig cell tumor

  d. Sertoli-Leydig tumor

36–23. A 30-year-old woman with the oral finding below is found to have a sex cord-stromal tumor. Which of the following is **FALSE**?

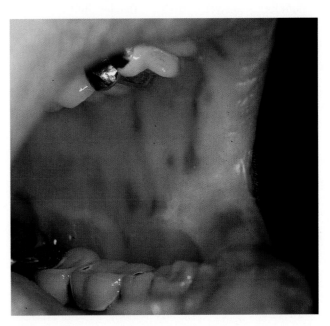

Reproduced, with permission, from Wolff K, Johnson RA (eds): Skin signs of systemic cancers. Fitzpatrick's Color Atlas and Synopsis of Clinical Dermatology, 6th ed. New York, McGraw-Hill, 2009, Figure 18-12.

  a. Her sex cord-stromal tumor is malignant.

  b. Her sex cord-stromal tumor is likely bilateral.

  c. She probably has hamartomatous polyps in her colon.

  d. She has a 15 percent chance of developing adenoma malignum.

36–24. Which of the following is **NOT** an appropriate adjuvant treatment for a patient with a stage III granulosa cell tumor?

  a. Whole pelvic radiotherapy

  b. Carboplatin and paclitaxel

  c. Bleomycin-etoposide-cisplatin chemotherapy

  d. All of the above are appropriate treatment options

36–25. Which of the following is a prognostic factor for sex cord-stromal tumors?

  a. Age

  b. Stage

  c. Amount of residual disease

  d. All of the above

Chapter 36   ANSWER KEY

Question number	Letter answer	Page cited	Header cited	Question number	Letter answer	Page cited	Header cited
36–1	b	p. 879	Introduction	36–15	a	p. 886	Chemotherapy
36–2	a	p. 879	Malignant Ovarian Germ Cell Tumors	36–16	b	p. 887	Epidemiology
				36–17	d	p. 887	Signs and Symptoms
36–3	b	p. 880	Signs and Symptoms	36–18	c	p. 889	Adult Granulosa Cell Tumors
36–4	a	p. 881	Table 36-1				
36–5	a	p. 882	Dysgerminoma	36–19	d	p. 889	Adult Granulosa Cell Tumors
36–6	a	p. 882	Dysgerminoma				
36–7	c	p. 882	Dysgerminoma	36–20	a	p. 890	Thecoma-Fibroma Group
36–8	a	p. 882	Dysgerminoma	36–21	a	p. 891	Fibromas-Fibrosarcomas
36–9	b	p. 883	Yolk Sac Tumors	36–22	d	p. 891	Sertoli-Leydig Cell Tumors
36–10	b	p. 883	Yolk Sac Tumors	36–23	a	p. 892	Sex Cord Tumors with Annular Tubules
36–11	d	p. 884	Immature Teratomas				
36–12	c	p. 884	Immature Teratomas	36–24	a	p. 893	Chemotherapy and Radiation
36–13	d	p. 884	Immature Teratomas				
36–14	d	p. 885	Malignant Transformation of Mature Cystic Teratomas	36–25	d	p. 894	Prognosis

CHAPTER 37

Gestational Trophoblastic Disease

37-1. Epidemiologic factors that carry a higher risk of gestational trophoblastic disease include all **EXCEPT** which of the following?

a. Older maternal age

b. Younger paternal age

c. Use of oral contraceptives

d. Native Americans living in the United States

37-2. By what factor is the risk of molar pregnancy increased with a prior history of spontaneous abortion?

a. Double

b. Triple

c. Quadruple

d. Risk is not increased.

37-3. With regard to molar pregnancies, what does the term *androgenesis* refer to?

a. Development of theca-lutein cysts

b. Absence of fetal tissue and amnion

c. Development of a zygote that contains only maternal chromosomes

d. Development of a zygote that contains only paternal chromosomes

37-4. All **EXCEPT** which of the following features are characteristic of complete hydatidiform molar pregnancies?

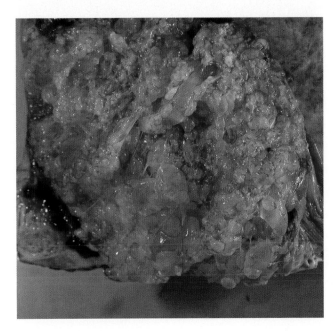

Photograph contributed by Dr. Brian Levenson.

a. Diploid karyotype

b. Absent fetal tissue

c. Focal villous edema

d. 15-percent risk of postmolar malignant sequelae

37-5. All **EXCEPT** which of the following signs or symptoms are typically seen in the presentation of a complete hydatidiform molar pregnancy?

a. Preeclampsia

b. Vaginal bleeding

c. Increased plasma thyroxine levels

d. Greater than expected serum β-human chorionic gonadotropin (β-hCG) levels

37–6. This finding, if found bilaterally in the adnexa of a patient with a molar pregnancy, increases the risk of which of the following?

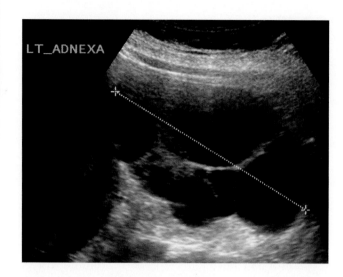

a. Preeclampsia

b. Thyroid storm

c. Hyperemesis gravidarum

d. Gestational trophoblastic neoplasia

37–7. All **EXCEPT** which of the following features are characteristic of partial hydatidiform molar pregnancies?

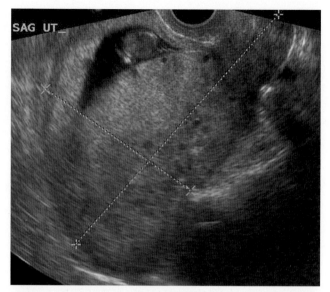

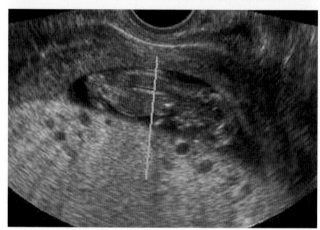

a. Triploid karyotype

b. Focal villous edema

c. Present fetal tissue

d. 25-percent risk of postmolar malignant sequelae

37–8. Which of the following signs or symptoms are typically seen in the presentation of a partial hydatidiform molar pregnancy?

a. Theca-lutein cysts

b. Higher than expected β-human chorionic gonadotropin (β-hCG) levels

c. Uterine enlargement in excess of gestational age

d. None of the above

37–9. Sonographic features of a complete mole (shown here) include which of the following?

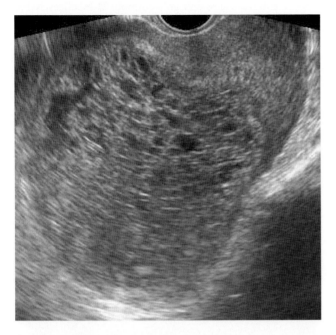

a. Absent fetal and amnionic tissues

b. Hydropic changes of the trophoblastic tissue

c. Inhomogeneous and echogenic endometrial mass

d. All of the above

37–10. Which of the following treatments is most appropriate for the patient with the sonographic findings in Question 37-9?

a. Observation

b. Hysterectomy

c. Suction curettage

d. Prostanoid induction

37–11. Your patient, who is pregnant with an estimated gestational age (EGA) of 7 to 8 weeks by last menstrual period, presents to the emergency department with heavy vaginal bleeding and passage of tissue. Sonography reveals no intrauterine pregnancy and an endometrial cavity filled with blood and tissue exhibiting inhomogeneous echoes and some hydropic changes. You perform a dilatation and curettage (D&C) with no complications. A week later, you receive the pathology report for the evacuated products of conception:

Specimen: uterine contents
DNA interpretation by image cytometry: diploid
Immunostaining: p57KIP2 positive

These histologic findings are consistent with which of the following diagnoses?

a. Partial mole

b. Complete mole

c. Spontaneous abortion

d. None of the above

37–12. All **EXCEPT** which of the statements below are true regarding surveillance practices following evacuation of a molar pregnancy?

a. Serial quantitative serum β-human chorionic gonadotropin (β-hCG) levels are the standard.

b. A single blood sample demonstrating an undetectable level of β-human chorionic gonadotropin (β-hCG) following molar evacuation is sufficient.

c. Serum β-human chorionic gonadotropin (β-hCG) levels should be monitored every 1 to 2 weeks until undetectable, after which monthly levels are drawn for the next 6 months.

d. None of the above

37–13. Which of the following statements is true regarding contraceptive practices after evacuation of a molar pregnancy?

a. Intrauterine devices should not be inserted until the β-human chorionic gonadotropin (β-hCG) level is undetectable.

b. Pregnancies that occur during the monitoring period increase the risk of progression to gestational trophoblastic neoplasia.

c. Hormonal contraception, such as oral contraceptive pills and injectable medroxyprogesterone acetate, should not be initiated until the β-human chorionic gonadotropin (β-hCG) level is undetectable.

d. None of the above

37–14. Gestational trophoblastic neoplasia (GTN) includes all **EXCEPT** which of the following histologies?

a. Invasive mole

b. Choriocarcinoma

c. Hydatidiform mole

d. Placental site trophoblastic tumor

37–15. Which of the following histologic types of gestational trophoblastic neoplasia (GTN) rarely develops metastases?

a. Invasive mole

b. Gestational choriocarcinoma

c. Epithelioid trophoblastic tumor

d. Placental site trophoblastic tumor

37–16. Evaluation of abnormal bleeding for more than 6 weeks following any pregnancy may include which of the following?

   a. Transvaginal sonography

   b. β-Human chorionic gonadotropin (β-hCG) levels to exclude choriocarcinoma

   c. Endometrial biopsy to exclude placental site trophoblastic tumor or epithelioid trophoblastic tumor

   d. All of the above

37–17. Compared with its postmolar gestational trophoblastic neoplasia (GTN) counterpart, which of the following is true for placental site trophoblastic tumor (PSTT)?

   a. Unlike choriocarcinoma, PSTT rarely follows a term pregnancy.

   b. Metastatic PSTT has a much better prognosis than metastatic choriocarcinoma.

   c. The pattern of metastasis for PSTT differs from that of gestational choriocarcinoma.

   d. Surgery is the primary treatment for PSTT due to its relative insensitivity to chemotherapy.

37–18. Serum β-human chorionic gonadotropin (β-hCG) criteria for the diagnosis of gestational trophoblastic neoplasia (GTN) include which of the following?

   a. Rise of β-hCG levels

   b. Plateau of β-hCG levels

   c. Persistent elevation of β-hCG levels

   d. All of the above

37–19. All **EXCEPT** which of the following tests should be part of the pretreatment assessment for gestational trophoblastic neoplasia (GTN)?

   a. Pelvic sonography

   b. Chest radiograph (CXR)

   c. Chest computed tomography (CT)

   d. Abdominopelvic computed tomography (CT)

37–20. According to the modified prognostic scoring system of the World Health Organization (WHO), patients with which of the following score category are assigned to the high-risk gestational trophoblastic neoplasia (GTN) group?

   a. 0 to 6

   b. 4 to 6

   c. 7 or higher

   d. 12 or higher

37–21. Following dilatation and curettage (D&C) for a complete mole, your patient is surveilled with serial β-human chorionic gonadotropin (β-hCG) levels. For the past 3 weeks, the β-hCG values have plateaued. Diagnostic evaluation reveals a metastatic lesion in the liver (shown here). Given the extent of the disease, what is the International Federation of Gynecology and Obstetrics (FIGO) stage?

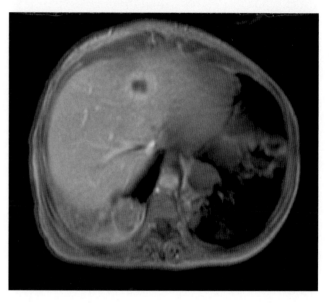

Photograph contributed by Dr. John Schorge.

   a. Stage I

   b. Stage II

   c. Stage III

   d. Stage IV

37–22. What is the approximate survival rate (percent) for women diagnosed with International Federation of Gynecology and Obstetrics (FIGO) stage III gestational trophoblastic neoplasia (GTN), that is, metastases to the lungs with or without genital tract involvement?

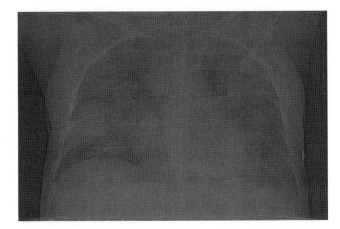

Photograph contributed by Dr. John Schorge.

a. 5
b. 25
c. 50
d. 100

37–23. What is the most common site of metastatic spread of choriocarcinoma?

a. Brain
b. Liver
c. Lungs
d. Vagina

37–24. Your patient has been diagnosed with postmolar choriocarcinoma gestational trophoblastic neoplasia (GTN). She is presently asymptomatic. What is the most appropriate treatment in her management?

a. Radiation
b. Chemotherapy
c. Hysterectomy
d. Dilatation and curettage (D&C)

37–25. Which of the following chemotherapeutic agents is most commonly used as primary treatment for low-risk gestational trophoblastic neoplasia (GTN)?

a. Etoposide
b. Pulse dactinomycin
c. Intravenous (IV) methotrexate
d. Intramuscular (IM) methotrexate

37–26. Which of the following symptoms is the most common side effect of methotrexate?

a. Pleurisy
b. Stomatitis
c. Pneumonitis
d. Pericarditis

37–27. Chemotherapy agents in the EMA/CO regimen for high-risk gestational trophoblastic neoplasia (GTN) include all **EXCEPT** which of the following?

a. Cisplatin
b. Etoposide
c. Methotrexate
d. Dactinomycin

37–28. Patients with brain metastases may present with which of the following symptoms?

a. Seizures
b. Headaches
c. Hemiparesis
d. All of the above

37–29. Compared with a molar pregnancy, how long are β-human chorionic gonadotropin (β-hCG) measurements used to monitor patients with gestational trophoblastic neoplasia (GTN) posttreatment?

a. Shorter amount of time (3 months)
b. The same length of time (6 months)
c. Longer amount of time (12–24 months)
d. β-hCG surveillance is not followed after treatment for GTN.

37–30. One year ago, your patient had a pregnancy affected by a histologically confirmed complete mole. Her β-human chorionic gonadotropin (β-hCG) levels have remained undetectable. What do you counsel her is the risk (percent) that she will have another mole in a subsequent pregnancy?

a. 1
b. 10
c. 25
d. 50

CHAPTER 37

37–31. Which of the following chemotherapeutic agents used for gestational trophoblastic neoplasia (GTN) therapy has been associated with an increased risk of certain cancers in patients who received the treatment?

    a. Etoposide

    b. Vincristine

    c. Dactinomycin

    d. Methotrexate

37–32. Heterophilic antibodies can interfere with serum β-human chorionic gonadotropin (β-hCG) immunoassays, causing false-positive results. Which of the following techniques can clarify the diagnosis?

    a. Perform serial dilution

    b. Perform a urine pregnancy test

    c. Perform specialized serum testing that blocks heterophilic antibodies

    d. All of the above

Chapter 37 ANSWER KEY

Question number	Letter answer	Page cited	Header cited	Question number	Letter answer	Page cited	Header cited
37–1	b	p. 898	Incidence	37–18	d	p. 907	Table 37-3
37–2	a	p. 899	Obstetric History	37–19	c	p. 907	Diagnostic Evaluation
37–3	d	p. 900	Karyotyping and Histology	37–20	c	p. 907	Staging
37–4	c	p. 899	Table 37-2	37–21	d	p. 908	Table 37-4
37–5	a	p. 901	Clinical Findings	37–22	d	p. 907	Staging
37–6	d	p. 901	Clinical Findings	37–23	c	p. 908	Metastatic Disease
37–7	d	p. 899	Table 37-2	37–24	b	p. 909	Surgical Management
37–8	d	p. 901	Partial Hydatidiform Mole	37–25	d	p. 910	Methotrexate
37–9	d	p. 902	Transvaginal Sonography	37–26	b	p. 910	Methotrexate
37–10	c	p. 903	Treatment	37–27	a	p. 911	Chemotherapy for High-Risk GTN
37–11	c	p. 902	Ploidy Determination				
37–12	d	p. 904	Surveillance Practices	37–28	d	p. 911	Brain Metastases
37–13	a	p. 904	Surveillance Practices	37–29	c	p. 911	Posttreatment Surveillance
37–14	c	p. 905	Gestational Trophoblastic Neoplasia; Table 37-1	37–30	a	p. 911	Subsequent Pregnancy Outcomes
37–15	a	p. 905	Histologic Classification	37–31	a	p. 911	Secondary Tumors
37–16	d	p. 905	Gestational choriocarcinoma	37–32	d	p. 911	Phantom β-hCGs
37–17	d	p. 906	Placental Site Trophoblastic Tumor				

ASPECTS OF GYNECOLOGIC SURGERY

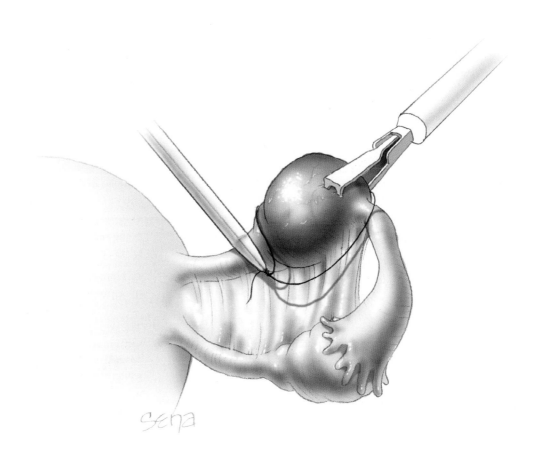

CHAPTER 38

Anatomy

38-1. Because of dermal fiber orientation, termed Langer lines, all **EXCEPT** which type of anterior abdominal wall incision leads to superior cosmetic results?

a. Cherney

b. Maylard

c. Pfannenstiel

d. Midline vertical

38-2. Camper and Scarpa fasciae of the anterior abdominal wall are not discrete layers but represent a continuum of the subcutaneous tissue layer. Which of the following best describes Camper fascia?

a. Deeper, more membranous

b. Deeper, predominantly fatty

c. Superficial, more membranous

d. Superficial, predominantly fatty

38-3. Below the arcuate line, the anterior rectus sheath represents the conjoined aponeuroses of which of the following muscles?

a. External and internal oblique

b. Rectus abdominis and external oblique

c. Transversus abdominis and pyramidalis

d. External and internal oblique plus the transversus abdominis

38-4. The fascia best recognized as the layer bluntly or sharply dissected off the anterior surface of the bladder during entry into the abdominal cavity is which of the following?

a. Camper

b. Arcuate

c. Superficial

d. Transversalis

38-5. The peritoneum that lines the inner surface of the abdominal walls is termed which of the following?

a. Rectus

b. Parietal

c. Transversalis

d. None of the above

38-6. Laceration of abdominal wall vessels can increase blood loss and risk of postoperative hematoma formation. The superficial epigastric, superficial circumflex iliac, and superficial external pudendal arteries all arise from which of the following?

a. Femoral artery

b. External iliac artery

c. Deep circumflex artery

d. Internal thoracic artery

38-7. The superficial epigastric vessels course diagonally toward the umbilicus and can be identified between which of the following structures?

a. Rectus fascia and skin

b. Peritoneum and Scarpa fascia

c. Transversalis and rectus fasciae

d. Internal and external oblique muscles

38-8. Damage to the *ilioinguinal nerve* during abdominal entry may cause loss of sensory function to the skin over which of the following?

a. Lower abdominal wall

b. Medial portion of the thigh

c. Upper portion of the labia majora

d. All of the above

38-9. The bony pelvis is comprised of the coccyx, the sacrum, and the two hip bones termed *innominate bones*. The *innominate bones* consist of all **EXCEPT** which of the following?

a. Ilium

b. Pubis

c. Ischium

d. Sacrotuberous

38-10. The U-shaped opening in the pelvic floor muscles through which the urethra, vagina, and rectum pass is termed which of the following?

a. Levator plate

b. Obturator canal

c. Urogenital hiatus

d. Greater sciatic foramen

38–11. The muscles colored yellow, green, and blue in the following figure indicate components of which of the following?

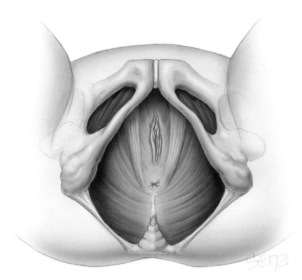

Image contributed by Ms. Marie Sena, CMI.

   a. Perineal body

   b. Levator ani muscle

   c. Iliococcygeal raphe

   d. None of the above

38–12. The levator ani muscle in the pelvic floor represents a critical component of pelvic organ support. The levator ani muscle is a complex unit that consists of all **EXCEPT** which of the following muscle components?

   a. Puborectalis

   b. Pubococcygeus

   c. Iliococcygeus

   d. Ischiocavernosus

38–13. The medial and inferior fibers of the levator ani muscle that arise on either side from the pubic bone and form a U-shaped muscle sling behind the anorectal junction may contribute to maintenance of fecal continence. This describes which of the following muscles?

   a. Puboanalis

   b. Puborectalis

   c. Pubovaginalis

   d. Puboperinealis

38–14. As shown by the red bracket in this figure, the *clinical term* used to describe the region between the anus and coccyx, formed primarily by the insertion of the iliococcygeus muscles, is which of the following?

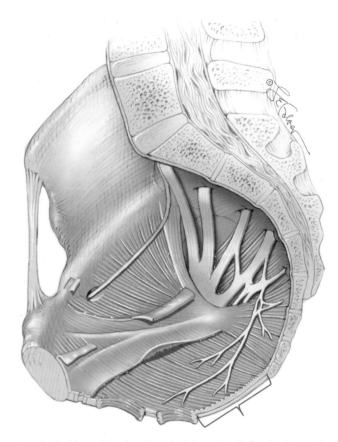

Reproduced, with permission, from Corton MM: Anatomy. In Hoffman BL, Schorge JO, Schaffer JI, et al (eds): Williams Gynecology, 2nd ed. New York, McGraw-Hill, 2012, Figure 38-7.

   a. Levator ani

   b. Levator plate

   c. Levator raphe

   d. Levator ligament

38–15. Which of the following approximate uterine measurements characterize the adult, nonpregnant woman?

   a. 7 cm length, 5 cm width at fundus

   b. 10 cm length, 5 cm width at fundus

   c. 10 cm length, 10 cm width at fundus

   d. 7 cm length, 10 cm width at fundus

38–16. The uterine cervix begins caudal to the uterine isthmus, consists primarily of fibrous tissue, and is approximately how many centimeters in length?

   a. 1

   b. 3

   c. 5

   d. 7

38–17. The lower border of the endocervical canal contains a transition from columnar epithelium of the cervical canal to squamous epithelium of the portio vaginalis and is termed which of the following?

    a. Endocervical os

    b. Squamoendocervix

    c. Portio supravaginalis

    d. Squamocolumnar junction

38–18. The main support of the uterus and cervix is provided by the interaction between the levator ani muscles and the connective tissue that attaches the walls of the cervix to the pelvic walls. The connective tissue that attaches lateral to the uterus is called the *parametria* and consists of what is known clinically as which of the following?

    a. Cardinal ligament

    b. Uterosacral ligament

    c. Transverse cervical ligaments

    d. All of the above

38–19. The broad ligaments are double layers of peritoneum that extend from the lateral walls of the uterus to the pelvic walls. Within the upper portion of these two layers lie which of the following?

    a. Fallopian tubes

    b. Round ligaments

    c. Utero-ovarian ligaments

    d. All of the above

38–20. In the image below, superior to the broad ligament, the double layer of peritoneum that drapes over the round ligament is termed which of the following?

    a. Mesoteres

    b. Mesovarium

    c. Mesosalpinx

    d. Mesosuspensus

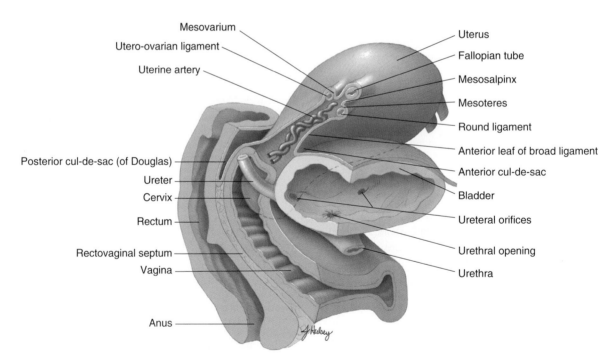

Reproduced, with permission, from Cunningham FG, Leveno KL, Bloom SL et al (eds): Williams Obstetrics, 23rd ed. New York, McGraw-Hill, 2010, Figure 2-8.

38–21. The blood supply to the uterine corpus generally arises from which of the following two arteries?

   a. Renal and ovarian

   b. Renal and uterine

   c. Uterine and ovarian

   d. External iliac and vaginal

38–22. The uterine artery approaches the uterus in the area of transition between the corpus and the cervix known as the *uterine isthmus*. In this area, the uterine artery courses over which of the following important structures?

   a. Ureter

   b. Round ligament

   c. Fallopian tube

   d. None of the above

38–23. Which of the following is true regarding the ovarian vessels?

   a. Both arteries arise from the aorta.

   b. Both veins drain into the vena cava.

   c. Right and left ovarian arteries arise from the right renal artery and aorta, respectively.

   d. Right and left ovarian veins drain into the right renal vein and vena cava, respectively.

38–24. The fallopian tube is a tubular structure that measures 7 to 12 cm in length and has four identifiable portions. In this figure, the arrow is pointing to which portion?

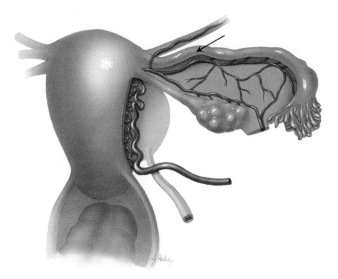

Reproduced, with permission, from Cunningham FG, Leveno KL, Bloom SL et al (eds): Williams Obstetrics, 23rd ed. New York, McGraw-Hill, 2010, Figure 2-15.

   a. Fimbria

   b. Ampulla

   c. Isthmus

   d. Interstitium

38–25. The walls of the vagina consist of three layers. Adjacent to the lumen, the first layer consists of which of the following?

   a. Smooth muscle

   b. Collagen and elastin

   c. Nonkeratinized squamous epithelium overlying a lamina propria

   d. None of the above

38–26. During the procedure shown here, which of the following vessels may commonly be lacerated?

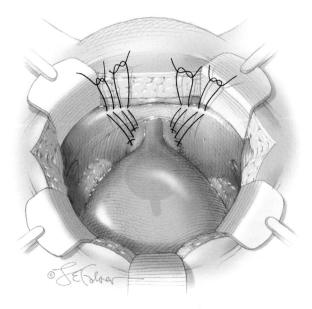

Reproduced, with permission, from Schaffer JI, Hoffman BL: Surgeries for female pelvic reconstruction. In Schorge JO, Schaffer JI, Halvorson LM, et al (eds): Williams Gynecology, 1st ed. New York, McGraw-Hill, 2008, Figure 42-2.2.

   a. Obturator vessels

   b. External iliac vessels

   c. Santorini venous plexus

   d. Deep circumflex iliac vein

38–27. The prepuce is the anterior fold that overlies the glans of the clitoris, and the frenulum is the fold that passes below the clitoris. These two folds comprise the apex of which of the following?

   a. Mons pubis

   b. Labia minora

   c. Labia majora

   d. Posterior fourchette

38–28. The pubic symphysis anteriorly, ischiopubic rami and ischial tuberosities anterolaterally, coccyx posteriorly, and sacrotuberous ligaments posterolaterally provide the boundaries for which of the following?

    a. Perineum

    b. Ischiorectal fossa

    c. Posterior anal triangle

    d. Anterior urogenital triangle

38–29. Measuring approximately 2 to 4 cm anterior-to-posterior as well as superior-to-inferior, this mass of fibromuscular tissue found between the distal part of the posterior vaginal wall and the anus is termed which of the following?

    a. Perineal body

    b. Posterior fourchette

    c. Bulbocavernosus muscle

    d. External anal sphincter

38–30. The vessels that drain vulvar and perineal structures, with the exception of the erectile tissue of the clitoris, drain into which of the following veins?

    a. Middle sacral

    b. Superior rectal

    c. Internal pudendal

    d. Superficial epigastric

Chapter 38   ANSWER KEY

Question number	Letter answer	Page cited	Header cited
38–1	d	p. 918	Skin
38–2	d	p. 918	Subcutaneous Layer
38–3	d	p. 918	Rectus Sheath
38–4	d	p. 920	Transversalis Fascia
38–5	b	p. 920	Peritoneum
38–6	a	p. 921	Femoral Branches
38–7	a	p. 921	Femoral Branches
38–8	d	p. 922	Nerve Supply
38–9	d	p. 922	Bony Pelvis and Pelvic Joints
38–10	c	p. 922	Pelvic Openings
38–11	b	p. 925	Pelvic Floor
38–12	d	p. 925	Levator Ani Muscles
38–13	b	p. 926	Puborectalis Muscle
38–14	b	p. 926	Iliococcygeus Muscle
38–15	a	p. 928	Uterus
38–16	b	p. 929	Cervix
38–17	d	p. 929	Cervix
38–18	d	p. 930	Uterine Support
38–19	d	p. 931	Broad Ligaments
38–20	a	p. 931	Broad Ligaments
38–21	c	p. 931	Uterine Blood Supply
38–22	a	p. 931	Uterine Blood Supply
38–23	a	p. 932	Ovaries
38–24	c	p. 933	Fallopian Tubes
38–25	c	p. 933	Vagina
38–26	c	p. 939	Prevesical Space
38–27	b	p. 941	Labia Minora
38–28	a	p. 942	Perineum
38–29	a	p. 945	Perineal Body
38–30	c	p. 945	Blood Vessels

CHAPTER 39

Perioperative Considerations

39-1. Which of the following is a significant risk for perioperative pulmonary complications?

   a. 25 pack-year smoking history

   b. Asthma well controlled with medication

   c. Community-acquired pneumonia 6 months ago

   d. All are significant risks

39-2. Preoperative chest radiography may be indicated in which of the following clinical settings?

   a. New-onset dyspnea

   b. 10 pack-year history of smoking

   c. American Society of Anesthesiologist (ASA) status 2

   d. All preoperative patients

39-3. Which of the following is true of methods to prevent postoperative pulmonary complications?

   a. A smoking-cessation duration of less than 6 months prior to surgery does not significantly alter complication rates.

   b. Routine use of nasogastric tube suctioning postoperatively is associated with higher complication rates compared with selective use.

   c. Postoperative intermittent positive-pressure breathing (IPPB) lowers complication rates to a greater degree than incentive spirometry.

   d. Early ambulation is as effective for pulmonary embolism prevention as intermittent pneumatic compression stockings in those with risk factors for thromboembolic disease.

39-4. Which of the following preventive measures related to cardiac disease lowers perioperative morbidity and mortality rates?

   a. Maintaining hemoglobin level above 10 g/dL in those with cardiac disease

   b. Intraoperative use of monopolar energy rather than bipolar energy in those with pacemaker devices

   c. Initiation of perioperative beta-blocker use for all with an elevated Revised Cardiac Risk Index (RCRI)

   d. Preoperative antibiotic endocarditis prophylaxis for those with valvular heart disease undergoing genitourinary procedures

39-5. In women with classic iron deficiency anemia, which of the following values is elevated?

   a. Serum iron level

   b. Serum ferritin level

   c. Mean corpuscular volume

   d. Total iron binding capacity

39-6. Which of the following regimens will most effectively correct the anemia shown here?

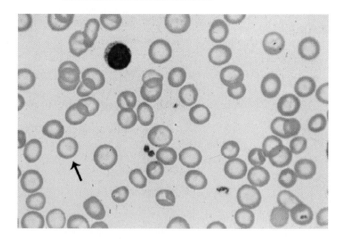

Reproduced, with permission, from Lichtman MA, Shafer JA, Felgar RE, et al (eds): Lichtman's Atlas of Hematology. New York, McGraw-Hill, 2007, Figure I.C. 80.

   a. Folate, 1 mg orally daily

   b. Cyanocobalamin, 1000 μg IM monthly

   c. Ferrous sulfate, 325 mg orally two times daily

   d. Ferrous fumarate, 200 mg orally three times daily

39-7. In patients with type 1 diabetes mellitus, postoperative insulin administration using a sliding scale should strive to maintain blood sugars below what level?

   a. 100 mg/dL

   b. 200 mg/dL

   c. 250 mg/dL

   d. 300 mg/dL

39-8. For those with adrenal insufficiency, which of the following is true regarding perioperative corticosteroid replacement?

   a. All patients chronically taking oral corticosteroids require replacement prior to all surgical procedures.

   b. All patients chronically taking oral corticosteroids require replacement only prior to major surgical procedures.

   c. Only those chronically taking 5 mg or more of prednisone daily require supplementation for all minor and major surgical procedures.

   d. None of the above

39-9. During informed consent, documentation of patient refusal for a specific procedure should include all **EXCEPT** which of the following?

   a. Documentation of the reason for the patient's refusal

   b. Documentation that the patient refused the recommended intervention

   c. Documentation that the intervention and its value were explained to the patient

   d. Documentation that the patient will be discharged from the provider's care following the refusal

39-10. Preoperative antibiotic prophylaxis is recommended for which of the following procedures?

   a. Total laparoscopic hysterectomy

   b. Ovarian cystectomy via laparotomy

   c. Hysteroscopic myomectomy of a type 0 lesion

   d. Laparoscopic tubal application of Filshie clips

39-11. Prior to total abdominal hysterectomy, all **EXCEPT** which of the following are suitable preoperative intravenous antibiotic prophylaxis regimens?

   a. Cefoxitin 2 g

   b. Clindamycin 600 mg

   c. Clindamycin 600 mg plus ciprofloxacin 400 mg

   d. Metronidazole 500 mg plus gentamicin 1.5 mg/kg

39-12. Risk factors for venous thromboembolism (VTE) include all **EXCEPT** which of the following?

   a. Pregnancy

   b. Tamoxifen therapy

   c. Copper intrauterine device

   d. Ovarian hyperstimulation syndrome

39-13. Of the thrombophilias, which is the most thrombogenic?

   a. Protein C deficiency

   b. Antithrombin deficiency

   c. Prothrombin G20210A mutation

   d. Activated protein C resistance (factor V Leiden mutation)

39-14. Of the thrombophilias, which is the most prevalent?

   a. Protein C deficiency

   b. Antithrombin deficiency

   c. Prothrombin G20210A mutation

   d. Activated protein C resistance (factor V Leiden mutation)

39-15. In evaluation of patients for thromboembolism prophylaxis, all **EXCEPT** which of the following are major considerations?

   a. Minor versus major surgery planned

   b. Coexistent venous thromboembolism risks

   c. General versus regional anesthesia planned

   d. Laparoscopic versus open surgical approach planned

39-16. According to the American College of Chest Physicians 2008 guidelines, for patients with no venous thromboembolism (VTE) risks who are undergoing major gynecologic surgery, all **EXCEPT** which of the following are suitable VTE prophylaxis?

   a. Low-molecular-weight heparin

   b. Low-dose unfractionated heparin

   c. Graduated compression stockings

   d. Intermittent pneumatic compression

39-17. Findings suggestive of a prerenal source for postoperative oliguria include all **EXCEPT** which of the following?

   a. Tachycardia

   b. Orthostatic hypotension

   c. Urine sodium of 15 mEq/L

   d. Fractional excretion of sodium greater than 3 percent

39–18. Eight hours following an uncomplicated total abdominal hysterectomy for large uterine leiomyomas, you notice that your patient has a temperature of 37.8°C during your postoperative check. She is asymptomatic, her pulse is 88, respiratory rate is 12, and her blood pressure is 132/78. Her lungs are clear during auscultation, her urine appears clear and copious, and her wound shows no bleeding or erythema. Which of the following is an appropriate response?

   a. Order a chest radiograph

   b. Initiate broad-spectrum antibiotics

   c. Order chest computed tomography angiography

   d. Encourage deep breathing and continue observation

39–19. All of the following organisms may commonly be the primary pathogen for hospital-acquired pneumonia, **EXCEPT** for which gram-negative coccobacillus shown here?

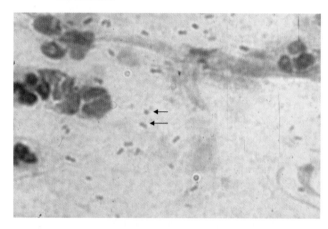

Reproduced, with permission, from Levinson W: Gram-negative rods related to the respiratory tract. In Review of Medical Microbiology and Immunology, 11th ed. New York, McGraw-Hill, 2010, Figure 19-1.

   a. *Escherichia coli*

   b. *Klebsiella pneumoniae*

   c. *Pseudomonas aeruginosa*

   d. *Haemophilus influenzae*

39–20. Following total abdominal hysterectomy for uterine leiomyomas, your patient complains of dyspnea on postoperative day 1. Her respiratory rate is 33, oxygen saturation is 88 percent on room air, pulse rate is 98, and her temperature is 38.3°C. She has no prior or family history of thromboembolism or thrombophilia. Her chest radiograph is shown below. Which of the following is the most appropriate next step?

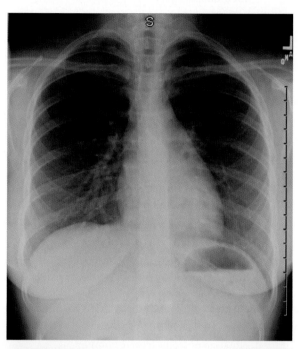

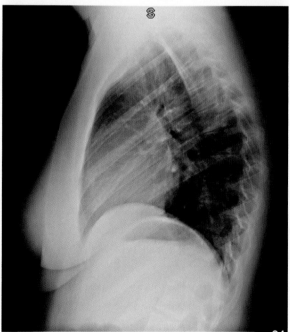

   a. D-Dimer measurement

   b. Chest computed tomographic (CT) angiography

   c. Initiate antibiotics with gram-negative coverage

   d. Encourage deep breathing and continue observation

39–21. Below is the computed tomographic (CT) angiogram from the patient in Question 39–20. You initiate pulmonary support and anticoagulation therapy. How long postoperatively should her anticoagulation therapy be continued?

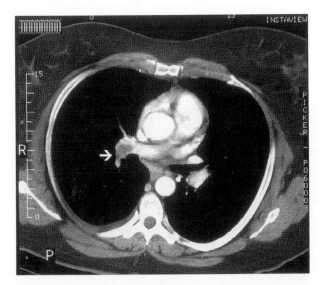

Reproduced, with permission, from Cunningham FG, Leveno KL, Bloom SL, et al (eds): Thromboembolic disorders. In Williams Obstetrics, 23rd ed. New York, McGraw-Hill, 2010, Figure 47-5.

a. 6 weeks

b. 3 months

c. 6 months

d. Indefinitely

39–22. Postoperatively, if deep-vein thrombosis is suspected, which of the following diagnostic tests (shown here) is initially preferred?

a. Venography

b. Duplex sonography

c. Magnetic resonance imaging

d. Impedance plethysmography

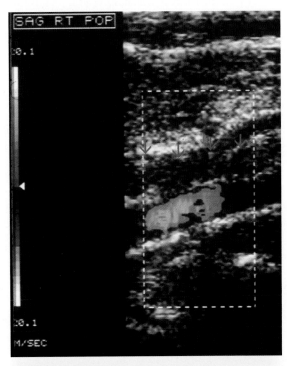

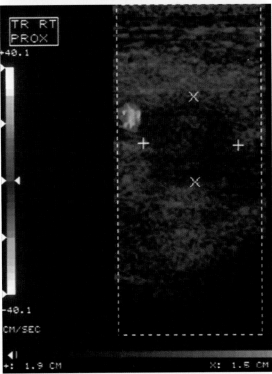

Reproduced, with permission, from Moschos E, Twickler DM: Techniques used for imaging in gynecology. In Schorge JO, Schaffer JI, Halvorson LM, et al (eds): Williams Gynecology, 1st ed. New York, McGraw-Hill, 2008, Figure 2-21.

39–23. Routine use of which of the following is an effective strategy in the treatment of ileus?

   a. Gum chewing

   b. Nasogastric tube suctioning

   c. Intravenous fluids and electrolyte repletion

   d. All of the above

39–24. In general, which of the following is the most common type of shock encountered in gynecology?

   a. Septic

   b. Neurogenic

   c. Hypovolemic

   d. Cardiogenic

39–25. For patient with hypovolemic shock, which of the following is selected for initial intravenous resuscitation?

   a. Whole blood

   b. Isotonic crystalloids

   c. Hydroxyethyl starch (hetastarch) colloid solution

   d. None of the above

39–26. Clinical signs of superficial wound infection commonly include all **EXCEPT** which of the following?

   a. Drainage from the wound

   b. Erythema surrounding the wound

   c. Petechial rash surrounding the wound

   d. Superficial separation of wound edges

39–27. Initial steps of superficial wound infection treatment include all **EXCEPT** which of the following?

   a. Antibiotic treatment

   b. Evacuation of hematomas

   c. Debridement of devitalized tissue

   d. Wound reapproximation with delayed-absorbable suture

39–28. Six days following total abdominal hysterectomy through a midline vertical incision, your patient presents with an erythematous wound with scant purulent drainage. During examination, the wound spontaneously opens (shown here) and copious foul serosanguinous fluid spills. Her temperature is 38.2°C. Because of concerns for fascial dehiscence, she is taken to the operating room for debridement of her incision and examination of the fascia. Integrity of the fascial incision is documented. Antibiotics selected for this patient should cover which of the following pathogens?

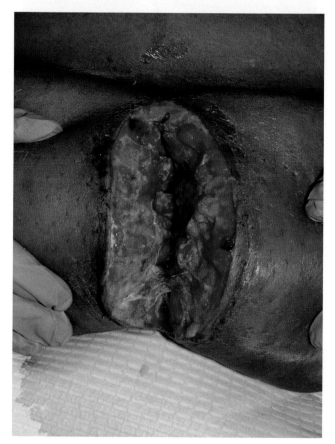

   a. Solely gram-positive bacteria

   b. Solely gram-negative bacteria

   c. Anaerobic and gram-positive bacteria

   d. Anaerobic, gram-positive, and gram-negative bacteria

39–29. The wound technology shown here offers which advantages?

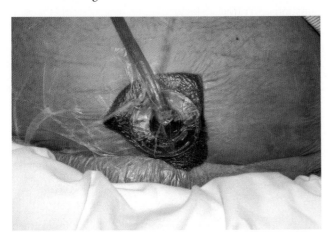

a. Removes exudates

b. Prompts wound retraction

c. Stimulates granulation tissue formation

d. All of the above

Reference

Geerts WH, Bergqvist D, Pineo GF, et al: Prevention of venous thromboembolism: American College of Chest Physicians Evidence-Based Clinical Practice Guidelines (8th Ed.). Chest 133(6 Suppl):381S, 2008.

CHAPTER 39

Chapter 39 ANSWER KEY

Question number	Letter answer	Page cited	Header cited	Question number	Letter answer	Page cited	Header cited
39–1	a	p. 949	Risk Factors for Pulmonary Complications	39–16	c	p. 962	Table 39-9
				39–17	d	p. 965	Oliguria
39–2	a	p. 950	Pulmonary Function Tests (PFTs) and Chest Radiography	39–18	d	p. 966	Atelectasis
				39–19	d	p. 967	Hospital-Acquired Pneumonia
39–3	b	p. 950	Prevention of Pulmonary Complications; Table 39-9	39–20	b	p. 968	Diagnosis and Treatment of Thromboembolism
39–4	a	p. 952	Prevention Strategies	39–21	c	p. 968	Diagnosis and Treatment of Thromboembolism
39–5	d	p. 954	Anemia				
39–6	d	p. 954	Anemia	39–22	b	p. 968	Diagnosis and Treatment of Thromboembolism
39–7	b	p. 956	Diabetes Mellitus				
39–8	d	p. 956	Adrenal Insufficiency	39–23	c	p. 969	Ileus
39–9	d	p. 958	Informed Consent	39–24	c	p. 971	Diagnosis of Hypovolemic Shock
39–10	a	p. 959	Table 39-6				
39–11	b	p. 959	Table 39-6	39–25	b	p. 971	Treatment of Hypovolemic Shock
39–12	c	p. 960	Table 39-8				
39–13	b	p. 960	Antithrombin Deficiency	39–26	c	p. 972	Wound Dehiscence
39–14	d	p. 961	Activated Protein C Resistance (Factor V Leiden Mutation)	39–27	d	p. 972	Wound Dehiscence
				39–28	d	p. 973	Wet to Dry Dressing Changes
39–15	c	p. 962	Table 39-9	39–29	d	p. 974	Negative-Pressure Wound Therapy

CHAPTER 40

Intraoperative Considerations

40–1. To achieve adequate blockade of Frankenhaüser plexus during paracervical blockade, injections should ideally be placed at what sites around the cervical base?

    a. 1 and 6 o'clock

    b. 2 and 10 o'clock

    c. 3 and 9 o'clock

    d. 4 and 8 o'clock

40–2. Classic signs of lidocaine toxicity include all **EXCEPT** which of the following?

    a. Seizure

    b. Tinnitus

    c. Petechial rash

    d. Perioral tingling

40–3. During the presurgical "time out," the entire surgical team should routinely reach consensus agreement on all **EXCEPT** which of the following?

    a. Patient identity

    b. Procedure planned

    c. Patient blood type

    d. Side of patient to be treated

40–4. Correct patient positioning can avert many intraoperative neurologic injuries. All **EXCEPT** which of the following patient or surgical characteristics is associated with an increased risk of such injury?

    a. Diabetes mellitus

    b. Body mass index (BMI) of 25

    c. 20 pack-year history of smoking

    d. Use of a self-retaining retractor

40–5. Malpositioning of a self-retaining retractor can injure the femoral nerve as it runs near the psoas major muscle, as shown here. Which of the following may be seen classically with a femoral neuropathy?

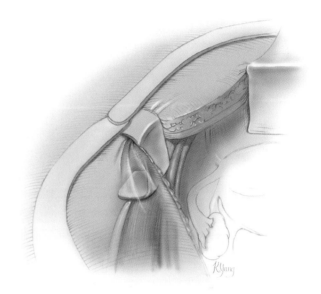

Reproduced, with permission, from Hamid CA, Hoffman BL: Intraoperative considerations. In Hoffman BL, Schorge JO, Schaffer JI, et al (eds): Williams Gynecology, 2nd ed. New York, McGraw-Hill, 2012, Figure 40-5.

    a. Absent patellar reflex

    b. Inability to flex the knee

    c. Inability to extend the hip

    d. Paresthesia over the posterior thigh

40–6. All **EXCEPT** which of the following procedures places the obturator nerve at risk of injury?

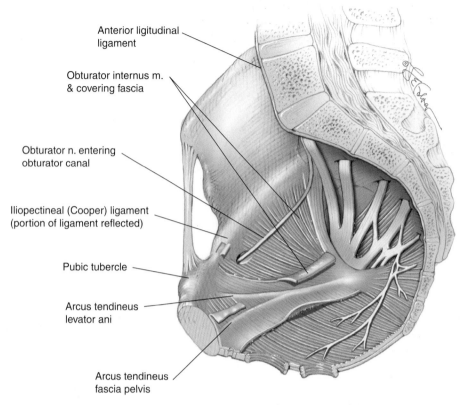

Anterior ligitudinal ligament

Obturator internus m. & covering fascia

Obturator n. entering obturator canal

Iliopectineal (Cooper) ligament (portion of ligament reflected)

Pubic tubercle

Arcus tendineus levator ani

Arcus tendineus fascia pelvis

Reproduced, with permission, from Corton MM: Anatomy. In Hoffman BL, Schorge JO, Schaffer JI, et al (eds): Williams Gynecology, 2nd ed. New York, McGraw-Hill, 2012, Figure 38-7.

a. Burch colposuspension

b. Abdominal sacrocolpopexy

c. Pelvic lymph node dissection

d. Resection of endometriosis adhered to the pelvic sidewall

40–7. In general, which of the following incisions for abdominal entry provides the **LEAST** operative space?

a. Cherney

b. Maylard

c. Pfannenstiel

d. Midline vertical

40–8. Which of the following is commonly used to lower postoperative wound infection and dehiscence rates?

a. Subcutaneous drain placement prior to skin closure

b. Closer of subcutaneous layer if greater than 2 cm deep

c. Wound irrigation with concentrated povidone-iodine solution prior to skin closure

d. All of the above

40–9. For most Pfannenstiel incisions, which of the following offers superior skin closure?

a. Staples

b. Subcuticular suturing

c. Octyl-2-cyanoacrylate (Dermabond)

d. All provide equivalent results

40-10. Which of the following blades would be preferred for incision and drainage of the cyst shown here?

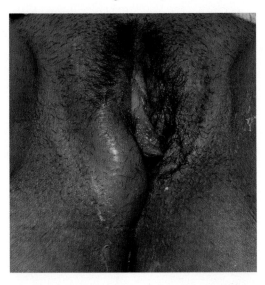

  a. No. 11 blade
  b. No. 10 blade
  c. No. 20 blade
  d. Beaver blade

40-11. Shown here, which of the following is traditionally used as a vaginal retractor?

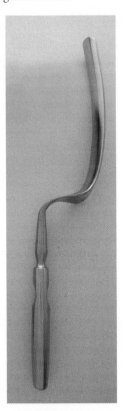

  a. Deaver retractor
  b. Richardson retractor
  c. Harrington retractor
  d. Breitsky-Navratil retractor

40-12. Placement of the grounding pad as shown here on the upper thigh prior to hysterectomy serves all **EXCEPT** which of the following goals?

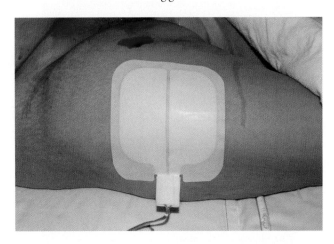

  a. Provides a flat surface to maximize the exit site for current
  b. Provides a small surface area on which to concentrate current
  c. Provides an exit site for current that is close to the operative site
  d. Aids prevention of electrical burns when using monopolar electrosurgery

40–13. Which of the following is true of cavitational ultrasonic surgical aspiration?

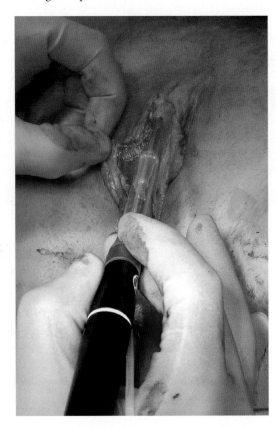

Reproduced, with permission, from Word L, Hoffman BL: Surgeries for benign gynecologic conditions. In Hoffman BL, Schorge JO, Schaffer JI, et al (eds): Williams Gynecology, 2nd ed. New York, McGraw-Hill, 2012, Figure 41-28.3.

   a. Requires a grounding pad for patient safety

   b. Is less disruptive to tissues with a high water content

   c. Disrupts tissue architecture using a process termed *reabsorption*

   d. May be selected to minimize nerve and blood vessel damage within affected tissues

40–14. To control bleeding from an isolated small vessel, sealing the vessel using electrosurgical energy offers all **EXCEPT** which of the following advantages compared with suture ligature?

   a. Is faster

   b. Avoids suture ligature slippage

   c. Creates less damage to surrounding tissues

   d. More easily reaches vessels in narrow spaces

40–15. Which of the following topical hemostats does **NOT** include coagulation cascade proteins?

   a. Fibrin sealants

   b. Active hemostats

   c. Flowable hemostats

   d. Mechanical hemostats

40–16. Mechanical hemostats aid control of bleeding by which of the following mechanisms?

   a. Create a pressure scaffold that entraps platelets

   b. Bind directly to von Willebrand factor to promote platelet aggregation

   c. Directly stimulate thromboxane-A synthase production of thromboxane

   d. Bind to prothrombinase complex to promote direct conversion of prothrombin to thrombin

40–17. Bleeding in the space of Retzius may complicate all **EXCEPT** which of the following procedures?

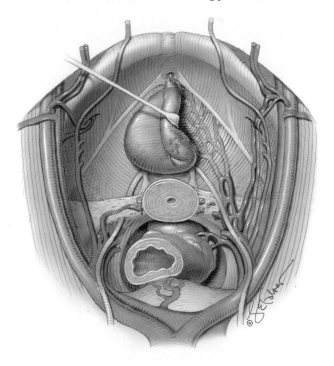

Reproduced, with permission, from Corton MM: Anatomy. In Hoffman BL, Schorge JO, Schaffer JI, et al (eds): Williams Gynecology, 2nd ed. New York, McGraw-Hill, 2012, Figure 38-24.

   a. Burch colposuspension

   b. Transobturator tape procedure

   c. Tension-free vaginal tape procedure

   d. Abdominal paravaginal defect repair

40–18. What is the blood volume of a 50-kg female?

   a. 2500 mL

   b. 3500 mL

   c. 4500 mL

   d. 5500 mL

40–19. What volume of blood typically can be lost by a 50-kg woman before tachycardia and blood pressure changes develop?

    a. 500 mL

    b. 1000 mL

    c. 1250 mL

    d. 1500 mL

40–20. Targets of fluid replacement include which of the following?

    a. Urine output of 30 mL/hr or more

    b. Heart rate less than 100 beats per minute

    c. Systolic blood pressure above 90 mm Hg

    d. All of the above

40–21. In those without significant heart disease, what is the threshold above which red blood cell transfusion is seldom required?

    a. 8 g/dL

    b. 9 g/dL

    c. 10 g/dL

    d. 11 g/dL

40–22. Side effects seen with an acute hemolytic transfusion reaction include all **EXCEPT** which of the following?

    a. Fever

    b. Dyspnea

    c. Acute tubular necrosis

    d. Fulminant liver failure

40–23. If acute hemolytic transfusion reaction is suspected, which of the following immediate steps is indicated?

    a. Halt transfusion.

    b. Initiate prompt diuresis with intravenous crystalloids and furosemide diuretic.

    c. Obtain a patient blood sample for the hematology laboratory to compare with the transfused bag.

    d. All of the above

40–24. Which of the following is true of packed red blood cell (RBC) transfusion?

    a. Each unit of packed RBCs provides 500 mL of volume.

    b. Each unit of packed RBCs has a hematocrit of approximately 70 percent.

    c. Each unit of packed RBCs typically increases the hemoglobin level by approximately 3 g/dL.

    d. Each unit of packed RBCs contains enough fibrinogen to raise the fibrinogen level by 10 g/dL.

40–25. Injury to the bladder during total abdominal hysterectomy may more commonly occur at which of the following surgical steps?

    a. Closing the vaginal cuff

    b. Opening the vesicovaginal space

    c. Dissecting the bladder off the cervix

    d. All of the above

40–26. Injury to the bladder may be identified using which of the following procedures?

    a. Cystoscopy

    b. Direct visualization of the Foley bulb

    c. Retrograde instillation of sterile milk

    d. All of the above

40–27. Injury to the ureter during total abdominal hysterectomy may more commonly occur at which of the following surgical steps?

    a. Closing the vaginal cuff

    b. Ligating the uterine artery

    c. Ligating of the infundibulopelvic ligament

    d. Opening the anterior leaf of the broad ligament

Chapter 40   ANSWER KEY

Question number	Letter answer	Page cited	Header cited
40–1	d	p. 980	Paracervical Blockade
40–2	c	p. 981	Toxicity
40–3	c	p. 981	Surgical Safety
40–4	b	p. 982	Patient Positioning
40–5	a	p. 982	Femoral Nerve Injury
40–6	b	p. 984	Obturator Nerve Injury
40–7	c	p. 983	Transverse Incisions
40–8	b	p. 986	Subcutaneous Adipose Layer
40–9	d	p. 987	Skin
40–10	a	p. 988	Scalpel and Blades
40–11	d	p. 992	Retractors Used in Vaginal Surgery
40–12	b	p. 1001	Patient Grounding
40–13	d	p. 1002	Cavitational Ultrasonic Surgical Aspiration
40–14	c	p. 1003	Suture Ligature
40–15	d	p. 1005	Table 40-6

Question number	Letter answer	Page cited	Header cited
40–16	a	p. 1004	Local Topical Hemostats
40–17	b	p. 1005	Space of Retzius
40–18	b	p. 1006	Fluid Resuscitation and Blood Transfusion
40–19	a	p. 1006	Fluid Resuscitation and Blood Transfusion
40–20	d	p. 1007	Fluid Resuscitation
40–21	c	p. 1008	Red Blood Cell Replacement
40–22	d	p. 1009	Acute Hemolytic Transfusion Reactions
40–23	d	p. 1009	Acute Hemolytic Transfusion Reactions
40–24	b	p. 1009	Table 40-8
40–25	d	p. 1011	Bladder and Urethra
40–26	d	p. 1011	Diagnosis
40–27	c	p. 1011	Ureteral Injury

ATLAS OF GYNECOLOGIC SURGERY

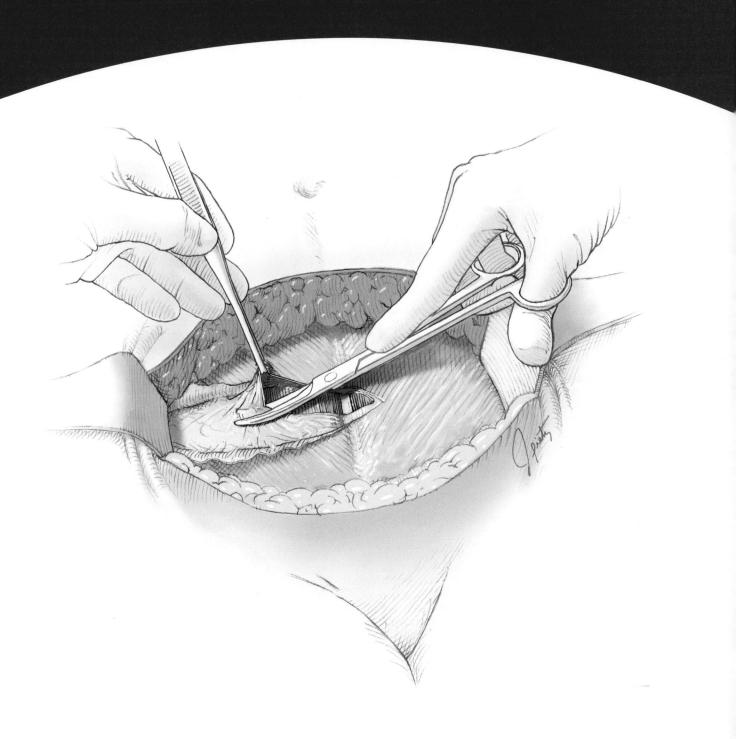

CHAPTER 41

Surgeries for Benign Gynecologic Conditions

41-1. Compared with a midline vertical incision, attributes of the Pfannenstiel incision include which of the following?

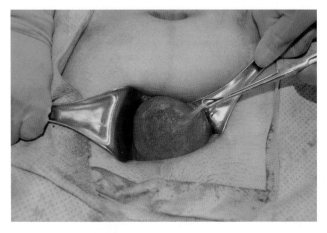

Photograph contributed by Dr. Marlene Corton.

    a. Inferior cosmetic results

    b. Greater access to the upper abdomen

    c. Fewer neurovascular structures encountered

    d. Lower rates of subsequent incisional hernia

41-2. With wide transverse incisions, improper self-retaining retractor placement may lead to injury of which of the following nerves?

    a. Femoral

    b. Pudendal

    c. Obturator

    d. Lateral femoral cutaneous

41-3. The Pfannenstiel, Cherney, and Maylard incisions are abdominal incisions used for gynecologic procedures. The Maylard incision differs mainly from the Pfannenstiel and Cherney incisions in which of the following ways?

    a. It is a transverse abdominal incision.

    b. The tendons of the pyramidalis muscle are transected.

    c. The tendons of the rectus abdominis muscle are transected.

    d. The bellies of the rectus abdominis muscle are transected.

41-4. During oophorectomy, the infundibulopelvic ligament is isolated prior to clamping, transection, and ligation. This ideally averts injury to the structure shown in the second image beneath the arrow.

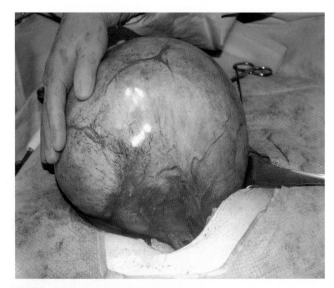

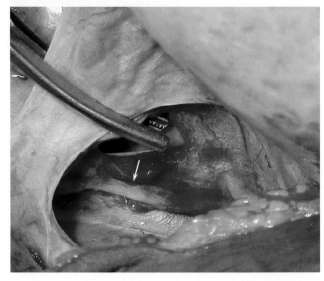

Photographs contributed by Dr. David Miller.

    a. Ureter

    b. Uterine artery

    c. Obturator nerve

    d. Genitofemoral nerve

41–5. The images below illustrate which interval partial salpingectomy method?

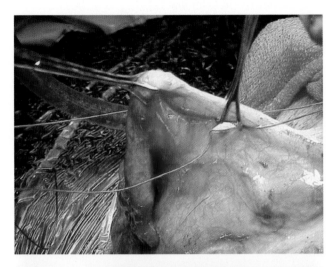

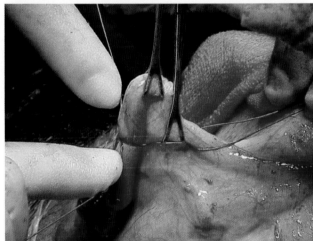

Reproduced, with permission, from Hnat MD: Tubal ligation at the time of cesarean section (update). In Cunningham FG, Leveno KL, Bloom SL, et al (eds), Williams Obstetrics, 22nd ed. Online, New York, McGraw-Hill, 2006, http://www.accessmedicine.com, Figures 5 and 6.

   a. Uchida

   b. Irving

   c. Pomeroy

   d. Parkland

41–6. The image below illustrates incision of the mesosalpinx, which is an early step performed in which of the following operative procedures?

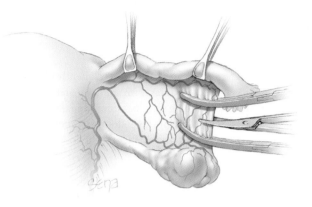

Reproduced, with permission, from Hoffman BL: Surgeries for benign gynecologic conditions. In Schorge JO, Schaffer JI, Halvorson LM, et al (eds): Williams Gynecology, 1st ed. New York, McGraw-Hill, 2008, Figure 41-25.1.

   a. Cystectomy

   b. Salpingostomy

   c. Salpingectomy

   d. Salpingoplasty

41–7. Gonadotropin-releasing hormone agonist (GnRH) use may benefit menorrhagia and anemia prior to myomectomy. Which of the following is an additional benefit of GnRH use preoperatively?

   a. Decreases uterine volume

   b. Increases uterine blood flow

   c. Increases leiomyoma vascularity

   d. None of the above

41–8. 8-Arginine vasopressin is effective in limiting uterine blood loss during myomectomy. Patients with which of the following health conditions may be poor candidates for 8-arginine vasopressin?

   a. Migraine

   b. Uncontrolled hypertension

   c. Chronic obstructive pulmonary disease

   d. All of the above

41–9. Which of the following has been shown to reduce the incidence of adhesion formation following myomectomy?

   a. Postoperative antibiotics

   b. Absorbable adhesion barriers

   c. Normal saline pelvic irrigation

   d. Postoperative transfusion for anemic patients

41-10. Of the hysterectomy types, which has the highest risk of bladder and ureteral injury?

   a. Vaginal hysterectomy

   b. Abdominal hysterectomy

   c. Supracervical hysterectomy

   d. Laparoscopic hysterectomy (LH)

41-11. Hysterectomy is one of the most frequently performed gynecologic procedures, with approximately 600,000 women undergoing this procedure annually in the United States. During this abdominal procedure, the figure below illustrates which of the following?

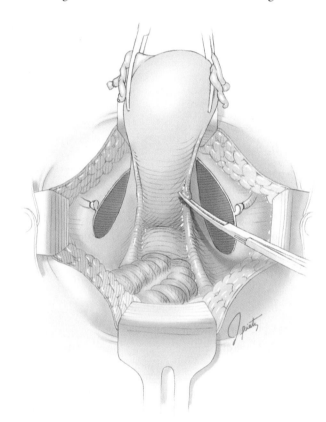

Reproduced, with permission, from Hoffman BL: Surgeries for benign gynecologic conditions. In Schorge JO, Schaffer JI, Halvorson LM, et al (eds): Williams Gynecology, 1st ed. New York, McGraw-Hill, 2008, Figure 41-19.9.

   a. Uterine artery transection

   b. Round ligament transection

   c. Cardinal ligament transection

   d. Uterosacral ligament transection

41-12. With anterior peritoneal cavity entry during vaginal hysterectomy, the final layer incised to gain entry is which of the following?

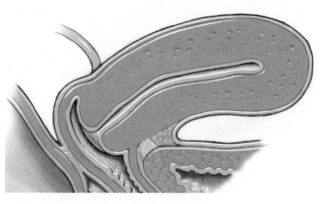

Reproduced and modified, with permission, from Corton MM: Anatomy. In Hoffman BL, Schorge JO, Schaffer JI, et al (eds): Williams Gynecology, 2nd ed. New York, McGraw-Hill, 2012, Figure 38-17.

   a. Vesicouterine fold

   b. Pubocervical fascia

   c. Cul-de-sac of Douglas

   d. Bladder fibrous bands

41-13. At the conclusion of the vaginal hysterectomy, to improve final suspension and support for the vaginal vault, which ligament is sutured to each lateral side of the vaginal cuff?

   a. Round

   b. Broad

   c. Uterosacral

   d. Infundibulopelvic

41-14. Nerve damage may occur from patient positioning for extended periods in the dorsal lithotomy position. Which of the following nerves are at greatest risk?

   a. Genitofemoral

   b. Common peroneal and femoral

   c. Ilioinguinal and iliohypogastric

   d. Abdominal extensions of the intercostals

41-15. With the resurgence of supracervical hysterectomy now performed via laparoscopy, rates of trachelectomy for benign causes are expected to rise in the future. Unlike vaginal hysterectomy, which of the following characterizes trachelectomy?

   a. Clear tissue planes are usually encountered.

   b. Entry into the peritoneal cavity is not required.

   c. During separation of the vaginal wall from the cervix, blunt, not sharp, dissection is preferred.

   d. None of the above

41-16. To decrease the risk of uterine perforation during sharp dilatation and curettage (D&C), which of the following is the first surgical step?

    a. Uterine sounding

    b. Uterine dilation

    c. Bimanual examination

    d. Transvaginal sonography

41-17. During suction dilatation and curettage (D&C), the rate of uterine perforation is greater with which of the following?

    a. A soft uterus

    b. A retroflexed uterus

    c. A dilated cervical os

    d. A cervical os that exhibits a healed obstetric tear

41-18. The main surgical goal following the incision and drainage of a Bartholin gland duct abscess includes steps to create which of the following?

    a. A new duct ostium

    b. Labia cosmetic reapproximation

    c. A blocked epithelialized tract

    d. All of the above

41-19. Compared with Word catheter placement, this treatment of a Bartholin gland duct cyst is associated with which of the following?

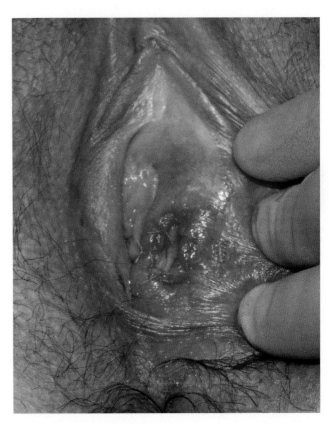

Photograph contributed by Dr. William N. Denson.

    a. Less operative pain

    b. Higher recurrence rates

    c. Smaller intraoperative incision

    d. None of the above

41–20. A 48-year-old patient returns with repetitive recurrence of a painless vulvar cyst shown in the image below. Appropriate management includes which of the following?

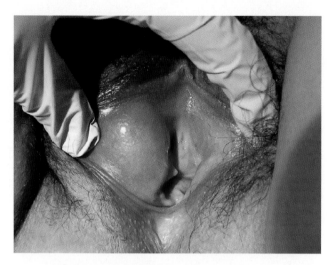

a. Sitz baths only

b. Incision and drainage of the cyst

c. An extended course of oral antibiotics

d. Incision and drainage of the cyst with biopsy of the cyst wall

41–21. Most cases of vulvodynia are managed conservatively, but for refractory cases, which of the following has been employed?

a. Perineoplasty

b. Vestibulectomy

c. Vestibuloplasty

d. All of the above

41–22. The most important factor for surgical success in treating vulvar pain is identifying the proper candidate. Which of the following coexists in approximately half of patients with vulvodynia and is associated with lower rates of postoperative pain relief?

a. Vaginismus

b. Vaginal atrophy

c. Chronic depression

d. A lichenoid epithelial process

41–23. Prior to correction of this condition, the consenting discussion should include which of the following points?

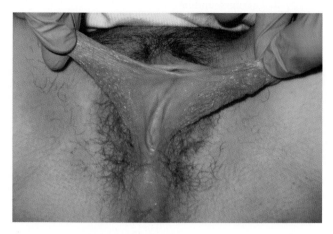

Photograph contributed by Dr. Ellen Wilson.

a. Postoperative dyspareunia is a common complication.

b. Patient expectations should be realistic as to the final size, shape, and color of the labia.

c. Wound complications including hematoma, cellulitis and incisional dehiscence are common complications.

d. All of the above

41–24. Creation of a functional vagina is the treatment goal for many women with congenital agenesis of the vagina. Which of the following surgical procedures is commonly employed in the United States?

a. Septum revision

b. McIndoe procedure

c. Vaginal dilatation

d. Septum reapproximation

41–25. Cryotherapy has been used for decades to safely and effectively eliminate cervical intraepithelial lesions (CIN). The image below illustrates the creation of an iceball. To ensure a necessary 5-mm lethal zone for epithelium cell death, to what distance should the iceball extend beyond the outer margin of the cryoprobe?

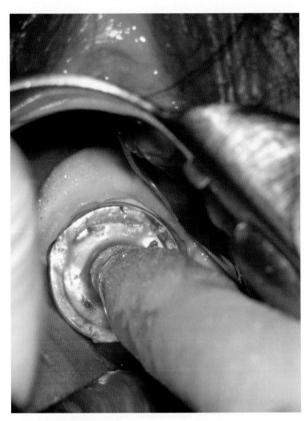

Photograph contributed by Dr. Claudia Werner. Reproduced, with permission, from Hoffman BL: Surgeries for benign gynecologic conditions. In Schorge JO, Schaffer JI, Halvorson LM, et al (eds): Williams Gynecology, 1st ed. New York, McGraw-Hill, 2008, Figure 41-13.3B.

a. 1 mm
b. 2 mm
c. 4 mm
d. 7 mm

41–26. Loop electrosurgical excision procedure (LEEP) uses electric current to generate energy waveforms through a metal electrode that either cuts or desiccates cervical tissue. During the patient consenting process, major complications may include bowel or bladder injury and hemorrhage. Of the following, what is the rate of major complications (percent)?

a. 0.5
b. 1.0
c. 5.0
d. 10

41–27. Compared to the loop electrosurgical excision procedure (LEEP), cervical cold-knife conization has a definitive greater risk of which of the following?

a. Cervical infection
b. Poor obstetric outcome
c. Cervical stenosis and bleeding
d. All of the above

41–28. A 55-year-old otherwise healthy patient presents with biopsy proven vulvar intraepithelial neoplasia (VIN) 2 as shown in the image below. Which of the following is the most appropriate management?

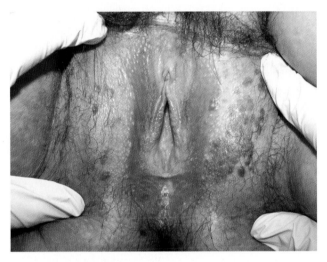

a. Wide local excision
b. Skinning vulvectomy
c. Continued surveillance
d. Combined wide local excision and laser ablation

41–29. Of the following, what is the recommended postprocedural colposcopic vulvar surveillance schedule for high-grade vulvar intraepithelial neoplasia (VIN)?

a. Annually
b. Every 3 months
c. Every 6 months for 3 years
d. Every 6 months for 1 year, then annually thereafter

Chapter 41   ANSWER KEY

Question number	Letter answer	Page cited	Header cited	Question number	Letter answer	Page cited	Header cited
41–1	d	p. 1022	Pfannenstiel Incision	41–18	a	p. 1063	Bartholin Gland Duct Incision and Drainage
41–2	a	p. 1024	Cherney Incision	41–19	d	p. 1065	Bartholin Gland Duct Marsupialization
41–3	d	p. 1025	Maylard Incision				
41–4	a	p. 1028	Oophorectomy	41–20	d	p. 1066	Bartholin Gland Duct Cystectomy
41–5	d	p. 1030	Interval Partial Salpingectomy	41–21	d	p. 1070	Vestibulectomy
41–6	c	p. 1033	Salpingectomy and Salpingostomy	41–22	a	p. 1070	Vestibulectomy
41–7	a	p. 1039	Abdominal Myomectomy	41–23	b	p. 1072	Labial Minora Reduction
41–8	d	p. 1039	Abdominal Myomectomy	41–24	b	p. 1075	McIndoe Procedure
41–9	b	p. 1039	Abdominal Myomectomy	41–25	d	p. 1078	Treatment of Preinvasive Ectocervical Lesions
41–10	d	p. 1045	Abdominal Hysterectomy				
41–11	d	p. 1045	Abdominal Hysterectomy	41–26	a	p. 1078	Treatment of Preinvasive Ectocervical Lesions
41–12	a	p. 1051	Vaginal Hysterectomy				
41–13	c	p. 1051	Vaginal Hysterectomy	41–27	c	p. 1083	Cervical Conization
41–14	b	p. 1051	Vaginal hysterectomy	41–28	d	p. 1086	Treatment of Vulvar Intraepithelial Neoplasia
41–15	b	p. 1055	Trachelectomy				
41–16	c	p. 1057	Sharp Dilation and Curettage	41–29	d	p. 1086	Treatment of Vulvar Intraepithelial Neoplasia
41–17	b	p. 1059	Suction Dilation and Curettage				

CHAPTER 42

Minimally Invasive Surgery

42-1. All **EXCEPT** which of the following are contraindications to the use of pneumoperitoneum during laparoscopy?

    a. Acute glaucoma

    b. Peritoneal shunt

    c. Second-trimester pregnancy

    d. Increased intracranial pressure

42-2. All **EXCEPT** which of the following may be used to effectively compensate for difficulties encountered during laparoscopy in an obese patient?

    a. Steeper Trendelenburg position to improve patient ventilation

    b. Veress needle insertion at an angle that is nearly perpendicular to the skin

    c. Placement of additional ancillary ports to assist in lifting a fattier omentum from the operating field

    d. Use of a gel pad beneath the patient and tucking of patient arms to limit patient slippage while in Trendelenburg position

42-3. The medial umbilical ligament and round ligament are ideally identified prior to ancillary trocar placement through the lower anterior abdominal wall. This assists in minimizing injury to which of the following vessels?

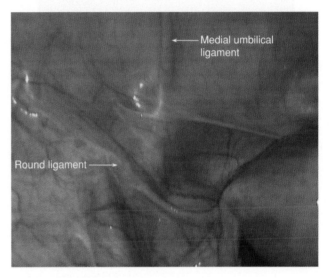

Photograph contributed by Dr. Mayra Thompson.

    a. Inferior epigastric artery

    b. Superior epigastric artery

    c. Superficial epigastric artery

    d. Superficial circumflex iliac artery

42-4. When used for entry at the umbilicus, which of the following abdominal entry methods is associated with the lowest rate of puncture injury?

    a. Open umbilical entry

    b. Optical access trocar entry

    c. Closed entry with Veress needle

    d. All have similar rates

42-5. With abdominal entry using the Veress needle, what threshold for initial abdominal pressure is used to reassure the surgeon regarding correct intraperitoneal needle placement?

    a. <3 mm Hg

    b. <8 mm Hg

    c. <15 mm Hg

    d. <20 mm Hg

42–6. Transillumination of the anterior abdominal wall (shown here) may assist in locating which of the following vessels prior to ancillary trocar placement?

   a. Inferior epigastric artery
   b. Superior epigastric artery
   c. Superficial epigastric artery
   d. Superficial circumflex iliac artery

42–7. Preoperative methods to prevent conception prior to laparoscopic sterilization include which of the following?

   a. Perform surgery in the luteal phase of the menstrual cycle
   b. Provide effective contraception well in advance of surgery
   c. Provide mifepristone 600 mg in a single dose prior to the surgical procedure
   d. All of the above

42–8. During sterilization counseling for tubal sterilization, all **EXCEPT** which of the following discussion points is correct?

   a. Tubal sterilization is surgically challenging and costly to reverse.
   b. Vasectomy is comparable in efficacy but is associated with fewer surgical complications.
   c. If pregnancy occurs following tubal sterilization, the risk of ectopic pregnancy is less than 5 percent.
   d. Risk of regret following sterilization is lower in those who are older at the time of surgery.

42–9. To ensure Filshie clip efficacy, which of the following is true?

   a. Two clips are placed on each fallopian tube.
   b. The clip must remain permanently around the tubal midsegment.
   c. Following clip placement, chromotubation should be performed to document tubal occlusion.
   d. Prior to clip application across the fallopian tube diameter, the tip of the lower jaw should be seen through the mesosalpinx.

42–10. At the time of hysterectomy, a Falope ring is seen loosely adhered to the fallopian tube. Which of the following is true regarding this method of sterilization?

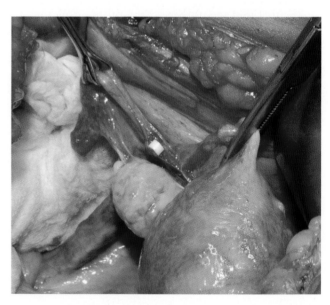

   a. Sterilization is achieved by necrosis and fibrosis of the tubal ends.
   b. A ring must remain around a midsegment loop of fallopian tube to sustain efficacy.
   c. These silicone-based rings are no longer used due to their link with autoimmune disease.
   d. In most cases, a Falope ring found in the cul-de-sac should be considered a dangerous foreign body.

42–11. Important care points for patients following salpingostomy for ectopic pregnancy include which of the following?

 a. Administration of Rh_O (D) immunoglobulin to all patients to prevent Rh sensitization

 b. Postoperative hysterosalpingogram on postoperative day 10 to document tubal patency on the affected side

 c. Administration of single-dose methotrexate 50 mg/m^2 on postoperative day 1 to prevent persistent trophoblastic tissue

 d. Measurement of a serum human chorionic gonadotropin level on postoperative day 1 to exclude persistent trophoblastic tissue

42–12. With laparoscopic oophorectomy, all **EXCEPT** which of the following are appropriate steps completed to anticipate the possibility of ovarian malignancy?

 a. Tumor markers are obtained preoperatively.

 b. Pneumatic compression hose are placed preoperatively.

 c. Pelvic washings are obtained following specimen removal to determine if any cyst contents have spilled.

 d. Preoperatively, patients are counseled regarding the steps of surgical cancer staging that would be performed if malignancy is found intraoperatively.

42–13. Ovarian drilling may be indicated for which of the following patients with polycystic ovarian syndrome (PCOS)?

 a. Those who choose to lower their risk of twins

 b. Those who fail to ovulate with clomiphene citrate

 c. Those with risk factors for ovarian hyperstimulation syndrome

 d. All of the above

42–14. In addition to an intraligamentous location, which of the following characteristics increases the risk of complications during laparoscopic myomectomy?

 a. Nulliparity

 b. Pedunculated leiomyoma

 c. More than three tumors requiring excision

 d. All of the above

42–15. All **EXCEPT** which of the following are suitable techniques to employ during laparoscopic myomectomy?

 a. Use of barbed suture to close the hysterotomy incision

 b. Delivery of the enucleated leiomyoma through a colpotomy incision

 c. Injection of dilute oxytocin into the myometrium to control bleeding during tumor enucleation

 d. Copious irrigation to float and allow removal of myometrium pieces dropped during morcellation

42–16. Women with which of the following characteristics are considered poor candidates for vaginal hysterectomy?

 a. Contracted pelvis

 b. Large adnexal pathology

 c. Suspected dense pelvic adhesions

 d. All of the above

42–17. For vessel occlusion during laparoscopic hysterectomy, which of the following is a suitable choice?

 a. Harmonic scalpel

 b. Bipolar electrosurgery instruments

 c. Monopolar electrosurgery instruments

 d. All of the above

42–18. Women with which of the following characteristics are considered poor candidates for supracervical hysterectomy?

 a. Those with high-grade endocervical dysplasia

 b. Those with endometrial hyperplasia with atypia

 c. Those unable to maintain routine Pap smear screening

 d. All of the above

42–19. Which of the following is true of morcellation of the uterine fundus following supracervical hysterectomy?

 a. Morcellated uterine fragments may be left intraabdominally with no harmful patient effects.

 b. A coring technique into the middle of the mass, rather than a peeling technique, is preferred.

 c. Tissue is held stable in the anterior cul-de-sac, and the morcellator is moved to the mass.

 d. None of the above

42–20. Uterine manipulators designed specifically for total laparoscopic hysterectomy may help with which of the following?

 a. Displacing the ureters laterally

 b. Maintaining pneumoperitoneum during colpotomy

 c. Delineating the cervicovaginal junction for colpotomy

 d. All of the above

42–21. Laminaria are shown before and after expansion. Alternatively, what other options may effectively ease cervical dilatation prior to hysteroscope insertion?

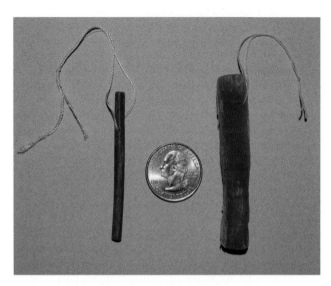

Reproduced, with permission, from Word L, Hoffman BL: Surgeries for benign gynecologic conditions. In Hoffman BL, Schorge JO, Schaffer JI, et al (eds): Williams Gynecology, 2nd ed. New York, McGraw-Hill, 2012, Figure 41-16.1A.

   a. Preoperative misoprostol orally

   b. Preoperative misoprostol vaginally

   c. Dilute vasopressin injected into the cervix intraoperatively

   d. All of the above

42–22. During which of the following hysteroscopic procedures does carbon dioxide serve best as a distension medium?

   a. Leiomyoma resection

   b. Uterine septum excision

   c. Diagnostic hysteroscopy

   d. Endometrial polyp resection

42–23. If excess fluid volume is absorbed during hysteroscopy, patients are at greatest risk of developing hyponatremia with which of the following?

   a. 5-percent mannitol

   b. 1.5-percent glycine

   c. Normal saline

   d. All have equivalent risk of producing hyponatremia

42–24. If gas embolism is suspected, all **EXCEPT** which of the following should be performed?

   a. Remove the hysteroscope

   b. Clamp the cervical os closed

   c. Place the patient in reverse Trendelenburg position

   d. Move the patient to a left lateral decubitus position

42–25. Sonographic and hysteroscopic images display the same endometrial polyp. Hysteroscopic removal can be accomplished by which of the following methods?

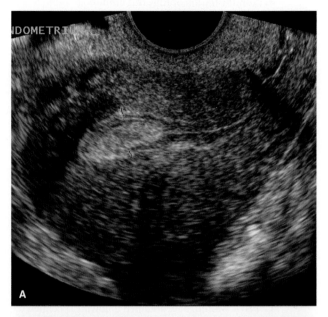

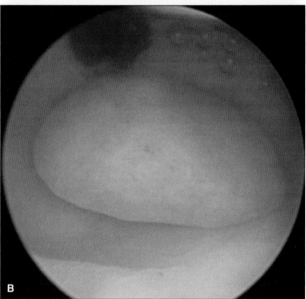

Photograph B contributed by Dr. Kimberly Kho.

   a. Resectoscope loop

   b. Hysteroscopic scissors

   c. Hysteroscopic morcellator

   d. All of the above

42–26. During saline-infusion sonography or hysteroscopy to evaluate leiomyoma characteristics prior to hysteroscopic myomectomy, leiomyomas may be grouped according to criteria from the European Society of Hysteroscopy. As shown here, which of the following classes is associated with the highest clinical success rate, lowest surgical risk, and an infrequent need for more than one surgical session to complete resection?

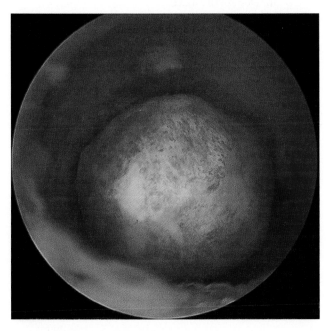

Photograph contributed by Dr. Karen Bradshaw.

- **a.** Class 0
- **b.** Class I
- **c.** Class II
- **d.** Class III

42–27. In addition to the degree of tumor penetration and tumor size, which of the following other leiomyoma characteristics increases the difficulty of hysteroscopic resection?

- **a.** Wide tumor base
- **b.** Tumors along the lateral wall
- **c.** Tumors in the upper portion of the cavity
- **d.** All of the above

42–28. Patients undergoing endometrial ablation for a bleeding abnormality should not be *guaranteed* amenorrhea as a treatment goal. In general, which of the following rates of amenorrhea (percent) is expected?

- **a.** 5–10
- **b.** 15–35
- **c.** 50-65
- **d.** 75-80

42–29. What obstetric problems are associated with pregnancy following endometrial ablation?

- **a.** Prematurity
- **b.** Malpresentation
- **c.** Abnormal adherent placenta
- **d.** All of the above

42–30. Endometrial ablation using this device is achieved by which of the following mechanisms?

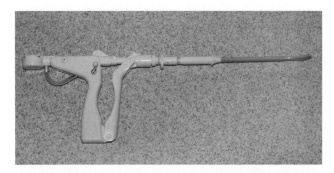

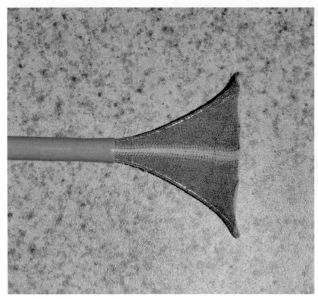

- **a.** Cryonecrosis
- **b.** Microwave energy
- **c.** Monopolar electrosurgical coagulation
- **d.** None of the above

42–31. This device achieves sterilization by which of the following methods?

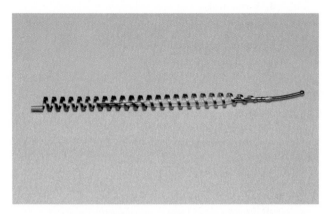

a. Lies within the cervical canal to secrete spermicide

b. Wraps around the fallopian tube to occlude the lumen

c. Is placed within the tubal ostia to promote occlusive tissue ingrowth

d. Is placed within the endometrial canal to agglutinate the endometrium

42–32. Which of the following statement is true of women following Essure microinsert placement?

a. Sterilization is immediate.

b. Hysterosalpingogram is recommended at 6 months following placement.

c. The device in Question 42–30 can be used safely in Essure patients at a later date if needed.

d. None of the above

42–33. Intrauterine adhesions called *synechiae* may develop following uterine curettage and less commonly from pelvic irradiation or tuberculous endometritis. The presence of these adhesions, also termed Asherman syndrome, may lead to increased rates of which of the following?

a. Menorrhagia

b. Infertility

c. Pelvic inflammatory disease

d. All of the above

Chapter 42   ANSWER KEY

Question number	Letter answer	Page cited	Header cited	Question number	Letter answer	Page cited	Header cited
42–1	a	p. 1095	Patient Factors	42–17	d	p. 1145	Laparoscopic Hysterectomy
42–2	a	p. 1096	Obesity	42–18	d	p. 1149	Laparoscopic Supracervical Hysterectomy
42–3	a	p. 1109	Superficial Landmarks to Retroperitoneal Structures	42–19	d	p. 1149	Morcellation
				42–20	d	p. 1154	Colpotomy
42–4	d	p. 1109	Abdominal Access	42–21	d	p. 1157	Cervical Dilatation
42–5	b	p. 1115	Port Placement	42–22	c	p. 1159	Carbon Dioxide
42–6	c	p. 1115	Ancillary Port Placement	42–23	b	p. 1159	Fluid Media
42–7	b	p. 1123	Concurrent Pregnancy	42–24	c	p. 1161	Gas Embolism
42–8	c	p. 1123	Consent	42–25	d	p. 1164	Hysteroscopic Polypectomy
42–9	d	p. 1124	Filshie Clip	42–26	a	p. 1166	Hysteroscopic Myomectomy
42–10	a	p. 1125	Falope Ring (Silastic Band)	42–27	d	p. 1166	Hysteroscopic Myomectomy
42–11	d	p. 1131	Laparoscopic Salpingostomy	42–28	b	p. 1169	Endometrial Ablation Procedures
42–12	c	p. 1137	Laparoscopic Salpingo-oophorectomy	42–29	d	p. 1169	Endometrial Ablation Procedures
42–13	d	p. 1139	Ovarian Drilling	42–30	d	p. 1169	Endometrial Ablation Procedures
42–14	c	p. 1140	Laparoscopic Myomectomy	42–31	c	p. 1172	Transcervical Sterilization
42–15	c	p. 1140	Laparoscopic Myomectomy	42–32	d	p. 1172	Transcervical Sterilization
42–16	d	p. 1145	Laparoscopic Hysterectomy	42–33	b	p. 1178	Lysis of Intrauterine Adhesions

Surgeries for Pelvic Floor Disorders

43–1. Mandatory components to a rigid cystoscope include all **EXCEPT** which of the following?

  a. Bridge

  b. Camera

  c. Sheath

  d. Telescope and light source

43–2. Which rigid telescope most easily permits visualization of the lateral, anterior, and posterior bladder walls during diagnostic cystoscopy?

  a. 0-degree lens

  b. 30-degree lens

  c. 70-degree lens

  d. 120-degree lens

43–3. In this figure, the retropubic space is shown with two sutures on either side of the urethra. The first sutures are at the level of the urethrovesical junction, and the second are near the proximal third of the urethra. These are tied to the ipsilateral iliopectineal ligament (Cooper ligament). All **EXCEPT** which of the following are true regarding this procedure?

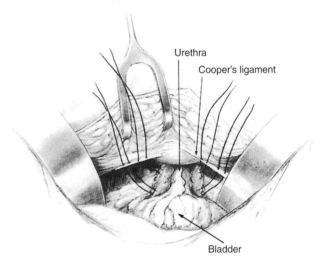

Reproduced, with permission, from Tarnay CM, Bhatia NN: Urinary incontinence. In DeCherney AH, Nathan L (eds): CURRENT Diagnosis & Treatment Obstetrics & Gynecology, 10th ed. New York, McGraw-Hill, 2007, Figure 45-6A.

  a. Brisk bleeding in this operative space is likely due to laceration of vessels within the plexus of Santorini.

  b. The patient is placed in candy-cane stirrups or Allen stirrups in high lithotomy position for this procedure.

  c. Symptomatic success or cure in treatment of stress urinary incontinence is achieved in approximately 85 percent of patients.

  d. Overcorrection of the urethrovesical angle (i.e., not leaving a suture bridge) has been suggested as a cause of postoperative voiding dysfunction.

43–4. Indications for the tension-free vaginal tape procedure include all **EXCEPT** which of the following?

  a. Urge urinary incontinence

  b. Prior failed anti-incontinence procedure

  c. Stress urinary incontinence related to urethral hypermobility

  d. Stress urinary incontinence related to intrinsic sphincteric deficiency

43-5. Risks associated with the transobturator tape sling include all **EXCEPT** which of the following?

a. Groin pain

b. Bleeding in the space of Retzius

c. Postoperative urgency incontinence

d. Postoperative voiding dysfunction, urinary retention

43-6. Which of the following statements regarding urethral bulking injection is correct?

a. It requires general anesthesia in the operating room.

b. Autologous fat is the most commonly used bulking agent.

c. Its success and cure rates for stress urinary incontinence are equivalent to those seen using midurethral slings.

d. None of the above

43-7. All **EXCEPT** which of these statements regarding urethrolysis are true?

a. The usual indication is bladder hypotonia.

b. Antibiotic prophylaxis is generally given.

c. Performing preoperative urodynamic studies is appropriate.

d. It may be performed transvaginally or abdominally depending on the route of the original anti-incontinence surgery.

43-8. Which of these is **NOT** an approach to urethral diverticulum repair?

a. Latzko vaginal repair

b. Spence marsupialization

c. Complete diverticulectomy

d. Partial diverticular ablation

43-9. In the United States, most vesicovaginal fistulas are associated with which of the following?

a. Obstetric trauma

b. Pelvic radiation therapy

c. Prior hysterectomy for benign causes

d. Hysterectomy related to gynecologic malignancy

43-10. Regarding the timing of vesicovaginal fistula repair identified after hysterectomy, which statement is correct?

a. Surrounding tissue infection or inflammation must be absent.

b. Repair may be completed within the first few days posthysterectomy.

c. Repair may be completed after a delay of 4 to 6 weeks after the initial surgery.

d. All of the above

43-11. Which surgical steps would be recommended for the transvaginal repair of the fistula demonstrated here?

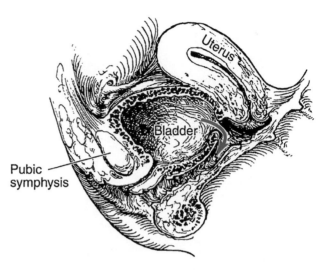

Reproduced, with permission, from Tanagho EA: Disorders of the bladder, prostate, and seminal vesicles. In Tanagho EA, McAninch JW (eds): Smith's General Urology, 17th ed. New York. McGraw-Hill, 2008, Figure 37-3.

a. Cystoscopy to demonstrate ureteral patency

b. Placement of ureteral stents if ureters are close to the fistula

c. Placement of a pediatric urethral catheter through the fistulous opening

d. All of the above

43-12. When attempting a transvaginal repair of a vesicovaginal fistula that resulted from prior irradiation and in which vaginal tissues are fibrotic, which of the following techniques is the most appropriate to consider?

a. Inject a fibrin sealant via the cystoscope

b. Use a vascular graft such as the bulbocavernosus fat pad

c. Minimize approximation of the vaginal fibromuscular layer

d. Create increased tension along a rapidly absorbable suture line

43-13. Sacral neuromodulation has all **EXCEPT** which of the following indications?

a. Urinary urgency

b. Urinary frequency

c. Urge urinary incontinence

d. Obstructive urinary retention

43-14. What is the key reason to consider preoperative urodynamic testing for a continent woman planning the anterior vaginal wall surgery pictured below?

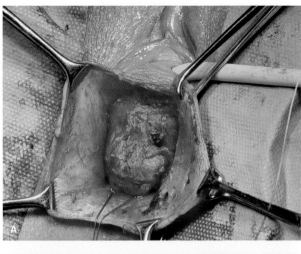
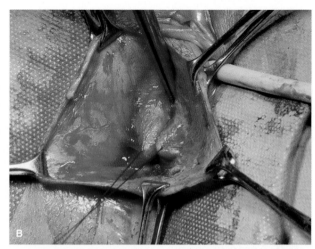
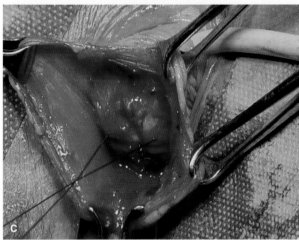
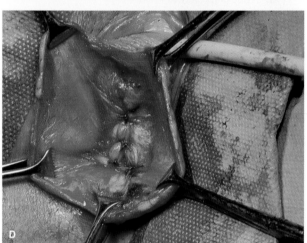

a. To predict those at highest risk for prolapse recurrence

b. To minimize the high risk of ureteral entrapment/injury that is associated with this procedure

c. To "unmask" those patients with "occult" incontinence so as to consider a concomitant anti-incontinence procedure

d. None of the above

43-15. Which of the following statements regarding the abdominal paravaginal repair is true?

a. It provides support to the distal anterior vagina.

b. It is an effective treatment for stress urinary incontinence.

c. It is useful for correction of midline defects in the anterior vaginal wall.

d. It is commonly performed in conjunction with the Burch colposuspension or other retropubic urethropexy.

43–16. The patient pictured below presents complaining of the need to manually reduce the bulge by pushing her fingers inside the vagina every time she has to defecate—especially when she is constipated. Which of the following statements regarding the procedure used to correct this defect is correct?

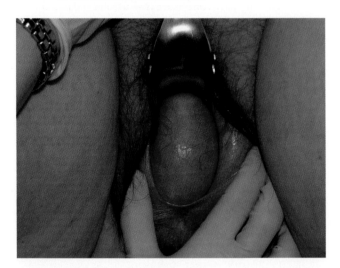

Photograph contributed by Dr. Marlene Corton.

  a. Concomitant perineorrhaphy is rarely necessary.

  b. There is significant risk of ureteral entrapment or injury.

  c. Placement of plication sutures too far laterally may result in dyspareunia.

  d. Correction of the bulge should reliably improve the patient's constipation.

43–17. Compared with traditional restorative transvaginal procedures for correcting apical vaginal prolapse, which of the following is true regarding the abdominal route pictured below?

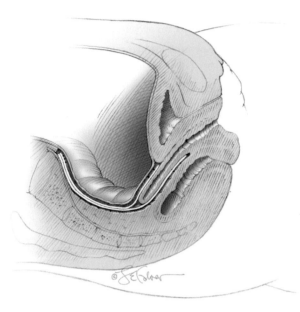

Reproduced, with permission, from Schaffer JI, Hoffman BL: Surgeries for female pelvic reconstruction. In Schorge JO, Schaffer JI, Halvorson LM, et al (eds): **Williams Gynecology**, 1st ed. New York, McGraw-Hill, 2008, Figure 42-17.7.

  a. Has a higher risk of failure

  b. Tends to shorten the vaginal length

  c. Creates a mobile vaginal apex, thereby possibly decreasing the risk of dyspareunia

  d. Should only be used for recurrent prolapse after other failed prolapse surgeries

43–18. Which of the following describes the best graft material for most patients undergoing abdominal sacrocolpopexy?

  a. Cadaveric fascia

  b. Monofilament synthetic mesh with large pore size

  c. Multifilament synthetic mesh with small pore size

  d. Autologous fascia such as fascia lata or rectus fascia

43–19. Risks associated with vaginal uterosacral ligament suspension may include which of the following?

  a. Ureteral kinking and injury

  b. Nerve injury and subsequent neuropathy

  c. Shortening and fixation of the upper vagina with postoperative dyspareunia

  d. All of the above

43-20. Which of the following is true of the sacrospinous ligament fixation procedure?

   a. May ultimately result in recurrent or de novo anterior compartment prolapse

   b. May lead to hemorrhage due to laceration of vessels within the plexus of Santorini

   c. Has a substantially higher anatomic success rate compared to uterosacral ligament suspension

   d. Has a longer operating time and more prolonged recovery compared with abdominal sacrocolpopexy

43-21. Which of these statements regarding obliteration of the cul-de-sac of Douglas is correct?

   a. These procedures are used to address cystoceles.

   b. Both the Moschcowitz and Halban approaches may be associated with ureteral kinking and injury.

   c. The transabdominal procedures are increasing in popularity due to their effective correction of apical prolapse.

   d. McCall culdoplasty is preferred to uterosacral or sacrospinous ligament fixation for addressing significant vaginal apical prolapse.

43-22. All **EXCEPT** which of the following procedures are commonly performed concomitantly with a Lefort partial colpocleisis?

   a. Cystoscopy

   b. Perineorrhaphy

   c. Vaginal hysterectomy

   d. Anti-incontinence procedure

43-23. Lefort colpocleisis is contraindicated in which of the following patients?

   a. Those with unexplained vaginal bleeding

   b. Those without a normal, recent Pap smear

   c. Those desiring future vaginal intercourse

   d. All of the above

43-24. Which of the following statements regarding anal sphincteroplasty is correct?

   a. Wound complications are rare.

   b. Muscle fibers may be identified using a nerve stimulator.

   c. Long-term continence rates to solid and liquid stool are excellent and approximate 80 percent.

   d. Attention is primarily directed to repair of the external anal sphincter muscle to address the resting tone of the anal canal.

43-25. The patient with the defect below complains of passing flatus from her vagina and of occasional brown malodorous discharge sometimes when wiping after voiding. All **EXCEPT** which of the following are appropriate perioperative interventions?

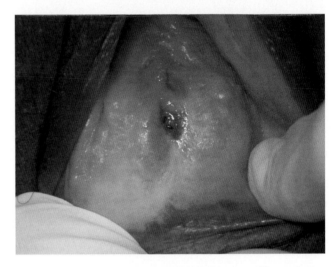

Reproduced, with permission, from Corton MM: Anal incontinence and functional anorectal disorders. In Schorge JO, Schaffer JI, Halvorson LM, et al (eds): Williams Gynecology, 1st ed. New York, McGraw-Hill, 2008, Figure 25-10.

   a. Preoperative bowel preparation

   b. Delaying defecation for several days postprocedure

   c. Avoiding constipation with liberal use of stool softeners postprocedure

   d. Antibiotic prophylaxis beginning 3 days before the reparative procedure

Chapter 43   ANSWER KEY

Question number	Letter answer	Page cited	Header cited
43–1	b	p. 1185	Diagnostic and Operative Cystoscopy and Urethroscopy
43–2	c	p. 1185	Diagnostic and Operative Cystoscopy and Urethroscopy
43–3	b	p. 1189	Burch Colposuspension
43–4	a	p. 1191	Tension-Free Vaginal Tape
43–5	b	p. 1194	Transobturator Tape Sling
43–6	d	p. 1198	Urethral Bulking Injections
43–7	a	p. 1200	Urethrolysis
43–8	a	p. 1203	Urethral Diverticulum Repair
43–9	c	p. 1206	Vesicovaginal Fistula: Latzko Technique
43–10	d	p. 1206	Vesicovaginal Fistula: Latzko Technique
43–11	d	p. 1206	Vesicovaginal Fistula: Latzko Technique
43–12	b	p. 1210	Martius Bulbocavernosus Fat Pad Flap
43–13	d	p. 1212	Sacral Neuromodulation
43–14	c	p. 1214	Anterior Colporrhaphy

Question number	Letter answer	Page cited	Header cited
43–15	d	p. 1217	Abdominal Paravaginal Defect Repair
43–16	c	p. 1219	Posterior Colporrhaphy
43–17	c	p. 1225	Abdominal Sacrocolpopexy
43–18	b	p. 1225	Abdominal Sacrocolpopexy
43–19	d	p. 1236	Vaginal Uterosacral Ligament Suspension
43–20	a	p. 1238	Sacrospinous Ligament Fixation
43–21	b	p. 1242	McCall Culdoplasty and Abdominal Culdoplasty Procedures
43–22	c	p. 1246	Lefort Partial Colpocleisis
43–23	d	p. 1246	Lefort Partial Colpocleisis
43–24	b	p. 1252	Anal Sphincteroplasty
43–25	d	p. 1255	Rectovaginal Fistula Repair

CHAPTER 44

Surgeries for Gynecologic Malignacies

44-1. What is the most common complication from a radical abdominal hysterectomy and lymph node dissection?

   a. Lymphocele

   b. Constipation

   c. Urinary retention

   d. Intraoperative hemorrhage

44-2. Which of the following is **FALSE** regarding type II radical hysterectomy?

   a. Postoperative bladder dysfunction is uncommon.

   b. The uterine vessels are ligated at their origin.

   c. The most common indication is stage IA2 cervical cancer.

   d. Less vaginal tissue is removed compared with a type III radical hysterectomy.

44-3. Which of the following is **NOT** an advantage of laparoscopic radical hysterectomy compared with an abdominal approach?

   a. Less blood loss

   b. Shorter procedure

   c. Shorter hospital stay

   d. Less postoperative pain

44-4. What steps can be taken during laparoscopy to minimize complications?

   a. Placement of Foley catheter

   b. Placement of nasogastric or orogastric tube

   c. Positioning of the patient flat, not in Trendelenburg position

   d. All of the above

44-5. What is the first step of a radical hysterectomy?

   a. Opening the paravesical and pararectal spaces

   b. Dividing the utero-ovarian ligaments if ovarian preservation is planned

   c. Dissecting the ureters from the peritoneum to the level of the uterine arteries

   d. Opening the rectovaginal septum and dissecting the rectum off the posterior vagina

44-6. What is the most common indication for performing a total pelvic exenteration?

   a. Recurrent vulvar cancer

   b. Stage IVA cervical cancer

   c. Recurrent endometrial cancer

   d. Centrally recurrent cervical cancer

44-7. What is the most common reason for aborting an exenteration?

   a. Sidewall involvement

   b. Peritoneal metastases

   c. Parametrial involvement

   d. Para-aortic lymph node metastases

44-8. What is the most common complication of an incontinent urinary conduit?

   a. Infection

   b. Anastomotic leak

   c. Ureteral stricture

   d. Electrolyte abnormalities

44-9. Which of the following statements regarding continent urinary conduits is **FALSE**?

   a. Obese women are ideal candidates for this surgery.

   b. Approximately 10 percent of patients will require surgical revision.

   c. A Miami pouch includes portions of the ileum, ascending colon, and transverse colon.

   d. Complications are common, and include pyelonephritis, urinary strictures, and difficulty with catheterization.

44-10. Which of the following flaps cannot be performed in a patient with a history of a Maylard incision?

   a. Rhomboid flap

   b. Gracilis myocutaneous flap

   c. Rectus abdominis myocutaneous flap

   d. Pudendal thigh fasciocutaneous flap

44–11. What is the structure identified by the arrow?

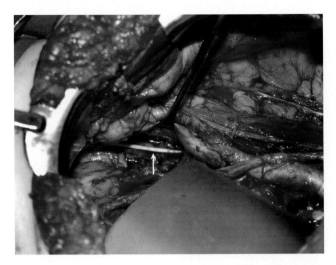

- **a.** Obturator vein
- **b.** Obturator nerve
- **c.** Obturator artery
- **d.** Genitofemoral nerve

44–12. Which of the following are the correct boundaries for a paraaortic lymphadenectomy for endometrioid adenocarcinoma of the uterus?

- **a.** Bifurcation of aorta, renal vein
- **b.** Mid-common iliac artery, renal vein
- **c.** Bifurcation of aorta, inferior mesenteric artery
- **d.** Mid-common iliac artery, inferior mesenteric artery

44–13. Which of the following is the **LEAST** common complication from para-aortic lymphadenectomy?

- **a.** Ileus
- **b.** Lymphocyst
- **c.** Ureteral injury
- **d.** Intraoperative hemorrhage

44–14. Which of the following is **NOT** an indication for omentectomy?

- **a.** Clinical stage I ovarian cancer
- **b.** Advanced ovarian cancer with omental involvement
- **c.** Papillary serous endometrial cancer clinically confined to the uterus
- **d.** Grade I endometrioid adenocarcinoma of the uterus clinically confined to the uterus

44–15. The organ to the right was removed with the omentum during cancer debulking surgery. Which of the following vaccines should be administered postoperatively?

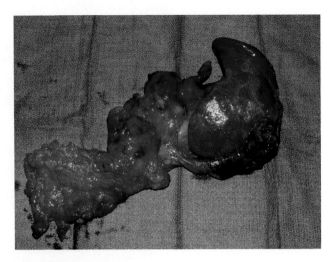

Photograph contributed by Dr. Jennifer Prats.

- **a.** Pneumococcal
- **b.** Meningococcal
- **c.** Haemophilus influenzae
- **d.** All of the above

44–16. Which of the following statements regarding diaphragm resection for ovarian cancer is **FALSE**?

- **a.** Chest tubes are typically required.
- **b.** The use of grafts for repair is uncommon.
- **c.** Pleural effusion is a common complication.
- **d.** In the setting of optimal debulking, it improves survival rates.

44–17. When is a loop colostomy **NOT** recommended?

- **a.** Colonic perforation during chemotherapy for ovarian cancer
- **b.** Large bowel obstruction in the setting of recurrent cervical cancer
- **c.** Protection of a low rectal anastomosis after ovarian cancer debulking
- **d.** Rectovaginal fistula after chemoradiation for cervical cancer, with no evidence of disease

44-18. Which of the following bowel segments is **NOT** directly supplied by a branch of the superior mesenteric artery?

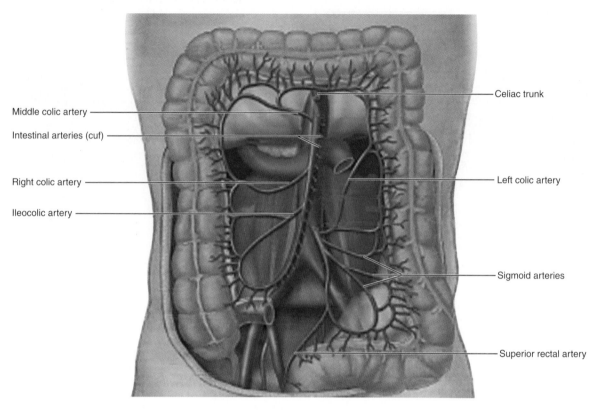

Reproduced, with permission, from McKinley M, O'Loughlin VD (eds): Vessels and circulation. In Human Anatomy. New York, McGraw-Hill, 2006, Figure 23-15.

a. Cecum

b. Ascending colon

c. Transverse colon

d. Descending colon

44-19. A 45-year-old woman has a history of stage IIB cervical cancer for which she completed chemoradiation therapy 12 months ago. She is admitted with a diagnosis of recurrent small bowel obstruction. Her computed tomography scan is shown below. Where is the most likely site of obstruction?

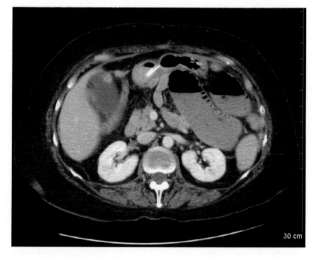

a. Jejunum

b. Distal ileum

c. Gastric outlet

d. Proximal ileum

44–20. Which of the following is a risk factor for anastomotic leak of a rectosigmoid anastomosis?

- **a.** Low anastomosis
- **b.** Albumin level less than 3 g/dL
- **c.** History of pelvic radiation
- **d.** All of the above

44–21. A 55-year-old woman with a history of cervical cancer and chemoradiation treatment undergoes an intestinal bypass for a nonresectable small bowel obstruction. She initially does well but then develops recurrent nausea, vomiting, and diarrhea. She continues to pass flatus. Which of the following is **NOT** part of this condition?

- **a.** Steatorrhea
- **b.** Bacterial overgrowth
- **c.** Small bowel obstruction
- **d.** Vitamin B_{12} malabsorption

44–22. In which of the following patients is an appendectomy during gynecologic surgery **NOT** indicated?

- **a.** A 25-year-old who undergoes a right salpingo-oophorectomy for a serous cystadenoma
- **b.** A 25-year-old who undergoes a right salpingo-oophorectomy for a mucinous low malignant potential tumor
- **c.** A 60-year-old with stage IIIC ovarian cancer undergoing cytoreductive surgery and with tumor involving the appendix
- **d.** A 40-year-old woman who is found to have extensive mucin in her abdomen and bilateral mucinous tumors of the ovaries

44–23. Which of the following statements regarding radical partial vulvectomy is **FALSE**?

- **a.** Local recurrence rate is approximately 10 percent.
- **b.** It is ideal for women with unilateral well-circumscribed lesions.
- **c.** The distal urethra may be removed without an increase risk in urinary incontinence.
- **d.** Survival is worse compared with patients undergoing complete radical vulvectomy, even if negative margins are achieved.

44–24. During inguinofemoral lymphadenectomy, which of the following may lower postoperative rates of chronic lymphedema?

- **a.** Sparing the saphenous vein
- **b.** Sparing the cribriform fascia
- **c.** Sartorius muscle transposition
- **d.** Jackson-Pratt drain placed prior to incision closure

44–25. During inguinofemoral lymphadenectomy, if the lymph nodes in the groin are grossly positive below the cribriform fascia, what is the most appropriate management?

- **a.** Do not resect them, and give postoperative chemoradiation
- **b.** Incise the cribriform fascia, and remove the lymph nodes
- **c.** Incise the cribriform fascia, remove the involved lymph nodes, repair the defect in the cribriform fascia, and consider a transposition of the sartorius muscle
- **d.** Incise the cribriform fascia, remove the involved lymph nodes, repair the defect in the cribriform fascia, transpose the sartorius muscle, and give postoperative chemoradiation

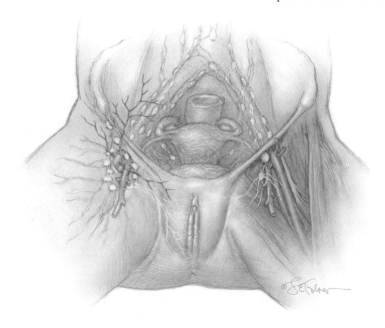

Chapter 44   ANSWER KEY

Question number	Letter answer	Page cited	Header cited
44–1	d	p. 1259	Radical Abdominal Hysterectomy
44–2	b	p. 1265	Modified Radical Abdominal Hysterectomy
44–3	b	p. 1267	Laparoscopic Radical Hysterectomy
44–4	d	p. 1267	Laparoscopic Radical Hysterectomy
44–5	a	p. 1272	Robotic Radical Hysterectomy
44–6	d	p. 1276	Total Pelvic Exenteration
44–7	b	p. 1276	Total Pelvic Exenteration
44–8	a	p. 1284	Incontinent Urinary Conduit
44–9	a	p. 1288	Continent Urinary Conduit
44–10	c	p. 1292	Vaginal Reconstruction
44–11	b	p. 1296	Pelvic Lymphadenectomy
44–12	d	p. 1299	Para-aortic Lymphadenectomy
44–13	b	p. 1306	Robotic Surgical Staging
44–14	d	p. 1313	Omentectomy
44–15	d	p. 1315	Splenectomy
44–16	a	p. 1317	Diaphragmatic Surgery
44–17	d	p. 1319	Colostomy
44–18	d	p. 1322	Large Bowel Resection
44–19	b	p. 1325	Small Bowel Resection
44–20	d	p. 1327	Low Anterior Resection
44–21	c	p. 1331	Intestinal Bypass
44–22	a	p. 1333	Appendectomy
44–23	d	p. 1337	Radical Partial Vulvectomy
44–24	a	p. 1343	Inguinofemoral Lymphadenectomy
44–25	d	p. 1343	Inguinofemoral Lymphadenectomy

Index

Thyrotropin-releasing hormone, 89
Total abdominal hysterectomy
    injury to bladder, 233, 234
    injury to ureter, 233, 234
    midline vertical incision, 226, 228
    preoperative intravenous antibiotic
        prophylaxis regimens, 223, 228
    for uterine leiomyomas, 224, 228
Total abdominal hysterectomy (TAH), 191,
    193, 195
Tranexamic acid, 46
Transobturator tape procedure, 232, 234
Transobturator tape sling, 250, 255
Transvaginal sonography, 38, 44
    advantages of, 43
Transverse cervical ligaments, 218, 221
Transverse vaginal septum, 105
Triple test, 69
Tubal obstruction, 58, 116
Tubal sterilization, 244, 249
Tuberous breasts, 81
Tuboovarian abscess, 54
Tumor cells susceptibility, chemotherapy for,
    154, 158
Tumor markers, 51, 55
Turner syndrome, 93, 94, 104
Type 1 diabetes mellitus, postoperative
    insulin administration, 222, 228
Type II radical hysterectomy, 256, 260

U

Umbilical ligament, 243, 249
Uncomplicated total abdominal
    hysterectomy, 224, 228
Unicornuate uterus, 106
Unilateral salpingooophorectomy (USO),
    203, 206
Ureter, 236, 242
Ureterovaginal fistula, 151, 152
    in developed countries, 150, 152
    diagnostic tools/techniques, 148, 152
Urethra integrity
    factors affecting, 132, 136
Urethral bulking injection, 251, 255
Urethral diverticula, 132, 136
    calculi development, 150, 152
    cystourethroscopy for, 150, 152
    and urethral cancers, 150, 152
    women with symptomatic, 150, 152
Urethral diverticulum, 25
    repair, 251, 255
Urethral stenosis, 151, 152
Urethrolysis, 251, 255
Urge incontinence, 130
Urinary conduit, 256, 260
Urinary cortisol measurement, 99
Urinary incontinence
    risk factor for, 130
Urinary leakage, 151, 152
Urinary luteinizing hormone (LH) kits,
    110
Urodynamic stress incontinence, 130

Uroflowmetry, 133, 136
Urogenital sinus, 103
U.S. Preventive Services Task Force, 6
U-shaped opening in pelvic floor muscles,
    216, 221
Uterine artery, anomalous distribution,
    106
Uterine artery embolization (UAE), 50
    contraindications to, 50
    MRI for, 12
Uterine bleeding, 120
Uterine cancer
    laparoscopy use, 187, 189
    photomicrograph, 186, 189
    in US, 184, 189
    woman's risk, 184, 189
Uterine cervix length, 217, 221
Uterine corpus, blood supply, 219, 221
Uterine didelphys, 107
Uterine isthmus, 219, 221
Uterine manipulators, 245, 249
Uterine sarcoma
    criteria, 192, 195
    imaging, 191, 195
    lymph node involvement, 193–4, 195
    oral progestin therapy, 194, 195
    proliferative phase endometrium,
        192, 195
    stage I or II, 194, 195
    symptom of women with, 190, 195
    TAH, 194, 195
    tumor histology, 194, 195
    types, 190, 195
Utero-ovarian ligaments, 218, 221
Uterosacral ligament, 218, 221
    suspension, 140, 142
Uterovaginal malformations, 103

V

Vagina, walls of, 219, 221
Vaginal adenocarcinoma, 181, 183
Vaginal bleeding, 33
    intermittent, 81
Vaginal cancer
    AFP level, 182, 183
    drugs for, 181, 183
    FIGO stage, 180, 183
    fused Müllerian tubes, 179, 183
    parts of vagina, 180, 183
    radiotherapy for, 180–1, 183
    Schiller-Duval body, 182, 183
    sole therapy for, 180, 183
    types, 179, 183
Vaginal conjugated estrogen cream, 126
Vaginal flora, 14
Vaginal hysterectomy, 245, 249
    ligament, sutured, 238, 242
Vaginal lichen planus, treatment of, 23
Vaginal melanoma, 182, 183
Vaginal mucosa, 14
Vaginal mucosal fluid secretions, 126
Vaginal pathogen, risk factors for, 18

Vaginal pH
    after menopause, 14
    normal range, 14
Vaginal reconstructive procedure, 140, 142
Vaginal retractor, 231, 234
Vaginal support levels, 138, 142
Vaginal uterosacral ligament suspension,
    253, 255
Vancomycin, adverse effects of, 15
Varenicline, 6
Varicocele, 109
Vasectomy, 29
Vasomotor symptoms, 120
    treatment of, 124
Venous thromboembolism (VTE), risk
    factors for, 223, 228
Vesicovaginal fistulas, 251, 255
    transvaginal repair of, 251, 255
Visceral pain, 61
Vitamin D deficiency, 125, 126
Vitiligo, 24
Voiding cystourethrography (VCUG), 10
Von Willebrand disease, treatment for, 45
Vulvar abscess, 16
Vulvar cancer
    lesion, 177, 178
    minimally invasive, 175, 178
    percentage of, 175, 178
    prognostic factor, 176, 178
    radical vulvectomy, 176, 178
    risk factor for, 175, 178
    risk of recurrence, 176, 178
    tests for, 175, 178
    in US, 174, 178
    vulvar mass, 177, 178
Vulvar cyst, 240, 242
Vulvar hygiene, 22
Vulvar intraepithelial neoplasia (VIN),
    241, 242
Vulvar lesions, 19
    antibody testing in, 16
Vulvar lesions, pathology of, 22
Vulvar pruritis, 175, 178
Vulvodynia, 25
    cases of, 240, 242
    diagnosis of, 25
    pain of, 25
    treatment for, 25

W

Women's Health Initiative (WHI), 123
Wound healing events, 148, 152
Wound retraction, 227, 228

X

Xenografts, 141, 142

Y

Y-chromosome deletions, 112

Z

Zona pellucida proteins, 90